Recent epidemiological studies indicate that around 10 per cent of children and young people suffer from developmental, emotional or behavioural problems. Building upon the success of the *Cambridge Monographs in Child and Adolescent Psychiatry*, this is the first in an affiliated programme of volumes which specifically address therapeutic and service issues.

Cognitive–behaviour therapy is a relatively new treatment approach which has a firm theoretical base and has been subject to empirical validation. It has been demonstrated to be an effective form of treatment for many childhood disorders. This volume uniquely provides a comprehensive account of cognitive–behavioural approaches to psychological problems in children, adolescents and their families. The text is structured developmentally, passing from pre-school through to adolescence. An introductory chapter outlines general principles and subsequent chapters describe the therapeutic approaches for each specific disorder. The authors of each chapter first provide a rationale for treatment and then proceed to describe assessment and therapy, including detailed case examples. The authors also highlight the context of multimodal therapy and their visions for future research.

Written by an international team of experts, this very practical handbook provides a valuable resource which will be welcomed by a wide range of individuals concerned with the mental health of the young.

Cognitive–Behaviour Therapy for Children and Families

Cambridge Child and Adolescent Psychiatry Series
Formerly known as *Cambridge Monographs in Child and Adolescent Psychiatry*

This series has focused to date on psychopathology, highlighting those topics for which growth of knowledge has had the greatest impact on clinical practice and on the treatment and understanding of mental illness in children and adolescents. An important aim for the series as a whole is to illustrate the scientific principles inherent in clinical practice. This can be best achieved by volumes that analyse particular therapeutic strategies in the treatment and management of developmental psychopathologies. For these reasons, the editors are pleased to announce the addition of new therapeutic volumes to the series. Each volume will be complete in its own right, but the volumes will also relate to each other and to the existing texts within the series on the scientific basis of mental disorder. Therapeutics volumes will set out to describe in detail particular treatment strategies, starting with the theoretical basis, and providing a clear description of their use with different forms of child psychiatric disorder and therefore providing an up-to-date description of clinical practice. The therapeutic volumes will appeal to a wide range of clinical practitioners including child psychiatrists, psychologists, nurses, social workers, psychotherapists and others working in child mental health practices both in community and hospital settings.

Cognitive–Behaviour Therapy for Children and Families

Edited by Philip Graham

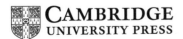

CAMBRIDGE
UNIVERSITY PRESS

PUBLISHED BY THE PRESS SYNDICATE OF THE UNIVERSITY OF CAMBRIDGE
The Pitt Building, Trumpington Street, Cambridge CB2 1RP, United Kingdom

CAMBRIDGE UNIVERSITY PRESS
The Edinburgh Building, Cambridge CB2 2RU, United Kingdom
40 West 20th Street, New York, NY 10011-4211, USA
10 Stamford Road, Oakleigh, Melbourne 3166, Australia

Cambridge University Press 1998

First published 1998

Printed in the United Kingdom at the University Press, Cambridge

Typeset in 10 on 13pt Times

A catalogue record for this book is available from the British Library

Library of Congress Cataloguing in Publication data

Cognitive–behaviour therapy for children and families / edited by
   Philip Graham.
       p.   cm. — (Cambridge monographs in child and adolescent
   psychiatry)
     Includes bibliographical references and index.
     ISBN 0 521 57252 5 (hc) – ISBN 0 521 57626 1 (pbk)
     1. Cognitive therapy for children. 2. Cognitive therapy for
   teenagers.   3. Family psychotherapy.   I. Graham, P. J. (Philip
   Jeremy)   II. Series.
   RJ505.C63C645   1998
   618.92'89142 – dc21   97-29374 CIP

ISBN 0 521 57252 5 hardback
ISBN 0 521 57626 1 paperback

Contents

Contributors

Veira Bailey, Department of Child and Adolescent Psychiatry, Thelma Golding Centre, 92 Bath Road, Hounslow TW3 3EL

Frank P. Deane, Department of Psychology, Massey University, Private Bag 11222, Palmerston North, New Zealand

Caroline Donovan, Department of Psychology, University of Queensland, Brisbane, Queensland 4072, Australia

Jo Douglas, Department of Psychological Medicine, Great Ormond Street Hospital for Children NHS Trust,Great Ormond Street, London WC1N 3JH

Julie E. Goodman, Department of Psychology, Dalhousie University, Halifax, Nova Scotia B3H 4J1, Canada

Philip Graham, The Developmental Psychiatry Section, Department of Psychiatry, University of Cambridge, 18b Trumpington Road, Cambridge CB2 2AH

Richard Harrington, Department of Psychiatry, Royal Manchester Children's Hospital, Pendlebury, Manchester M27 4HA

Martin Herbert, Department of Psychology, University of Exeter, Washington Singer Laboratories, Perry Road, Exeter EX4 4QG

A.E. Koning, Paedologisch Instituut, PO Box 10545, 6500 MB Nijmegen, The Netherlands

Patrick J. McGrath, Departments of Psychology, Pediatrics, Psychiatry and Occupational Therapy, Dalhousie University, Pain and Palliative Care Service, IWK Grace Health Centre, Halifax, Nova Scotia B3H 3J1, Canada

H. Oosterbaan, Paedologisch Instituut, PO Box 10545, 6500 MB Nijmegen, The Netherlands

S. Perrin, Institute of Psychiatry, De Crespigny Park, London SE5 8AF

Kevin R. Ronan, Department of Psychology, Massey University, Private Bag 11222, Palmerston North, New Zealand

Tammie Ronen, The Bob Shapell School of Social Work, Tel Aviv University, Tel Aviv 69978, Israel

Ulrike Schmidt, Department of Psychiatry, Maudsley Hospital, Denmark Hill, London SE5 8AZ

Roz Shafran, Psychology Department, 2136 West Mall, University of British Columbia, Vancouver, British Columbia V6T 1Z4, Canada

P. Smith, Institute of Psychiatry, De Crespigny Park, London SE5 8AF

Susan H. Spence, Department of Psychology, University of Queensland, Brisbane, Queensland 4072, Australia

Jeremy Turk, Department of Child and Adolescent Psychiatry, St George's Hospital Medical School, Cranmer Terrace, London SW17 0RE

Henck van Bilsen, Auckland Institute for Cognitive and Behavioural Therapies, 75c Goodall Street, 2Hillsborough, Auckland, New Zealand

R. J. van der Krol, Paedologisch Instituut, PO Box 10545, 6500 MB Nijmegen, The Netherlands

Chrissie Verduyn, Department of Psychiatry, Royal Manchester Children's Hospital, Pendlebury, Manchester M27 4HA

S.D. Weller, Paedologisch Instituut, PO Box 10545, 6500 MB Nijmegen, The Netherlands

Miriana Wilke, Auckland Institute for Cognitive and Behavioural Therapies, 75c Goodall Street, Hillsborough, Auckland, New Zealand

Alison Wood, Department of Psychiatry, Royal Manchester Children's Hospital, Pendlebury, Manchester M27 4HA

W. Yule, Department of Psychology, Institute of Psychiatry, De Crespigny Park, London SE5 8AF

Series preface

The editors of the Cambridge Monographs in Child and Adolescent Psychiatry are extremely pleased to release this, the first volume on therapeutics in this series. Whilst we will continue to publish volumes on specific syndromes, the editors recognise a growing need for a broader topic coverage of the 'how' of child mental health practice. Philip Graham has produced such a volume on cognitive–behaviour therapy. We look forward to further additions to this monograph series on issues in clinical practice.

William Parry-Jones   *Ian M. Goodyer*

Preface

The drive towards evidence-based clinical practice in child mental health continues. Just as in other branches of psychology, psychiatry and medicine, managers increasingly ask clinicians in the field of child and family psychiatry to justify the methods they use. In a recent authoritative review of the evidence of effectiveness for different forms of therapy in this field, Wallace *et al.* (1996) refer to cognitive–behavioural therapy (CBT) as having a place based on evidence (albeit nearly always incomplete) in the treatment of most psychological conditions suffered by children and adolescents. In their recent review of the effectiveness of psychological therapies in the treatment of such disorders, Target and Fonagy (1996) conclude that, though the findings may be open to challenge, at a general level behavioural treatments are more effective than non-behavioural or family treatments. Bearing in mind the immense literature devoted to family therapy and psychodynamic therapies in the treatment of childhood disorders, it seemed timely to bring out a book dedicated to this relatively new form of therapy.

I first became aware of the lack of published material on cognitive–behaviour therapy for children and familes outside the USA in late 1994, when I organised a meeting on the subject in London. A not very well-publicised conference drew a large audience eager for more information. The idea for this book arose from that meeting.

Invitations to contribute were sent to authorities in different parts of the world, and I am delighted that it was possible to secure collaboration from authors working in Australia, New Zealand, Israel, the Netherlands, and Canada, as well as the United Kingdom. Unfortunately, three American authors declined the invitation. However, despite the lack of American contributors, I do hope that there will be American readers who will find the book helpful. The contribution of American psychologists and psychiatrists to this field has been enormous (Kendall, 1991).

Apart from Tammie Ronen, who wrote the introductory chapter, the contributors were all given the same brief. They were asked to focus on a particular disorder. They should open with a brief description of the condition, with a rationale for using cognitive–behaviour therapy as a useful form of therapy. Techniques of assessment and treatment should then be described. These should be illustrated with a small number of case examples, of which perhaps two could demonstrate success and one failure (in order to demonstrate problems still to be addressed). There should then be a section discussing the use of the therapy as part of a multimodal approach, followed by a discussion of existing evidence for the effectiveness of CBT in the condition in question. Finally, the relevant current research issues should be addressed.

I hope readers will agree that the contributors have all succeeded admirably in meeting the difficult challenge set for them. The idea was to present material that would be practically useful for clinicians, but would also provide them with an intellectually satisfying theoretical framework for their interventions. Therapy cookbooks suffer from the disadvantage that unless the problem facing the therapist is exactly the same as that in the book (and it never is), the information provided is relatively useless. On the other hand, accounts of the therapy that are purely theoretical and only suggest interventions in very general, vague terms, are also unhelpful. I hope readers will agree that the contributors to this book have safely and usefully found a middle way.

The book has been structured as far as possible using a developmental framework. Following the introductory chapter, those contributions referring to pre-school children have been placed first, then those mainly dealing with children in their middle school years, and finally those mainly concerned with adolescents.

One question that had to be addressed was the definition of cognitive–behavioural therapy. How does CBT differ from behaviour therapy, interpersonal therapy, or psychodynamic psychotherapy? In an earlier publication, Sue Spence, one of the contributors to this volume, points to common features of cognitive therapies. Cognitive therapies assume that overt behaviour and affect are driven by cognitive events and processes, that cognitive events and processes can be changed directly, and that such change results in behavioural and affect change. Cognitive therapies focus on teaching cognitive skills to rectify cognitive deficits, and on modifying faulty cognitive processing (Spence, 1994). In contrast, behaviour therapy, while also focusing on the here and now, considers overt behaviour without reference to cognitions and aims to produce change entirely by influencing antecedents and consequences. Interpersonal therapies aim to change behaviour and affect by improving the quality of social relationships. Such improvement is brought about by education, clarification, and enhancement of problem-solving skills (Mufson *et al.*, 1993). While it is difficult to summarise the specific features of psychodynamic therapies, in general they emphasise the way the past is influencing the here and now rather than tackling the here and now directly. They use special techniques, especially the understanding of the client–therapist relationship, to bring unconscious cognitions and affects into consciousness. All the same, these different therapies have much in common, and no attempt has been made in this book to draw any hard and fast distinctions between CBT and other forms of psychotherapy.

The intention was that the book should be comprehensive, and, very broadly speaking, it is. Various issues have not been considered because they are already comprehensively discussed elsewhere. For example, the application of CBT to marital or adult partnership problems has been discussed by Schmaling, Fruzzetti and Jacobson (1989).

Finally, I would like to thank the editorial staff of Cambridge University Press for their extremely competent help during the preparation of this book.

References

Kendall, P.C. (1991). *Child and adolescent therapy: cognitive–behavioural therapies.* Guilford Press, New York.

Mufson, L., Moreau, D., Weissman, M. & Klerman, G. (1993). *Interpersonal psychotherapy for depressed adolescents.* Guilford Press, New York.

Schmaling, K.B., Fruzzetti, A.E. & Jacobson, N.S. (1989). Marital problems. In *Cognitive behaviour therapy for psychiatric problems* (ed. K. Hawton, P.M. Salkovskis, J. Kirk & D.M. Clark, pp. 339–69. Oxford Medical Publications, Oxford.

Spence, S.H. (1994). Cognitive therapy with children and adolescents: from theory to practice. *Journal of Child Psychology and Psychiatry*, **35**, 1191–228.

Target, M. & Fonagy, P. (1996). The psychological treatment of child and adolescent psychiatric disorders. In *What works for whom?* (ed. A. Roth & P. Fonagy), pp. 263–320. Guilford Press, New York, London.

Wallace, S.A., Crown, J., Cox, A.D. & Berger, M. (1996). *Epidemiologically based needs assessment: child and adolescent mental health.* Radcliffe Medical Press, Oxford.

Philip Graham   Cambridge

1

Linking developmental and emotional elements into child and family cognitive–behavioural therapy

Tammie Ronen

Cognitive–behavioural therapy (CBT) with children and families necessitates the adaptation of basic cognitive–behavioural principles to children's developmental and emotional needs and abilities. Recent epidemiological studies indicate that from 17 per cent to 22 per cent of children and young people under 18 years of age suffer from developmental, emotional or behavioural problems (Kazdin, 1993). Clearly there is a need for effective evidence-based therapies. CBT is a therapeutic approach which is rooted in theory and subject to rigorous empirical validation. It aims to offer effective means for achieving the main goals of child therapy: to decrease behaviours that appear too often (aggressiveness, hyperactivity, impulsivity); to increase behaviours that are too infrequent (social skills, self-evaluation, avoidance disorders due to anxiety, etc.); to remove anxieties that disturb the child's functioning (test anxiety, fear of social activities); and to facilitate developmental processes (self-control enhancement, assertiveness training, elimination of childish behaviour, etc.).

This chapter highlights the unique features of CBT with children and families that differentiate it from CBT with adults, as well as from other modes of child therapy. Emphasis is placed on incorporating the treatment of the child within his or her family and on integrating developmental and emotional elements into children's therapy. The interplay between cognitive, developmental and emotional components may be viewed as crucial in the planning of appropriate treatment for individual children with specific problems.

The basic view of cognitive–behavioural therapy

Cognitive–behavioural therapy is a purposeful attempt to preserve the demonstrated efficiencies of behaviour modification within a less doctrinaire context and to incorporate the cognitive activities of the client within the effort to produce therapeutic change (Kendall & Hollon, 1979). This therapeutic mode is based on the assumption that affect and behaviour are largely determined by the way in which the individual structures the world (Beck, 1976; Mahoney, 1991).

Cognitions – based on attitudes or assumptions (schemata) developed from previous experiences (Beck *et al.*, 1979) – are considered the most important links in the chain of events leading to disordered behaviour and psychological dysfunctions. There are complex interactions between cognitive events, processes, products and structures, affects, overt behaviours, and environmental contexts and experiences that contribute to various facets of dysfunctional behaviour (Braswell & Kendall, 1988). CBT focuses on helping the client to monitor cognitions (e.g. negative, automatic thoughts); to recognise the connections between cognitions, affects and behaviours; to examine the evidence for and against distorted automatic thoughts; to substitute more reality-oriented interpretations for these biased cognitions; and to learn to alter dysfunctional beliefs that predispose the client to distort his or her experiences (Beck *et al.*, 1979). Although CBT encompasses a variety of strategies and procedures, all share the tenet that learning plays a central role in the maintenance of behaviour, and the learning involves the manner in which the individual processes information cognitively (Hart & Morgan, 1993). CBT, therefore, is a structured, time-limited, problem-oriented psychotherapy aimed at modifying the faulty information-processing activities evident in psychological disorders (Rush *et al.*, 1977).

Cognitive–behavioural therapy with children as distinct from with adults

The above description emphasises the fact that cognitive therapy in adults is viewed as a broad theory for understanding and changing human functioning, depending largely on the client's ability to engage in philosophical disputation, logical analysis and abstract thinking. These components, however, appear too complicated for children younger than adolescence, who show a concrete way of thinking and difficulties with abstract, composite notions and concepts. For many years, children have been considered to be unable to benefit from CBT, and cognitive therapists working with children have focused on behavioural rather than on cognitive elements.

As applications of cognitive therapy with children have progressed, the field has developed differently from that of CBT with adults. CBT with children has not been based on a unified theoretical model to assess and address childhood disorders as well as to provide a framework for evaluating the proposed techniques (Ronen, 1995). Instead, CBT has become an umbrella term for different treatment techniques that can be offered in many different sequences and permutations. Most of the work being utilised with children either addresses one specific problem (e.g. fear of going out at night, thinking before starting a test, improving reading skills – see Kanfer, Karoly & Newman, 1975; Copeland, 1982; Kendall & Braswell, 1985), or makes use of one specific technique, in which children are taught to use cognitive mediational strategies to guide their behaviour and thus improve their adjustment (e.g. self-talk or self-recording – Durlak, Fuhrman & Lampman, 1991). CBT applications thus far have not adequately converged to provide a comprehensive compilation of assessment and treatment techniques to deal with the multiple aspects and components of prevalent childhood disorders such as attention-deficit/hyperactivity or anxiety disorders.

Child cognitive–behavioural therapy as compared to other modes of child therapy

Traditional child psychotherapies (e.g. psychodynamic and Adlerian approaches) have targeted the amelioration or resolution of neurosis, emotional disturbance, or undesirable behaviour in order to promote the child's general adjustment. In behavioural therapy, treatment goals have focused on altering specific behaviours or areas of functioning (Kovacs & Lohr, 1995), without regard to accompanying cognitive processes. Indeed, it has been thought important by behavioural therapists to ignore such cognitions.

In contrast, CBT pinpoints cognitive deficits and imparts children with needed skills within a treatment model that directly links assessment, intervention and evaluation. Through a careful assessment process, information that is directly relevant to treatment is obtained in order to achieve criteria for behaviour change. Therefore, the therapy involves an ongoing and self-evaluating process of assessment, facilitating a process of self-therapy while accentuating the maintenance and generalisation of learned skills to the child's external environment.

Cognitive–behavioural therapy with children is different from other children's therapies in its view of the child as an equal partner for intervention (Gelfand & Hartmann, 1984). The child is seen as someone who can be an active partner in decision making concerning the aims of therapy, establishing criteria for target behaviours, and making decisions about the kinds of techniques to be used. The child is not a passive receptor of treatment, but rather can learn and know about the techniques needed for behaviour change, understand their rationale, and take responsibility for their practice and application. The child is conceived as a scientist who studies his or her own behaviour, learns to identify its components, tests his or her belief system, and seeks out effective techniques to achieve change (Kanfer, 1977).

The focus of CBT with children lies in treating the children within their own natural environment, whether referring to the family, school or peer group. The relationship between children and their social systems cannot be overemphasised, the environment both affecting and being affected by the child's behaviour. Children's difficulties can be attributed on the one hand to the family and wider environment influencing their development and, on the other hand, to children themselves – their individual ways of thinking, coping, and dealing with their own internal cues as related to those of the environment (Kendall & Morris, 1991).

The wide range of CBT techniques with children points to the many roles of the cognitive therapist who combines the task of a consultant striving to develop skills, a diagnostician integrating data and judging against a background of a different knowledge area, and an educator promoting the learning of behaviour control, cognitive skills and emotional growth (Kendall & Lochman, 1994). CBT, therefore is conceived as an educational–therapeutic approach for achieving change.

As mentioned before, CBT with children is a combination of strategies, including behavioural performance-based procedures as well as cognitive interventions to produce change in thinking, feeling and behaviour. The model places great emphasis on learning processes and the influences of the social environment as well as on individual differences (Kendall & Lochman, 1994). One of the major characteristics of therapists is their ability to adjust their methods and techniques to individual problems while taking into account individual differences. They have developed a range of treatment techniques such as self-control training for helping children cope with fears (Kanfer *et al.*, 1975; Ronen, 1993b), school problems (Ronen, 1994) and impulsive behaviour (Kendall & Braswell, 1985); social skills training for helping children overcome loneliness, social deficit and aggressiveness (Bierman & Furman, 1984; Gresham, 1985); problem-solving methods for addressing interpersonal problems of relationships (Gresham, 1985; Pellegrini, 1994); self-instructional and self-talk training for modifying children's fears, obedience disorders and hyperactivity (Copeland, 1982; Kanfer *et al.*, 1975; Dush, Hirt & Schroeder, 1989) etc. Mash and Terdal (1988) have highlighted some unique features of CBT with children as compared to other therapies. For example, CBT with children is based on conceptualisations of personality and abnormal behaviour that target the child's thoughts, feelings and behaviours as they occur in specific situations, rather than as manifestations of some global underlying traits or dispositions. The therapy is predominantly idiographic and individualised, directed toward understanding the individual child and family, rather than toward nomothetic comparisons that attempt to describe individuals primarily in relation to dimensions derived from group norms. Unlike other therapies which emphasise the consistency of behaviour over time, concomitant with the stable and enduring nature of underlying causes, CBT underscores instability – the constantly changing nature of child and family behaviour over time. The focus is on contemporaneous controlling variables rather than historical causes, and on behaviours, cognitions and affects as direct samples of the domains rather than as signs of some underlying or remote causes. Kratochwill and Morris (1993) added a distinction between traditional therapies and CBT regarding the identification of the underlying agents of change that determine intervention planning. While traditional therapies are implemented directly with children, usually via non-verbal, indirect modes of intervention, CBT is most often implemented indirectly (by consulting teachers, counsellors or parents using a direct verbal mode of intervention), or at least is administered to the child within his or her family unit.

While the above description stresses the differences between CBT and other therapies, many areas of similarity exist. All psychotherapeutic approaches with children are based on developmental processes, requiring certain emotional and social supports to foster healthy, normal developmental needs. Consensus also exists that some affects, behaviours and thoughts are transient, whereas others are much more commonly persistent (Kazdin, 1994). The fact that many adult referrals to mental health services are rooted in childhood disorders (Kazdin, 1988) indicates the value of early intervention with children in need. All psychotherapies are designed to decrease distress, symptoms and maladaptive behaviour and to improve adaptive and prosocial functioning. In all psychotherapies, the focus of treatment may be dictated in part by the age of the child, and the techniques used are determined in part by the child's developmental stage.

The unique nature of cognitive–behavioural therapy with children

Cognitive models view individuals as actively involved in constructing their reality (Beck, 1963; Beck *et al.*, 1979; Mahoney, 1991). Thus all perceiving, learning, and knowing are products of an information-processing system which actively selects, filters and interprets environmental and other sensory input that impinges on the organism (Clark, 1995).

Cognitive–behavioural therapy with children is based on the assumption that children with deviant behaviour suffer from deficiencies in particular processes or from an inability to use or to apply cognitive skills (Kendall & Braswell, 1985). Examples may be an impulsive cognitive style, deficits in taking the perspective of others, or mis-attributions of others' intentions (Kazdin, 1988). CBT with children aims to help them to select appropriate behaviour for everyday life, focusing on the process rather than on the outcome, teaching them to engage in a step-by-step approach for solving problems, and combining behavioural and cognitive methods to lead them to an effective solution (Kazdin, 1988).

The need to integrate cognitive components into children's therapy is supported by evidence of the cognitive deficits characterising childhood disorders. Specific groups of children with different psychological problems have been shown to: generate fewer alternative solutions to interpersonal problems; focus on ends or goals rather than on the intermediate steps toward attaining them; see fewer consequences associated with their behaviour; fail to recognise the cause of other people's behaviour; and exhibit less sensitivity to interpersonal conflict (Kazdin, 1988; Ronen, 1992).

As described above, cognitive–behavioural treatments emphasise the link between the person and the social environment, viewing environment as strongly influencing behaviour, emotions and thoughts, as well as the reverse. Whenever a child is concerned, the family is involved, and most treatment settings include the child within his or her family. CBT with children and families in particular underscores situational influences on behaviour (Mash & Terdal, 1988). The therapy is system oriented, describing and understanding the characteristics of the child and the family, the context in which such characteristics are expressed, and the structural organisations and functional relationships that exist between situations and behaviours, thoughts and emotions (Mash & Terdal, 1988).

Cognitive–behavioural therapy has been considered a promising treatment strategy for a wide range of children with problems (Gresham, 1985; Dush, Hirt & Schroeder, 1989), as long as the therapist is able to adapt techniques to the children's developmental needs (Ronen, 1992). Adapting cognitive techniques to children depends, to a large extent, on the therapist's ability to translate cognitive concepts and techniques in a way which is clear, understandable and sensible to children and their parents (Ronen, 1992, 1993a; Knell, 1993). CBT with children requires an adaptation of the basic cognitive model to include assessment of developmental factors such as age, gender, cognitive level, and the kind of problems referred which can contribute to the selection of the most suitable treatment mode (Ronen, 1993a; 1997).

Developmental considerations in child cognitive–behavioural therapy

Development refers to the changing structure of behaviour over the lifespan, indicating not only changing degrees of organismic complexity, but changes in the biological and psychological substructures emerging and unfolding in social surroundings (Shapiro, 1995). Many child disturbances involve developmental considerations. Only through knowledge of normal developmental processes can one begin to understand deviations in development and their importance for assessment and intervention (Forehand & Weirson, 1993). While developmental considerations (age, gender and cognitive stages) influence child therapy in general, they have a crucial role in cognitive–behavioural treatments, where verbal and cognitive skills are of great importance.

Children's age, gender and cognitive stage influence therapy approaches. Our theoretical understanding and the basic research available on development indicate that, at different ages and stages of development and differentially for boys and girls, specific processes and opportunities may emerge in domains such as cognitive comprehension, exposure to new experiences, establishing relationships, perceiving and expressing emotions, etc. Research on cognitive development, the influence of peers, and transition periods (e.g. transferring to another school) suggests the need for different sorts of intervention to achieve change (Kazdin, 1993).

Developmental components are an integral part of making decisions about children's therapy throughout the entire process of intervention. However, their importance is pivotal at three main points in the assessment and treatment process: during the initial stage while assessing whether the problem needs to be treated at all; while making a decision about who should be treated; and while selecting and adapting the best techniques for the child's needs and abilities (Ronen, 1997).

Wenar (1982) contended that when problems occur in children, the effect can best be described as 'normal development gone awry'. Many researchers (e.g. Doleys, 1977) have asserted that as children have a high rate of spontaneous recovery, a large proportion of problematic children will solve their problems even without intervention. The children may quickly show mastery, with little evidence that the challenge was other than momentary. Other studies have emphasised the fact that children exhibit transient difficulties while struggling to deal with the challenges of normal development. Kazdin (1988) stated that only a small proportion of children in need will be referred for therapy and that referred children do not necessarily comprise that group in greatest need.

In contrast to traditional therapists, cognitive–behaviour therapists stress that clients are not treated because of their disorders but because of the way they cope with these disorders (Kanfer & Schefft, 1988). This is especially true with children, who experience disorders as a natural, integral part of their normal developmental processes. This normative basis for common childhood phenomena (e.g. fears and anxieties, enuresis, aggressiveness, learning difficulties, obsessive–compulsive rituals, social deficits, eating problems) hinders the differentiation between a normal developmental reaction and a behavioural dysfunction.

The integration of developmental theory into CBT should lead to two major shifts in the field. First, the understanding of normal development should be considered critical for assessment: placing symptoms into a developmental context can determine whether a specific behaviour is age-normal or age-deviant. Second, knowledge of developmental tasks facing children might help in explaining the aetiology of the referred problem, as well as the need to adapt assessment considerations to the child's age (Forehand & Weirson, 1993).

Age as a mediator in child therapy

Age criteria are often crucial in determining when a behaviour previously considered normal becomes maladaptive. For example, enuresis, fear of separation, lack of self-control, crying and shyness are natural behaviours for children during the first three years of their lives. As children grow up, they are expected to gain control of their bladders; they are expected to learn that their parents always come back and to stop crying when they leave; and they are expected gradually to gain self-control skills, develop assertiveness and an ability for self-evaluation, and learn to conduct verbal communication and negotiation instead of crying whenever they wish for something. Each of the above behaviours which are normal at age three will be problematic if children continue to exhibit them at age six (Ronen, 1997). However, it is impossible to assess a dysfunctional behaviour in relationship only to chronological age. With children, one can often expect discrepancies between chronological, emotional, cognitive and behavioural ages (Sahler & McAnarney, 1981). Such incongruities create a challenge for the therapist attempting to assess and diagnose an individual child referred for therapy.

In order to reach a decision regarding the need for treatment, the therapist should make a prediction based not only on general knowledge regarding spontaneous recovery rates for the specific area of difficulty, but also on the pace and development of the specific child's problem up to the time of assessment (Mash & Terdal, 1988). How old is the child? Is the behaviour normal for the child's age? Is it characteristic of the child's environment? Has the problem recently emerged or recently become aggravated? What is the probability of the problem disappearing? Will it remain stable, improve or become worse? Will its frequency increase, remain stable or decrease?

Age is crucial not only in determining whether or not to treat the problem, but also for decision making as to who should be treated. Children develop different roles at each childhood age/stage, requiring a specific treatment plan best suited to facilitating the new roles (Forehand & Weirson, 1993). For example, when children are young and dependent on their caregiver, therapy usually has primary prevention aims (i.e. preventing future risk and reducing the incidence of disorder – Graham, 1994) and takes the form of counselling and supervising parents in educating and rearing their children (Ronen, 1997). As children grow up and start school, therapy should be directed to the child within his or her natural environment (parents, teachers and friends) and toward educational–therapeutic assignments (i.e. secondary prevention, which prevents existing problems from worsening and reduces the duration of the disorder – Graham, 1994). As children enter adolescence, therapy should be directed toward the children themselves and focus on tertiary prevention (i.e. therapy aims to solve an already existing problem, prevent future risks, and impart skills for decreasing its frequency; it covers rehabilitative activities and reduces the disability arising from an established disorder – Graham, 1994).

Understanding developmental issues is critical not only in assessing the need for treatment and selecting the setting for intervention, but also during the intervention itself. Age should be a primary consideration in identifying the best technique for a specific child. Dush et al. (1989) found a positive relationship between age and treatment outcome, with older children benefiting more from cognitive treatments. The best results were found for adolescents (aged 13 to 18 years), and good outcomes were also shown for pre-adolescents (aged 11 to 13), but less success was demonstrated with younger children (aged 5 to 11) (Durlak et al., 1991). These outcomes suggest that different techniques in cognitive therapy should be considered for children of different ages. Young children need simple, specific instructions and can enjoy more behavioural techniques or cognitive techniques which are based on simple instructions (such as self-talk). Older children can benefit more from cognitive therapy and techniques such as changing automatic thoughts, rational analysis, and cognitive restructuring.

Gender as a mediator in child therapy

Basic cognitive and social learning research findings suggest that biological elements (genes and hormones) set the process of sex differentiation into motion but that environmental conditions, information-processing models, and parental influences maintain this process (Vasta, Haith & Miller, 1995).

Gender differences may be explained by several factors, such as social norms or a variation in maturation processes. On the one hand, girls as a group mature more quickly than boys, so one can expect fewer disorders with an important developmental component among them. On the other hand, role taking influences girls by allowing them to talk more freely about anxieties and fears than do boys, so that reports of anxiety are usually higher among girls (Kazdin, 1988; Ronen, 1997).

The development of sexual identity among children emerges in three stages: first, children develop gender identity (categorise themselves as male or female); then gender stability emerges (awareness that usually boys grow up to be men and girls grow up to be women); and, finally, gender consistency is attained (the recognition of the gender group to which the child belongs and an understanding of the implications) (Kohlberg & Ullian, 1974).

Gender influences development, and has an impact on behavioural dysfunction, by influencing social expectation. For example, in general, patterns of play and social relations are different among boys and girls (Raviv et al., 1990). Girls are tied more to one or two significant friends of their own age and sex, while boys play in large same-sex groups. Girls find it more difficult to make new friends than boys do. So, sex mediates social relationships, and to some degree predicts social adjustment to new environments (Raviv et al., 1990), and contributes to assessment and intervention processes.

Gender has a greater influence as children grow up and enter the adolescent stage, acquiring specific sex roles. Studies point to greater differences between the sexes as children mature. For example, in research on moving to a new house, girls were found to report more stress (feelings of loneliness, sadness and confusion) as compared with boys (Offer, Ostrov & Howard, 1981; Raviv et al., 1990).

The assessment process and decision making about the best form of treatment should take gender issues into account with respect not only to children's sex differences but to the parents' and therapist's sex and their combinations (mother with son, mother with daughter, father with son, female therapist with male child, etc.). Children are usually referred and escorted to therapy by their mothers. Mothers may have a different view of their children's disorders than do fathers; they are often more concerned and tend to see a greater need for therapy, whereas fathers more commonly tend to see dysfunctional disorder as normal and wish to wait for the child to grow out of it (Angold et al., 1987).

Finally, the treatment itself should also be influenced by gender-related considerations. Women, for instance, generally have a greater willingness to seek and receive help than do men, and girls, like women, can more easily accept help in times of crisis (Nadler, 1986). In addition, girls' greater expressiveness and ability to share their feelings with others may have important ramifications in the planning of treatments for both sexes. Boys are more likely to enjoy computer games and may more easily co-operate with exposure treatments, paradoxical techniques, and gradual assignment techniques. Over the last decade, cognitive therapy has begun to pinpoint not only the 'overcoming' techniques but also the 'living with' techniques that foster the accept-ance of negative emotions (Rosenbaum, 1993). Experiential techniques (accepting emo-tions, living with fears, self-talk, and imagination; see Rosenbaum, 1993; in press) might be easier to design for girls, who are less afraid of being thought weak and 'feeling bad' (Nadler, 1986).

Assessment for child therapy needs to be conducted to substantiate clinical observa-tions regarding the influence of gender on treatment (including the dissimilar responses of boys and girls of different ages to different therapeutic settings and techniques, the role of the therapist's sex in relation to the child's, etc.) and on the efficacy of treatment.

The cognitive approach to gender-role development focuses not so much on the sociobiological differences between the genders as on the kind of gender schemata each child develops. Basically there are 'masculine', 'feminine', and 'androgynous' schemata, each of which can be held by a child regardless of his or her gender. The 'androgynous' schemata may be most adaptive to the norms and mores of Western society, because they enable children to accept both the 'feminine' and 'masculine' parts of their personality. The role of the cognitive therapist is to discover the gender sche-mata of the child, and help him or her to develop healthy and functional gender schemata.

Cognitive stage as a mediator in child therapy
The need to integrate the child's cognitive capacities into CBT has implications for interviewing methods, assessment activities, therapeutic interpretations, and treatment techniques. An awareness of the child's cognitive level, strengths and limitations enables the therapist to devise the cognitive processes and techniques in a way that will appro-priately meet the child's developmental needs (Knell, 1993) and influence the design of intervention strategies (Bierman & Furman, 1984; Knell, 1993). There is general agree-ment about the need for a good match between the developmental level of the child and the level of complexity of the selected intervention. Questions arise as to how can one assess a child's cognitive level and what considerations should be taken into account.

The traditional view of child cognitive development was based on Piaget (1926), who described four cognitive developmental stages: the sensorimotor stage (infants and very young children), the pre-operational stage (school years), the concrete operational stage (the years leading to puberty), and the formal operational stage (pre-adolescence and adolescence). Each stage is characterised by different motoric, cognitive and language skills which result in different abilities to understand complex concepts.

Recent developmental and cognitive theories have opposed Piaget's view of children as being epistemologically weak, philosophically naïve, and empirically wrong (Brainerd, 1978; Modgil & Modgil, 1982; Siegal, 1991). Some opposed the rigid classification of stages that does not take into account individual differences in development (Brown & Desforges, 1977; Case, 1992). They suggested that children are capable of understanding complex concepts at earlier ages than Piaget proposed. In addition, they claim that developmental processes do not end at the end of adolescence: people continue to develop their cognitive abilities throughout life.

Focusing on children's cognitive development in the light of developmental tasks, Forehand and Weirson (1993) delineated the most appropriate cognitive interventions for each age. During infancy, the developmental task consists of shifting from dependence on the caregiver to increased independence and self-regulation. It follows that problems in gaining initial achievements in autonomy at this stage usually derive from, depend on, and relate to the way the parent educates his or her child. Understanding those cognitive-stage-dependent problems determines the kind of setting, strategies and techniques which could be employed with children. The major developmental task of early childhood is to begin mastery of academic and social situations. Hence, interventions at this age should involve parents' and teachers' supervision in how to use behavioural principles with children, as well as social skills training and group intervention. From middle childhood to early adolescence the main task consists of individual identity development and acquiring self-control. Therefore therapy should be based on social skills training and training in self-control methods (i.e. self-talk, self-reinforcement). The task of individuation from the family and moving toward independence in middle adolescence requires interventions based on problem-solving skills and self-control training.

Therapists need to be keenly aware of the child's language in order to use it for communication in therapy. This includes tuning into the child's specific interests and day-to-day experiences to provide content areas familiar to the child, that will serve as a reference base in therapeutic communication with the child. To engage the child's enthusiastic involvement, drawing, playing or talking may be employed. These communication requirements mean that child therapists must identify the important figures in the child's life, and be flexible in the use of different methods for helping the child. The decision about who should reinforce the child depends on developmental considerations, in view of the fact that at different ages and cognitive skill levels the child is likely to be influenced by different figures – parents with young children, teachers and peers during adolescence (Forehand & Weirson, 1993).

Thus age, gender, cognitive functioning and the nature of the presenting problem all have an impact on selecting the therapeutic mode. Age and phase competencies will dictate the type of intervention possible, and such knowledge will also determine the length of intervention and the baseline expectation of change points (Shapiro, 1995).

The role of emotion in child cognitive–behavioural therapy

'Behavioural and early cognitive therapies assumed that people behave first and then think about and (re)conceptualize their behaviour' (Dowd, in press). Cognitive–behavioural treatments have concentrated on problem solving and coping. In his early work on cognitive therapy for depression, Beck (1963) emphasised the role of emotion as an outcome of thinking processes and pointed to the need to change one's emotions by learning to identify and change automatic thoughts into controlled thoughts. Emotions have been conceived as the outcome of negative automatic thoughts, which need to be changed in order to achieve behaviour change. The aggressive child, for instance, has been taught to control behaviours such as hitting (e.g. using self-talk or imagination), but the feelings of frustration, anger and helplessness which underlie and elicit the aggressiveness have not, until recently, been regarded as central to therapy.

In the last few years, there has been a dramatic increase in interest in the role of emotion in therapy in general, and in CBT in particular, bringing the issues of emotions into clear focus in therapy. Emotions are no longer considered as being a 'by-product' or an 'outcome of' but rather as a necessary and an integral function of human beings. They are both the cause and the outcome of cognition (Mahoney, 1991). The human mind is no longer conceived as an information-processing organ but as one that actively constructs reality through its interaction with impinging stimuli and its interpretation and classification of these stimuli based on the individual's perception of the world (Guidano, 1987; Dowd, in press).

Affect is thus a core constituent of human self and establishes the link between self and environment and organises self-experiences (Greenberg, Rice & Elliott, 1993). Affects, therefore, are viewed both as a product of, and as a process in, social interaction (Parke, 1994) and everyday experiences. Modern cognitive therapists, and especially those using constructive therapy, no longer think of cognition and emotion as distinct and separate entities (Mahoney, 1991). Feelings are laden with cognitions, involving, among other processes, attentional allocation and automatic evaluation (Greenberg et al., 1993).

Children are frequently referred for psychotherapy because of problems with emotions, and many childhood disorders can be viewed as involving difficulties with the experience, expression or regulation of emotions (Shirk & Russell, 1996). To help children cope with, experience and be able to express emotions, we need to understand the role of emotion in behaviour in general, and its role in the acquisition, maintenance and change processes.

In the course of development, children are increasingly able to demonstrate signs of emotions, talk about emotions, show comprehension of emotional terms, understand situations which elicit emotions, induce emotions in themselves and others, understand emotional cues, and integrate successive or simultaneous emotions (Terwogt & Olthof, 1989).

The emergence of emotional expression is primarily guided by biological processes, but is subsequently tied to cognitive learning and influenced by the social environment (i.e. being learned through modelling and reinforcement processes). Like other modes of development (age, gender development, and cognitive development), emotions also develop in stages, from diffuse, intense emotional states in infancy, to a rudimentary awareness and discernment of some affects, to a capacity to regulate some of one's own emotions, and gradually to a more mature differentiation between subtleties in affective experience and an increased level of control. Social understanding of emotions develops from the first stage, where babies relate especially to facial expressions, to an ability to understand the emotions being expressed by others, through the stage where expectations start playing a central role (Vasta *et al.*, 1995). Unlike other modes of development, emotional processes are not linear, being impinged upon by stress and a multitude of experiences that can easily cause regression to an earlier stage.

Emotions are elicited through the development of an attachment to significant figures from the first few months, through the second year of life when specific attachment bonds become clearest and fear begins to emerge as a dominant emotion, including wariness of strangers and separation protests, and up to the age of 11 years and above when children are already more likely to attribute emotional arousal to internal causes rather than to external events (Thompson, 1989). Thus, with increasing age, children not only develop a broader range of emotional concepts, but also increasingly appreciate the psychological dimensions of emotional experience which help them to interpret their own emotional experiences in more sophisticated ways. This new perceptiveness fosters more accurate interpretations of the direct emotional displays of others and increases children's competences at inferring emotions in others when direct cues are lacking (Thompson, 1989).

Young children are likely to rely on cognitively uncomplicated outcome-dependent emotions such as happiness or sadness, which are developed early and easily understood (e.g. 'I hurt my knee, so I'm sad'). Not long afterwards, children begin mastering more complex concepts of emotion related to attributional understanding (Thompson, 1989) (e.g. 'Since I feel sad and scared when I hurt myself, Mum must also be feeling sad and scared right now because she hurt herself'). As cognitive functions mature, new emotions emerge and become available to children as experiences, and children can comprehend differential attributions (e.g. 'Maybe my mother feels differently from me when she gets hurt – maybe she's angry,' or 'Look, Mum feels sad and scared, and she didn't even hurt herself – there's another reason'). Psychologists identify cognitive–developmental transitions as preconditions for a child to be able to think about emotion (Gordon, 1989).

Studies linking emotion to cognition have focused on several issues. The first is related to vicarious, induced emotions and their relation to social behaviour. A central role in this development concerns empathy-based reactions and their relation to prosocial behaviour, with an attempt to arrive at a distinction between sympathy (as involving other-oriented, altruistic motivation) and personal distress (as associated with the self-oriented motive of alleviating one's own distress (Murphy, 1937; Eisenberg & Fabes, 1995). Before children gain the ability to feel empathy for others, it is difficult to train them in cognitive techniques involving problem solving or checking alternative solutions, which necessitate discerning what others feel and what others might do.

Studies have also illuminated how emotions that emerge early begin to grow in sophistication and scope throughout the childhood years, contributing to knowledge about others and oneself (Thompson, 1989). Helping the child understand emotions is a vital part of cognitive therapy, involving the identification of internal cues, differentiating between thoughts and emotions, and learning how emotions elicit behaviour.

Studies have investigated emotional reactions as a factor in children's behaviour during social interaction. The way children accept and understand the emotional cues of others as well as their own emotional responses can be a primary impetus for their behaviours toward peers. The fact that children's behavioural responses (e.g. anger, aggressiveness, patience) are directed by their emotions highlights the important role of treatment in teaching children to understand their emotional responses as a cue for learning about their internal thoughts, sensations and wishes. In society there is a need to modify the fixed relation between situations and emotional reactions to these situations, via a sensitivity to internal stimuli, so that emotions can be simulated and emotional reactions can be withheld or acted out more or less deliberately (Terwogt & Olthof, 1989).

A closer look at the way children learn, understand and enhance emotion clarifies the role of cognitions in affective development and regulation. In order to understand and express emotion, children must learn to take another's perspective and to access information from memory (Eisenberg & Fabes, 1995). Older children are likely to have a wider knowledge of the causes and the time course of emotions, which contribute to an ability for emotional self-control (Harris & Saarni, 1989). An understanding of emotions (which depends on children's schemata) contributes to an ability to predict another person's actions (Harris & Saarni, 1989) and to gain knowledge about the conditions that precede an emotional response. Important aspects of emotional knowledge include what goal is being pursued, the value of the goal, the feeling about the goal, and the probability of achieving it (Stein & Trabasso, 1989).

Cognitive–behavioural therapy is targeted toward the self-control of emotions, whether to suppress or express them. Controlling and regulating emotions enable flexibility in social behaviour, in communication, and in achieving the appropriate response to specific situations (Smiley & Huttenlocher, 1989; Terwogt & Olthof, 1989). Control of emotion cannot be learned by means of trial and error but rather requires modelling, reinforcing and mirroring. In order to control emotions, children need knowledge of when to control and how to control. Young children are rigid in the extent of control they apply, often demonstrating overcontrol or undercontrol in emotional functioning. Reinforcement, cognitions and knowledge obtained throughout the childhood years influence the process of appraising, dealing with, and regulating emotions.

Viewed in this light, the process of affective self-regulation will depend on the child's introspective abilities. The control of emotion may operate on two levels: on the one hand, the process of introspective self-reflection as critical to self-regulation for inter-rupting the automatic link between situational and subjective experiences; and, on the other hand, the socially mediated learning which helps in controlling overt affective displays (Harris & Saarni, 1989).

Cognitive therapy focuses on the importance of the person's schemata for the devel-opment of basic belief systems, automatic thoughts, and behaviours (Beck, 1976). With children, emotional experiences and the interpersonal frame of reference within which that experience develops are crucial for understanding the way children appraise a situation, evaluate it, and choose to deal with it. Children's egocentric thinking up to adolescence, and their limited means for appraising reality (in terms of its coincidence with their goals and their basic need for attachment), all influence their ability not only to participate in cognitive activities but also to achieve emotional understanding and regulated responding as well.

Summary

This introductory chapter highlights the role of developmental considerations (age, gender and cognitive stages) and emotional development and understanding in cogni-tive–behavioural therapy. Awareness of how a child expresses emotions and which kinds of affects are manifested, as well as the cognitive stage (that enables the child to deal with those emotions at a specific level), will make success in therapy more likely.

The focus in this chapter is on several principles underlying assessment and cognitive behavioural treatment. The importance of taking development cues, emotional as well as cognitive views into account has been stressed. The gender of the child and therapist may also influence the choice of therapeutic approach.

Acknowledgement

The author wishes to thank Dee B. Ankonina for her editorial contribution.

References

Angold, A., Weissman, M., Merikangas, J.K., Prusoff, B., Wickramaratne, P., Gammon, G. & Warner, B. (1987). Parent and child reports of depressive symptoms in children at low and high risk of depression. *Journal of Child Psychology and Psychiatry*, **28**, 901–15.

Beck, A.T. (1963). Thinking and depression. *Archives of General Psychiatry*, **9**, 324–33.

Beck, A.T. (1976). *Cognitive therapy and the emo-tional disorders*. Meridian Books, New York.

Beck, A.T., Rush, A.J., Shaw, B.F. & Emery, G. (1979). *Cognitive therapy of depression*, Guilford Press, New York.

Bierman, K.L. & Furman, W. (1984). The effects of social skills training and peer involvement on the social adjustment of preadolescents. *Child Development*, **55**, 151–62.

Brainerd, C. (1978). *Piaget's theory of intelligence*. Prentice-Hall, Englewood Cliffs, NJ.

Braswell, L. & Kendall, P.C. (1988). Cognitive-behavioral methods with children. In *Handbook* of cognitive-behavioral therapies (ed. K.S. Dobson), pp. 167–213. Guilford Press, New York.

Brown, G. & Desforges, C. (1977). Piagetian theory and education: Time for revision. *British Journal of Educational Psychology*, **47**, 7–17.

Case, R. (1992). *The mind's staircase*. Erlbaum, Hillsdale, NJ.

Clark, D.A. (1995). Perceived limitations of standard cognitive therapy: A consideration of efforts to revise Beck's theory and therapy. *Journal of Cognitive Psychotherapy: An International Quarterly*, **9**, 153–72.

Copeland, A.P. (1982). Individual difference factors in children's self-management: Toward individualized treatments. In *Self-management and behavior change: From theory to practice* (ed. P. Karoly & F.H. Kanfer), pp. 207–39. Pergamon Press, New York.

Doleys, D.M. (1977). Behavioral treatments for nocturnal enuresis in children: A review of the recent literature. *Psychological Bulletin*, **84**, 30–54.

Dowd, E.T. (in press). The evolution of the cognitive psychotherapies. In *Handbook of cognitive psychotherapies* (ed. I. Caro). Paidos, Barcelona.

Durlak, J.A., Fuhrman, T. & Lampman, C. (1991). Effectiveness of cognitive-behavior therapy for maladaptive children: A meta-analysis. *Psychological Bulletin*, **110**, 204–14.

Dush, D.M., Hirt, M.L. & Schroeder, H.E. (1989). Self-statement modification in the treatment of child behavior disorders: A meta-analysis. *Psychological Bulletin*, **106**, 97–106.

Eisenberg, N. & Fabes, R.A. (1995). The relation of young children's vicarious emotional responding to social competence, regulation, and emotionality. *Cognition and Emotion*, **9**, 203–28.

Forehand, R. & Weirson, M. (1993). The role of developmental factors in planning behavioral intervention for children. Disruptive behavior as an example. *Behavior Therapy*, **24**, 117–41.

Gelfand, D.M. & Hartmann, D.P. (1984). *Child behavior analysis and therapy*. Pergamon Press, New York.

Gordon, S.L. (1989). The socialization of children's emotions: Emotional culture, competence, and exposure. In *Children's understanding of emotion* (ed. C. Saarni & P.L. Harris), pp. 319–44. Cambridge University Press, New York.

Graham, P. (1994). Prevention. In *Child and adolescent psychiatry: Modern approaches*, 3rd edn (ed. M. Rutter, E. Taylor & L. Hersov), pp. 815–28. Blackwell, Oxford.

Greenberg, L.S., Rice, L.N. & Elliott, R. (1993). *Facilitating emotional change: The moment-by-moment process*. Guilford Press, New York.

Gresham, F.M. (1985). Utility of cognitive-behavioral procedures for social skills training with children. A critical review. *Journal of Abnormal Child Psychology*, **13** 411–23.

Guidano, V.F. (1987). *Complexity of the self: A developmental approach to psychopathology and therapy*. Guilford Press, New York.

Harris, L. & Saarni, C. (1989). Children's understanding of emotion: An introduction. In *Children's understanding of emotion*, (ed. C. Saarni & P.L. Harris), pp. 3–24. Cambridge University Press, New York.

Hart, K.J. & Morgan, J.R. (1993). Cognitive-behavioral procedures with children. In *Cognitive-behavioral procedures with children and adolescents*, (ed. A.J. Finch, W.M. Nelson & E.S. Ott), pp. 1–24. Allyn & Bacon, Boston.

Kanfer, F.H. (1977). The many faces of self-control, or behavior modification changes its focus. In *Behavioral self-management*, (ed. R.B. Stuart), pp. 1–48. Brunner/Mazel, New York.

Kanfer, F.H., Karoly, P. & Newman, A. (1975). Reduction of children's fear of the dark by confidence-related and situational threat-related verbal cues. *Journal of Consulting and Clinical Psychology*, **43**, 251–8.

Kanfer, F.H. & Schefft, B.K. (1988). *Guiding the process of therapeutic change*. Research Press, Champaign, Ill.

Kazdin, A.E. (1988). *Child psychotherapy: Developing and identifying effective treatments*. Pergamon Press, New York.

Kazdin, A.E. (1993). Psychotherapy for children and adolescents: Current progress and future directions. *American Psychologist*, **48**, 644–56.

Kazdin, A.E. (1994). Psychotherapy for children and adolescents. In *Handbook of psychotherapy and behavior change*, 4th edn (ed. A.E. Bergin & S.L. Garfield), pp. 543–94. Wiley, New York.

Kendall, P.C. & Braswell, L. (1985), *Cognitive behavioral therapy for impulsive children*. Guilford Press, New York.

Kendall, P.C. & Hollon, S.D. (eds.) (1979). *Cognitive-behavioral interventions: Theory, research, and procedures*. Academic Press, New York.

Kendall, P.C. & Lochman, J. (1994). Cognitive-behavioural therapies. In *Child and adolescent psychiatry: Modern approaches*, 3rd edn (ed. M. Rutter, E. Taylor, & L. Hersov), pp. 844–57. Blackwell, Oxford.

Kendall, P.C. & Morris, R.J. (1991). Child therapy: Issues and recommendations. *Journal of Consulting and Clinical Psychology*, **59**, 777–83.

Knell, S.M. (1993). *Cognitive behavioral play therapy*. Jason Aronson, Northvale, NJ.

Kohlberg, L. & Ullian, D.Z. (1974). Stages in development of psychosexual concepts and attitudes. In *Sex differences in behavior*, (ed. R.C. Friedman, R.M. Richart & R.L. VandlWiele). Wiley, New York.

Kovacs, M. & Lohr, W.D. (1995). Research on psychotherapy with children and adolescents: An overview of evolving trends and current issues. *Journal of Abnormal Child Psychology*, **23**, 11–30.

Kratochwill, T.R. & Morris, R.J. (1993). Introductory comments. In *Handbook of psychotherapy with children and adolescents*, (ed. T.R. Kratochwill & R.J. Morris), pp. 3–9. Allyn & Bacon, Boston.

Mahoney, M.J. (1991). *Human change processes: The scientific foundations of psychotherapy*. Basic Books, New York.

Mash, E. & Terdal, L.G. (1988). Behavioral assessment of child and family disturbance. In *Behavioral assessment of childhood disorders*, 2nd edn (ed. E.J. Mash & L.G. Terdal), pp. 3–65. Guilford Press, New York.

Modgil, S. & Modgil, C. (1982). *Jean Piaget: Consensus and controversy*. Holt, Rinehart & Winston, London.

Murphy, L.B. (1937). *Social behavior and child personality*. Columbia University Press, New York.

Nadler, A. (1986). Self-esteem and the seeking and receiving of help: Theoretical and empirical perspectives. *Experimental Personality Research*, **14**, 115–63.

Offer, D., Ostrov, E. & Howard, K. (1981). *The adolescent: A psychological self-report*. Basic Books, New York.

Parke, R.D. (1994). Progress, paradigms, and unresolved problems: Recent advances in our understanding of children's emotions. *Merrill-Palmer Quarterly*, **40**, 157–69.

Pellegrini, D.S. (1994). Training in interpersonal cognitive problem-solving. In *Child and adolescent psychiatry: Modern approaches*, 3rd edn (ed. M. Rutter, E. Taylor & L. Hersov), Blackwell, Oxford.

Piaget, J. (1926). *The language and thought of the child*. Routledge & Kegan Paul, London.

Raviv, A., Keinan, G., Abazon, Y. & Raviv, A. (1990). Moving as a stressful life event for adolescents. *Journal of Community Psychology*, **18**, 130–40.

Ronen, T. (1992). Cognitive therapy with young children. *Child Psychiatry and Human Development*, **23**, 19–30.

Ronen, T. (1993a). Decision making about children's therapy. *Child Psychiatry and Human Development*, **23**, 259–72.

Ronen, T. (1993b). Self-control training in the treatment of sleep-terror disorders. *Child and Family Behavior Therapy*, **15**, 53–63.

Ronen, T. (1994). Imparting children self-control skills in the school setting. *Child and Family Behavior Therapy*, **16**, 1–20.

Ronen, T. (1995). From what kind of self-control can children benefit? *The Journal of Cognitive Psychotherapy: An International Quarterly*, **9**, 45–61.

Ronen, T. (1997). *Cognitive-developmental therapy with children*. Wiley, Chichester.

Rosenbaum, M. (1993). The three functions of self-control behavior: Redressive, reformative and experiential. *Journal of Work and Stress*, **7**, 33–46.

Rosenbaum, M. (in press). The self-regulation of experience: Openness and constructions. In *Coping and health in organizations* (ed. P. Dewe, T. Cox & A.M. Leiter). Taylor & Francis, London.

Rush, A.J., Beck, A.T., Kovacs, M. & Hollon, S.D.M. (1977). Comparative efficacy of cognitive therapy and pharmacotherapy in the treatment of depressed outpatients. *Cognitive Therapy and Research*, **1**, 17–37.

Sahler, O.J.Z. & McAnarney, E.R. (1981). *The child from three to eighteen*. Mosby, London.

Shapiro, T. (1995). Developmental issues in psychotherapy research. *Journal of Abnormal Child Psychology*, **23**, 31–44.

Shirk, S.R. & Russell, R.L. (1996). *Change process in child psychotherapy*. Guilford Press, New York.

Siegel, M. (1991). *Knowing Children*. Erlbaum, Hillsdale, NJ.

Smiley, P. & Huttenlocher, J. (1989). Young children's acquisition of emotion concepts. In *Children's understanding of emotion* (ed. C. Saarni & P.L. Harris), pp. 27–48. Cambridge University Press, New York.

Stein, N.L. & Trabasso, T. (1989). Children's understanding of changing emotional states. In *Children's understanding of emotion* (ed. C. Saarni & P.L. Harris), pp. 50–77. Cambridge University Press, New York.

Terwogt, M.M. & Olthof, T. (1989). Awareness and self-regulation of emotion in young children. In *Children's understanding of emotion* (ed. C. Saarni & P.L. Harris), pp. 209–37. Cambridge University Press, New York.

Thompson, R.A. (1989). Causal attributions and children's emotional understanding. In *Children's understanding of emotion* (ed. C. Saarni & P.L. Harris), pp. 117–50. Cambridge University Press, New York.

Vasta, R., Haith, M.M. & Miller, S.A. (1995). *Child psychology: The modern science*. Wiley, New York.

Wenar, C. (1982). Developmental psychopathology: Its nature and models. *Journal of Clinical Child Psychology*, **11**, 192–201.

2

Therapy for parents of difficult pre-school children

Jo Douglas

The pre-school period is one of dramatic change in physical, cognitive and emotional development for the child. It is equally a period of stress, change and adjustment for the parents. Some parents find considerable difficulty in managing the demands and behaviour of their young children. This may be due to lack of confidence or to lack of knowledge about parenting skills. Parents who have experienced poor and inadequate parenting themselves in childhood may have considerable difficulties in demonstrating affection or setting appropriate boundaries and limits for their children. Social isolation and marital discordance are also important factors in families with difficult children.

Classification of young children's behaviour problems

Parents frequently express concern about their child's behaviour during the pre-school period and require reassurance and guidance about normal variations in behavioural development for the child's age.

It is often inappropriate to classify young children's behaviour problems as pathological as they can often be transient and the symptomatology may vary as the child grows older. Difficulties with separation, sleeping, eating and toileting will often fluctuate as the child develops. But parents may experience considerable stress in negotiating these periods and require psychological support in developing strategies for coping with their child's behaviour (Douglas, 1989a). There is also the risk that repeated problems in coping with these developmental transitions in the young child's life may have an additive effect in undermining the parents' confidence or ability to manage their child's behaviour appropriately.

In a study by Richman, Stevenson & Graham (1982), a quarter of the pre-school population studied showed behaviour problems, with 7 per cent showing moderate to severe problems and 15 per cent mild problems. These early problems were not usually transient: 63 per cent of three year olds with behaviour problems still had behaviour problems at eight years of age. The severity of the behaviour problems was related to the likelihood of the problems continuing. Three quarters of the children with severe problems at three years continued to show them at eight years, while only half of the children with mild problems continued to have problems. The type of problem also predicted continuity, with a combination of restlessness and oppositional behaviour most likely to persist.

Campbell (1990) has provided a valuable guide to when young children's behavioural problems can be considered clinically significant. The problems should include several components:

a pattern or constellation of symptoms;

a pattern of symptoms with at least short-term stability that goes beyond transient adjustment to stress or change;

a cluster of symptoms that is pervasive across settings and with people other than the parents;

a cluster of symptoms that is relatively severe;

symptoms that interfere with the child's ability to negotiate developmental challenges and reflect some impairment in functioning.

Attempts to classify pre-school behaviour problems and to provide some association with descriptions of behaviour problems later in childhood have led to separating them into externalising and internalising groups (Achenbach, Edelbrock & Howell, 1987). Problems with non-compliance, aggression, attention and self-regulation tend to co-occur as externalising symptoms; whereas withdrawal, anxiety and depression tend to co-occur as internalising symptoms.

Factors contributing to early childhood behaviour problems

A number of interrelating factors contribute to the development of early childhood behaviour problems and there remains much debate in the literature about the direction of the effects (Shaw & Bell, 1993). Most of the effects appear to be reciprocal and transactional. The nature of any mother–child interaction will be the result of the specifics of the ongoing interaction as well as of the history of the relationship (Campbell, 1995).

The effect of parental mental health on parenting skills

There is a strong association between the prevalence of young children's behavioural problems and maternal depression and family/marital dysfunction. This does have significant implications for the development of treatment approaches. Several routes have been identified relating depression and mental health problems in parents, including maternal depression and family/marital dysfunction, to childhood behaviour problems (Rutter & Quinton, 1984). These can be via:

genetic transmission;

adverse effects on the parent–child relationship, i.e. child-rearing practices, quality of attachment;

family disruption and breakdown;

marital discord.

The direct effect of the parent's depression on the child through emotional unavailability or insensitivity and thinking processes of depression is also important (Cummings & Davies, 1994). It has been proposed that the impact of the mother's behaviour may influence the infant's ability to regulate its own emotional arousal (Field, 1987). Negative social cognitions, lowered self-esteem, reduced sense of control and unrealistic expectations characterise depressed thinking patterns, with parents appraising their children's behaviour more negatively and in turn developing more critical and coercive parenting practices (Webster-Stratton & Hammond, 1988).

Low levels of self-efficacy in depressed mothers have been proposed as the primary mediator between parenting difficulties and stresses in the family and environment (Teti, Gelfand & Pompa, 1990). A mother who feels unable to affect her environment or achieve any sense of control in her life is likely to feel helpless in managing her young child's demands. She may avoid conflict by submitting to child non-compliance and use ineffective management techniques (Forehand et al., 1986).

The impact of the parents' emotional state on their parenting skills is significant. Depressed mothers have been reported to be negative, unsupportive and intrusive with their children (Gordon et al., 1989), and depressed mothers of two year olds show criticism and disengagement, with lack of responsivity to the child's cues and low warmth (Cox et al., 1987). They also engage in escalating cycles of coercion, and are less likely to use explanations, persuasion and reasoning in their attempts to manage their children (Cox et al., 1987). Coercive but lax and inconsistent parenting styles increase non-compliance and aggression in children.

Patterson (1982) proposed the coercive hypothesis to explain the escalation of aggression and violence and the effects of negative reinforcement in the interchanges between parents and children. As the child becomes increasingly aggressive or violent during an interchange, eventually the parent acts in a neutral or positive manner to escape the conflict. This process of escaping reinforces the child for being aggressive, and so the process is repeated in future conflicts.

A lethargic, preoccupied and depressed parent will be more inclined to use short-term approaches to management in order to minimise the amount of effort and energy expended in coping with their child's demands. Conversely, a parent who is volatile and has poor anger control can provoke coercive interchanges every time their own aggressive and violent behaviour towards their child causes the child to comply.

The effect of the child's temperament and characteristics on parenting skills

A child's temperamental characteristics – at least partly heritable (Emde *et al.*, 1992) – can also have a significant effect on the mother's mental state and affect her parenting skills, as one part of a transactional effect. Difficult early behaviour and perinatal problems are associated with the development of problems in young children, but only in the context of environmental adversity (Campbell, 1995). A child who is restless, shows poor rhythmicity, or who is easily over-aroused presents a more difficult parenting task than a child who relates positively, is calm in mood and regular in habits of eating and sleeping.

Parenting skills

Parenting skills have a direct effect on the child's behaviour. The evidence suggests that authoritative and supportive parenting, which is characterised by warmth and involvement in the context of clear, consistent and reasonable limit setting and control, is associated with higher levels of child competence and pro-social behaviour. Authoritarian and over-controlling styles of parenting, characterised by arbitrary and harsh limit setting, is associated with social withdrawal and anxiety or aggressive and explosive behaviour in the child, particularly when the parent expresses little warmth to the child (Denham, Renwick & Holt, 1991; Hart *et al.*, 1992).

Observations of parenting styles of parents with difficult children have identified four key management practices that are related to the development of problem behaviour in children:

(i) failure to provide consistent and effective discipline when the child is disobedient;
(ii) poor monitoring of the whereabouts of the child;
(iii) a low level of positive response when the child is showing sociable behaviour;
(iv) poor problem solving (Patterson, 1982).

Changing these features forms the basis of cognitive–behavioural intervention techniques with parents of difficult pre-schoolers.

A model of factors contributing to early childhood behaviour problems

A proposed model of interrelating effects on children's behaviour (Fig. 2.1) can provide a guideline to the types and goals of intervention that may be therapeutic. Cognitive behavioural intervention can occur at many different levels in the family system.

Intervention in parenting skills

For a simple or single behavioural problem like sleep difficulties in pre-schoolers, it is possible to provide direct cognitive–behavioural intervention targeted at the parents in order to change their management strategies of the child's sleeping pattern at Level 1 (Douglas & Richman, 1984). This impacts directly on their parenting skills.

Case illustration
Jenny (aged two years) was waking five to six times per night and could only be pacified by breast-feeding. Her mother was exhausted, irritable and desperate for help. She had another little boy aged five years who was lively and demanding and she felt unable to offer him the attention and stimulation that he required. Her husband was very supportive but felt helpless as he was unable to settle Jenny due to her dependence on breast-feeding. The parents had allowed Jenny to sleep in their bed in an effort to reduce the waking, but this had not helped. Both parents were devoted to their children, providing a supportive, warm and accepting atmosphere at home.

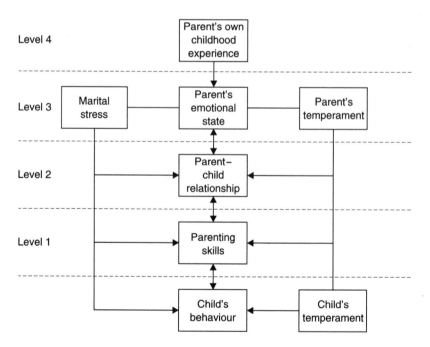

Figure 2.1. Levels of therapeutic intervention in families with difficult pre-school children.

Jenny completely dominated her mother during the day with her demands for breast-feeds, often latching on just for a five-minute comfort suck or lying across her mother's lap for up to an hour and not letting her move. Mother had not wanted to stop the breast-feeding as she felt that Jenny still needed it and would stop on her own eventually.

Initial discussion focused on the level of control that Jenny was exerting over her parents and how they could parent her more effectively. Mother finally agreed that giving in to the continual demands for breast-feeding was creating an impossible situation. Jenny's appetite for food was poor, she was generally irritable, her language was slightly delayed, she slept badly and additional stresses were being exerted on the marital relationship and the mother's relationship with the other sibling.

A plan to reduce demand breast-feeding commenced, initially focusing on the daytime feeds in order to increase Jenny's appetite for food and to build up mother's confidence that she could resist the demands. Successful resolution on set targets led on to a second plan to reduce the night-time feeds. Father was keen to co-operate and agreed to take over the management of Jenny at night as mother felt unable to resist the demands when she was tired. Mother agreed to sleep on the settee, while father settled Jenny by cuddling and soothing. He carried out a graded withdrawal of physical contact and attention at night, and also managed to get Jenny to sleep in her own bed in her own room before mother was allowed back into the parent's room. Within two months the problems had resolved entirely. Jenny was successfully weaned from the breast, she was eating well, her language had improved and she was less irritable. The parents were greatly relieved and less exhausted. Mother finally agreed that setting limits for Jenny's behaviour was necessary and beneficial.

Intervention in the parent–child relationship

In a family in which a child is showing generalised behaviour problems, a poor parent–child relationship may need to be addressed at Level 2, prior to behaviour management strategies being implemented. Forehand and McMahon (1981) in the Child's Game approach have described how to increase the use of parental reinforcement prior to the use of time-out procedures.

Case illustration

Dean, aged four years, was described as uncontrollable at home by his single mother. He was a tough, aggressive little boy who was strong, had poor expressive language and was generally non-compliant. His mother admitted that most of the time she hated him as he made her life a misery. She admitted to losing her temper with him frequently and often hitting him in desperation, and wanted to know of effective ways of punishing him. She could find little positive to say about him and it was clear that their relationship was volatile and poor.

The initial focus of intervention was to develop the positive elements of their relationship by focusing on play and developing a simple monitoring programme during the play interaction, with mother tracking and commenting on his play positively. She was to ignore provocative behaviour by him during these sessions. This was practised initially in the clinic playroom setting where play activities were set out and Dean and his mother were watched and prompted for quarter of an hour play sessions. She was asked to do this every day at home and, after feeling initially uncomfortable with this new style of activity, she became used to it and Dean would look forward to their 'playtime'. The aim was to enhance mother's reinforcing value to Dean so that her non-contingent positive attention could eventually be used contingently to increase his pro-social and compliant behaviour. Over the course of a couple of months, mother became better at playing with Dean and began to enjoy the sessions; she learned to use her attention positively with him and gained confidence once she was successful in getting him to clear up his toys before bed, get washed and changed without a fight and go to bed on time. These simple tasks were a great relief to her and as her confidence grew she was able to progress onto managing his aggressive and confrontational behaviour more appropriately.

Intervention in the parents' emotional state

At Level 3, parents who are depressed may require CBT to cope with depression as well as strategies to improve their relationship with their children and their parenting skills.

Case illustration

Chris (aged three years) was referred because of poor weight gain and selective eating. His mother was observed to be very caring but emotionally distant and tense. She was flat in her affect and often broke down into tears, describing Chris as difficult to manage, not affectionate, and self-willed. She had received antidepressants from her GP but had not found them to be of use. She admitted to feeling low and depressed most of the time, she felt helpless and dreaded mealtimes as these led to confrontations and repetition of her feelings of failure and being a poor parent.

She recognised that her relationship with Chris was poor and attributed this to his first two years of life when he had been repeatedly ill and had difficulty with feeding. She felt rejected by him and incompetent as a mother. Her expectations of her first baby were very high: a demand for perfection in the baby and herself. She felt driven to live up to the high expectations of her parents, whom she felt blamed her for her lack of ability to feed Chris and increased her feelings of stress and tension.

Management approaches to coping with Chris' eating difficulties were not successful until his mother recognised the root of her unrealistically high expectations of herself and of Chris. Her primary social support was her parents, who continually reinforced her view of herself as a poor mother. She was ambivalent about wanting them to take over and remove the problem from her, but was not prepared to pass over responsibility totally to them. The therapeutic plan was to reduce contact with them, to stop talking to them about Chris' eating problems, to focus only on positive elements about Chris, and to join a parent support group locally in order to hear how other mothers coped with similar problems in their children.

Cognitive re-structuring that emphasised Chris' avoidance of eating as due to unpleasant associations with feeding as an infant enabled her to stop blaming herself for his problem. She was then able to stop feeling anxious at meals and began to provide positive support for his eating so that he could eat more and a wider range of foods. Once she learned to focus on small goals of change in Chris' behaviour and genuinely praise him for these achievements, improvements started to occur not only in Chris' eating pattern but also in his relationship with his mother. He became more talkative with her, joined in games and wanted to be with her and to cuddle her.

Intervention related to marital dysfunction

Therapeutic intervention to alleviate the consequences of marital discord could have a direct positive effect on the parents' emotional state, the parent–child relationship, parenting skills and the child's behaviour by reducing the level of tension, distress and emotional arousal in the child.

Case illustration

John (aged three years) was referred for severe selective eating (he had eaten only spaghetti hoops and had drunk only milk since weaning). His mother was observed to be extremely competent, very close to him, with a warm relationship, but was unable to confront him about his eating pattern as she felt it would stress him unduly. She was unable to use any behavioural management advice about his eating until the depths of her marital problem had been revealed. She admitted that she was on the verge of leaving her husband after an unhappy, volatile marriage of four years. She realised the immense level of stress that John was suffering with the continual atmospheres and rows, and was reluctant to oppose him in any way in case he could not cope with the strain.

John's father was very critical of him and had a poor relationship with him. He was disappointed that John was a sensitive, quiet boy and often bullied him. John was anxious, socially shy and undemanding to anyone except his mother. He easily cried and whenever he did this she gave in to him immediately. She had evolved a system of allowing John to eat whatever he wanted to avoid stress on him and on herself.

Following counselling to help her decide about her marriage, she started divorce proceedings and was then able to focus on building up John's confidence and his ability to cope. She started to set small targets for John to achieve in tasting new foods and textures. As each small step was successful, the range of food that he would eat increased slowly and steadily.

Intervention directed at the child's temperamental characteristics

A child who is disobedient and overactive may be showing attention-deficit hyperactivity disorder (ADHD). Intervention in parenting skills may have some effect and may ameliorate many of the daily management problems, but therapy directed at the child's temperamental state, for example with medication or dietary management, may have a dramatic effect not only on the child's behaviour but also on parenting styles, parents' emotional states, and family functioning.

Case illustration

Lucia, aged two years, was referred because of hyperactive behaviour, aggression and poor sleeping. She was an only child, with two much older foster siblings. Her mother had always fostered children and enjoyed having children around the house but found that she could not manage Lucia, which was distressing as she felt that she was a competent and caring mother.

Lucia, on observation, was continually on the move. She would not settle to play with toys, she climbed on furniture, touched all objects in the room and if she was restrained she had a temper tantrum, hitting her mother and throwing herself around on the floor. Her mother commented that at home she could ignore this behaviour and let Lucia recover, but this approach seemed to have no effect on the frequency or intensity of these outbursts.

At night Lucia's mother had let Lucia cry for hours at a time and had carried out an 'extinction' approach to manage her night waking correctly, but this had not worked. Lucia still woke regularly, demanding bottles of milk during the night. She drank a lot during the day and yet still had a good appetite.

Lucia showed a very short attention span for her age, was very active and was continually irritable. It was clear that her mother had tried a number of approaches to managing Lucia, to no effect. Her mother reported that she carefully avoided all additives, preservatives and colouring in Lucia's diet and prided herself that the children always ate freshly cooked food with no manufactured food. Sweets were always carefully selected to be additive free as she had suspected that Lucia was hyperactive.

Every behavioural therapeutic strategy tried for managing the sleep problem and the daytime behaviour appeared to have no effect, until one session when Lucia seemed to be considerably better. This coincided with her father being away at work for three weeks. During this time the foster children, who were Iranian, undertook a religious fast and only ate steamed fish and rice. Lucia had joined them as she liked the food and her mother had stopped cooking the meat and two vegetable meals that she always provided for her husband and the children. It became apparent that her mother always used instant gravy granules with the roast dinner and had not realised that they contained additives. When her father returned, Lucia continued not to have gravy granules, and the behavioural improvement was maintained.

The therapist needs to assess the importance of varying influences on the child's behaviour and to anticipate the effect of any intervention. At times it is possible to intervene at a lower level to affect a change at a higher level, e.g. simple behavioural management strategies in parenting which are successful and create a positive change in the child's behaviour can impact positively on the parent–child relationship and on the parent's emotional state.

The therapist should assess at which point the intervention needs to be addressed in order to gain maximum effect on the child's behaviour problem and to be most cost efficient in the use of therapeutic time.

Cognitive–behavioural therapy strategies for parents

Parent training programmes for aggressive and non-compliant pre-school children

Parent training programmes have shown successful results over the last 20 years in reducing young children's levels of aggression and non-compliance. These programmes have focused on changing parents' behaviour towards their children in order to establish better control over antisocial and non-compliant behaviour. This may occur with individual families or in parent training groups.

The approach entails direct coaching of the parent during parent–child play sessions, with sequential training in the use of differential social attention and time out. Parents learn to alter the reinforcement contingencies they provide for their child. The Parent–Child Game has been a successful model of individual parent training in the clinic

(Forehand & McMahon, 1981) and Webster-Stratton (1990, 1994) has developed video-taped training packages for groups of parents.

Sutton (1992) found that there was no real difference between the efficacy of training parents using social-learning and behavioural principles in a small study that compared group training, home visits, or telephone contact. All three of the active interventions demonstrated clinical improvement compared to a waiting list control.

Successful short-term results have been shown in parents' and children's behaviour and in parental perceptions of child adjustment from parent training programmes (Webster-Stratton, 1984, 1985). Long-term follow-up of later adolescents who participated in parent training with their mothers when they were young, non-compliant children found that they were functioning as well as non-clinic individuals when examined on measures of delinquency, emotional adjustment, academic progress and relationship with parents (Long *et al.*, 1994).

A direct approach to address parenting skills is therefore a useful and effective treatment method. The elements of this approach usually include:

giving information to the parents by teaching them strategies of behaviour management – this may be done via talking with them or providing written material to read;

modelling and prompting improved behaviour management techniques via videos or direct contact;

setting tasks for the parents to carry out at home with the child;

using charts to record the child's behaviour and the parents' responses.

This approach has also been demonstrated to be successful with parents of pre-schoolers with ADDH (Pisterman *et al.*, 1992). There was a significant increase in the percentage of compliance in the children, and the parents gave more appropriate commands and more consistently reinforced compliance. In addition, the parents gave fewer directive statements and increased the proportion of positive feedback to their children. The parents were better at directing their children's attention to a task but the children's attention span did not improve. The authors concluded that to achieve specific improvement in attention, pharmacological treatment with stimulants may need to be included alongside the training programme.

Parent training programme for communication and anger management

Some parents do not respond to standard parent training packages. Characteristics such as marital distress, spouse abuse, lack of a supportive partner or family, maternal depression and high life stress are associated with treatment relapses or poorer outcome in many studies, although, as the above examples demonstrate, they do not preclude success. When treatment approaches are not successful, it is important to reconsider the factors that are influencing the existing state (see Fig. 2.1). Treatment approaches that impact on these areas then need to be considered.

Eyberg and Boggs (1989) describe a programme in which additional play therapy techniques and problem-solving skills are added to the basic parent training. The specific goals are to teach parents how to build a warm and mutually rewarding relationship with their pre-schooler, to teach their child desirable pro-social behaviours, and to decrease their child's inappropriate behaviours. Small-scale studies have demonstrated that these techniques are effective in reducing behaviour problems in the children and that parental attitudes alter positively.

Webster-Stratton (1994) has identified features of a more general relational deficit in communication, conflict resolution skills and affect regulation. She considers that, in these circumstances, the focus of the typical parent training programme may be too narrow and does not alter the parents' negative communication pattern, anger management difficulties and poor problem-solving techniques, all of which are still continuously modelled for the children at home. She developed a set of six videos plus group discussion to cover personal self-control, communication skills, problem-solving skills between adults, teaching children to problem solve, strengthening social support, and self-care, and used these in addition to her standard video parent training package. This only modestly improved outcome, with significant improvement in parents' problem solving, communication, collaboration skills and children's problem solving, but made no difference to parents' self-reports of marital satisfaction, anger, stress level or children's behaviour at short-term follow-up. The lack of difference may be due to delayed effects of the improved relational skills, a ceiling effect of the basic parent training programme which was already creating improvement in these areas, or inadequate application of the approach.

From a therapist's perspective, it is evident that in some families the parents require marital help or personal help for their own personality and emotional difficulties before they can effectively parent their children, but it is also evident that success in managing their children's behaviour using behaviour management methods can enhance parents' own self-esteem and confidence in a manner which may help to resolve many of their own problems and stresses.

Parent training programme for interpersonal problem solving

Other training approaches have focused on teaching parents how to develop problem solving and pro-social skills in their young children. Shure and Spivak (1978, 1980) developed a programme that enabled parents to teach their pre-schoolers social problem solving. Children at age four years show differences in their cognitive ability to solve typical interpersonal problems with peers and adults. Two processes of thought called Interpersonal Cognitive Problem Solving (ICPS) skills are significant predictors of social adjustment and interpersonal competence in this age group. The strongest predictors appear to be:

the ability to offer a variety of solutions to problems concerning peers or authority;

the ability to anticipate potential consequences to an interpersonal act.

Independent of IQ, children who show good ICPS skills are better liked by their peers and show greater awareness and concern to someone in distress, whereas children who are low in these skills are impulsive and disinhibited.

Shure and Spivak's programme emphasises teaching children to recognise their own and others' feelings, to generate alternative solutions to conflicts with other children or adults, and to identify the best solution. The emphasis is on 'how' to think rather than on 'what' to think. This approach requires parents to change their way of talking to and reacting to their children. Trained mothers have shown improvements in their problem-solving thinking about mother–child and child–child problems. The improvements in the children were also detectable by kindergarten teachers who were blind to the treatment conditions (Shure & Spivak, 1978). A review of the literature in this field concludes that ICPS training is an effective remediation strategy and secondary prevention strategy for children at risk (Pellegrini & Urbain, 1985).

A community approach to parent training

Parents who are economically disadvantaged, socially isolated, single or depressed are least likely to participate in individual clinic-based parent training programmes and so community-based approaches may be more effective in reaching this group of parents. Cunningham, Bremner and Boyle (1995) describe such a programme in which they used a coping, modelling and problem-solving model where parents of difficult pre-schoolers formulated their own solutions by identifying videotaped child management errors, discussing the consequences of these mistakes, suggesting alternative solutions and considering their advantages. Large-group discussion, modelling and role playing were supplemented by homework planning. The community groups created an opportunity to build networks between the families and time was also devoted to informal supportive interaction, opportunities to exchange information about the community resources, and activities designed to increase local personal networks.

Outcome measures indicated that the community group generated a wider number of management options and a greater improvement in behaviour problems at home compared to the individual parent training. The clinic-based parent training provided a greater parental sense of competence than community parent training between pre-tests and post-tests, but the community group showed a greater sense of competence in the follow-up. The community groups were also much more cost effective.

Parent training for sleep problems in pre-school children

Sleep problems are a common and stressful experience for many parents of young children. Behavioural management training for parents has been demonstrated to be effective in reducing the amount of night-time disturbance they experience (Richman *et al.*, 1985; Douglas, 1989b; Minde *et al.*, 1993). Increasing parents' sense of confidence about how to cope with the problem and enabling them to make decisions about how to improve settling to sleep and night waking in the most effective manner are crucial elements to this approach. A variety of behavioural management techniques is useful for teaching the child to settle without parental contact. Rapid improvement is common once the techniques are put into action by the parents.

Conclusion

Cognitive–behaviour interventions constitute a valuable and effective approach when helping parents of difficult pre-school children. The basic strategies of behaviour management have remained consistent over the past ten years and research has tended to examine routes of application rather than ways of altering the basic approach. The problem remains of how best to approach parents in families where there are multiple emotional, behavioural and environmental problems. The most alienated and deprived group of children and parents is the most difficult to access and appears to show the least change. It is with this group that there is the greatest need for research and service development.

References

Achenbach, T.M., Edelbrock, C. & Howell, C.T. (1987). Empirically based assessment of the behavioural/emotional problems of 2 and 3 year old children. *Journal of Abnormal Child Psychology*, **15**, 629–50.

Campbell, S.B. (1990). *Behaviour problems in pre-school children: clinical and developmental issues*. Guilford Press, New York.

Campbell, S.B. (1995). Behaviour problems in pre-school children: a review of recent literature. *Journal of Child Psychology and Psychiatry*, **36**, 113–51.

Cox, A.D., Puckering, C., Pound, A. & Mills, M. (1987). The impact of maternal depression in young people. *Journal of Child Psychology and Psychiatry*, **28**, 917–28.

Cummings, E.M. & Davies, P.T. (1994). Maternal depression and child development. *Journal of Child Psychology and Psychiatry*, **35**, 73–113.

Cunningham, C.E., Bremner, R. & Boyle, M. (1995). Large group community based parenting programs for families of preschoolers at risk for disruptive behaviour disorder: utilization, cost effectiveness and outcome. *Journal of Child Psychology and Psychiatry*, **36**, 1141–59.

Denham, S.A., Renwick, S.M. & Holt, R.W. (1991). Working and playing together: Prediction of pre-school emotional competence from mother–child interaction. *Child Development*, **62**, 242–9.

Douglas, J. (1989a). *Behaviour problems in young children*. Tavistock/Routledge, London.

Douglas, J. (1989b). Training parents to manage their child's sleep problem. In *Handbook of parent training* (ed. C.E. Schaeffer & J.M. Briemeister), pp. 36–66. Wiley, New York.

Douglas, J.E. & Richman, N. (1984). *My child won't sleep*. Penguin, Harmondsworth.

Emde, R.N., Plomin, R., Robinson, J.L., Corley, R., DeFries, J., Fulker, D.W., Reznick, J.S., Campos, J., Kagan, J. & Zahn-Waxler, C. (1992). Temperament, emotion and cognition at 14 months: The MacArthur Longitudinal Twin Study. *Child Development*, **63**, 1437–55.

Eyberg, S. & Boggs, S.R. (1989). Parent training for oppositional-defiant preschoolers. In *Handbook of parent training* (ed. C. Schaeffer & J.M. Briemeister). Wiley, New York.

Field, T.M. (1987). Affective and interactive disturbances in infants. In *Hanbook of infant development*, 2nd edn (ed. J.D. Osofsky), pp. 972–1005. John Wiley, New York.

Forehand, R., Lautenschlager, G.J., Faust, H.J. & Graziano, W.G. (1986). Parent perceptions and parent–child interactions in clinic referred children: a preliminary investigation of the effects of maternal depressive moods. *Behavior Research and Therapy*, **24**, 73–5.

Forehand, R. & McMahon, R. (1981). *Helping the non-compliant child: a clinician's guide to parent training*. Guilford Press, New York.

Gordon, D., Burge, D., Hammen, C., Adrian, C., Jaenicke, C. & Hirito, D. (1989). Observations of interactions of depressed women with their children. *American Journal of Psychiatry*, **146**, 50–5.

Hart, C.H., DeWolf, D.M., Wozniak, P. & Burts, D.C. (1992). Maternal and paternal disciplinary styles: relations with preschoolers' playground behavioural orientation and peer status. *Child Development*, **63**, 879–92.

Long, P., Forehand, R., Wierson, M. & Morgan, A. (1994). Does parent training with young non-compliant children have long term effects? *Behavior Research and Therapy*, **32**, 101–07.

Minde, K., Popiel, K., Leos, N., Falker, S., Parker, K. & Handley-Derry, M. (1993). The evaluation and treatment of sleep disturbances in young children. *Journal of Child Psychology and Psychiatry*, **34**, 521–33.

Patterson, G.R. (1982). *Coercive family process*. Castalia Press, Eugene, OR.

Pellegrini, D.S. & Urbain, E.S. (1985). An evaluation of interpersonal cognitive problem solving training with children. *Journal of Child Psychology and Psychiatry*, **1**, 17–41.

Pisterman, S., Firestone, P., McGrath, P., Goodman, J.T., Webster, I., Mallory, R. & Goffin, B. (1992). The role of parent training in treatment of preschoolers with ADDH. *American Journal of Orthopsychiatry*, **62**, 397–408.

Richman, N., Douglas, J., Hunt, H., Lansdown, R. & Levere, R. (1985). Behavioural methods in the treatment of sleep disorders – a pilot study. *Journal of Child Psychology and Psychiatry*, **26**, 581–90.

Richman, N., Stevenson, J. & Graham, P. (1982). *Pre-school to school: a behavioural study*. Academic Press, London.

Rutter, M. & Quinton, D. (1984). Parental psychiatric disorder: effects on children. *Psychological Medicine*, **14**, 853–80.

Shaw, D.S. & Bell, R.Q. (1993). Developmental theories of parental contributors to antisocial behaviour. *Journal of Abnormal Child Psychology*, **21**, 493–518.

Shure, M.B. & Spivak, G. (1978). *Problems solving techniques in child rearing*. Jossey-Bass, San Francisco.

Shure, M.B. & Spivak, G. (1980). Interpersonal problem solving as a mediator of behavioural adjustment in preschool and kindergarten children. *Journal of Applied Developmental Psychology*, **1**, 29–43.

Sutton, C. (1992). Training parents to manage difficult children: a comparison of methods. *Behavioural Psychotherapy*, **20**, 115–39.

Teti, D.M., Gelfand, D.M. & Pompa, J. (1990). Depressed mothers' behavioural competence with their infants: demographic and psycho-social correlates. *Development and Psychopathology*, **2**, 259–70.

Webster-Stratton, C. (1984). Randomised trial of two parent training programs for families with conduct disordered children. *Journal of Consulting and Clinical Psychology*, **52**, 666–78.

Webster-Stratton, C. (1985). Predictors of treatment outcome in parent training for conduct disordered children. *Behaviour Therapy*, **16**, 223–43.

Webster-Stratton, C. (1990). Enhancing the effectiveness of self-administered videotape parent training for families with conduct problem children. *Journal of Abnormal Child Psychology*, **18**, 479–92.

Webster-Stratton, C. (1994). Advancing videotape parent training: a comparison study. *Journal of Consulting and Clinical Psychology*, **62**, 583–93.

Webster-Stratton, C. & Hammond, M. (1988). Maternal depression and its relationship to life stress, perceptions of child behaviour problems, parenting behaviours, and child conduct problems. *Journal of Abnormal Child Psychology*, **16**, 299–315.

3
Attention-deficit hyperactivity disorder

R.J. van der Krol, H. Oosterbaan, S.D. Weller and A.E. Koning

Introduction

This chapter starts with an overview of the symptoms of attention-deficit hyperactivity disorder (ADHD), and of the factors that underlie it. Next, the various treatment modes for ADHD are discussed. The authors favour a multi-modal treatment approach. This implies the application of more than one treatment mode, preferably both at home and at school. Such a multi-modal approach can have an effect exceeding the sum of its parts (Kendall, Panichelli-Mindel & Gerow, 1995). The way CBT can be integrated within a multi-modal treatment arrangement is highlighted. A training programme by means of which parents are taught how to apply cognitive–behavioural principles in the rearing of their children with ADHD is described (Koning *et al.*, 1993a). Finally, the practicability and significance of CBT within a multi-modal ADHD approach are discussed.

What is attention-deficit hyperactivity disorder?

Attention-deficit hyperactivity disorder (American Psychiatric Association, 1995) consists of three main categories: inattention, hyperactivity and impulsivity. *Inattention* is revealed in poor selective attention (attending to irrelevant or distracting stimuli and ignoring relevant stimuli), and lack of sustained attention (the ability to keep paying attention over time) (Douglas, 1972). Children with this disorder are easily distracted and avoid tasks that require paying attention for a long timespan. *Hyperactivity* is reflected by enhanced motor activity. Children with ADHD seem unable to suppress their activity in situations which require them to do so. They move excessively, do not sit still, are permanently 'on the go', cannot play quietly, and often fidget with their hands or feet. *Impulsivity* is expressed in a lack of control in situations that require controlled attention or a structured approach. Children with ADHD are inclined to respond to the first thought that enters their mind, they do not consider sufficiently the effects of their behaviour, and find it difficult to delay the fulfilment of their needs. These three main characteristics of ADHD are not necessarily displayed at the same time nor to the same degree.

Attention-deficit hyperactivity disorder has a wide impact on the development of children – in learning, speech and language development – and is associated with a multitude of problems, such as sleeping, emotional, relational, and behaviour problems, and problems in sensory and motor activities. Sometimes these associated problems are so prominent that they obscure the existence of ADHD. In the current version of the DSM classification system (DSM-IV, APA, 1995), ADHD, together with oppositional defiant disorder and conduct disorder, comprise the cluster Attention-Deficit and Disruptive Behavior Disorders. The comorbidity of these three disorders is high (Hinshaw, 1994), and it is often difficult to decide diagnostically between them.

The causes of ADHD are not fully known, hence explanations have a tentative character. The literature suggests that in many cases biological–genetic factors are involved (Compernolle, 1996). It is hypothesised that children with ADHD suffer from an underactivity of the brain's behavioural inhibition system (Quay, 1989), or from an impairment in delayed responding, similar to patients with frontal–orbital lesions (Barkley, 1994). Goodman and Stevenson (1989) found that the concordance of ADHD is higher in monozygotic than in dizygotic twins. This supports the notion that genetic factors are significant causally. Environmental causes may also be involved. For instance, it has been reported that an insufficiently structured environment can enhance ADHD symptoms (Prins, 1994). It is unclear, though, whether the behaviour of parents should be considered as a cause of, or as a reaction to, the disruptive behaviour of the child. Usually, numerous different factors interact in any one affected child.

Treatment

The main established forms of treatment for ADHD are setting up and maintaining a structured environment, behaviour therapy, CBT, and medication.

Since children with ADHD lack stimulus control, the first step in the process of treatment is to create an orderly, *well-structured environment*. This reduces the probability of eliciting overactive and impulsive behaviour in the child. In order to compensate for their lack of stimulus control, Prins (1994) reports that children with ADHD should receive more prompts, cues and reinforcements than normal children. An environment providing for a large amount of structure – a so-called prosthetic environment – has a beneficial effect on the children's behaviour and should be maintained indefinitely.

Specific behaviour problems can then be addressed by *behaviour therapeutic* interventions. These comprise mainly operant techniques such as 'token' rewards, response–cost, and time-out. It is noted, however, that although operant procedures can bring about behaviour improvements, at home as well as at school, transfer to other situations and stability over time are generally poor (Prins, 1994).

From a *cognitive–behavioural* perspective, Kendall and co-workers (1995) point out that children with ADHD demonstrate a lack of information processing. They do not take the time to pay attention to and process social cues and information, to think about a situation and to plan for it. The aim of CBT is to provide the children with more self-control and with strategies that help them to manage and cope by themselves (Kendall, 1993). In effect, the ultimate goal of ADHD treatment is to enable the children to cope on their own with the situations and problems they encounter during life. This goal cannot be attained by medication alone or by the children learning rules by heart. It can only be accomplished by teaching the children strategies for dealing with people and tasks, which help in everyday functioning. Most CBTs can be characterised as stop–think–and–do trainings. They are usually conducted by a professional therapist (Camp & Bash, 1981; Kendall, 1992; Lauth & Schlottke, 1995), although sometimes they are carried out by the parents, who have been trained to conduct the programme with their child (Braswell & Bloomquist, 1991; Koning *et al.*, 1993a, 1993b; Petersen, 1995). The child is taught to tackle tasks and problems in a logical, stepwise fashion. This can be accomplished by cognitive modelling techniques, in which an adult demonstrates self-guiding verbalisation to the child. The first step to be learned is to stop, look and listen in order to understand what the problem is. The next step is to consider all possible solutions. The third step consists of executing the chosen solution. In the final step, the child evaluates the process as well as the result of the actions undertaken. In this way the child gradually learns to make use of general and specific strategies, which help him or her to cope with problem situations and to keep out of trouble.

Medication has proven to be highly effective in the temporary amelioration and normalisation of ADHD symptoms (Abikoff & Klein, 1992; Barkley, 1994). Gunning (1996), for example, demonstrated that the probability of a clinically significant effect of methylphenidate (Ritalin) is 70 per cent. However, even after careful dose adjustment, medication may have unwanted side-effects. Methylphenidate, for example, can cause irritability and problems in falling asleep. Therefore, medication should only be given after a thorough evaluation of all pros and cons.

Deciding which treatment to use is not simply a matter of making the right choice from a set comprised of setting up a structured environment, traditional behaviour therapy, CBT or medication. Rather, the issue is to find out which is the best mix for the child. One reason for this is that any one of the components affects the ADHD symptoms in its own way (Gunning, 1996). A second reason is that no single component has clinically relevant effects by itself (Prins, 1994). As Kendall and co-workers (1995) emphasise, children with ADHD have multiple problems, which can only be dealt with by a broad approach.

Figure 3.1 shows a tentative conceptual framework of the treatment modes, and of the way they are related to each other. Besides being helpful in selecting treatments for individual cases, it can also be used for purposes of (further) protocol development. The latter is currently an important issue in research as well as in clinical practice. In the authors' clinical setting, the framework is used in structuring and tuning treatment.

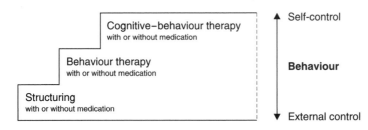

Figure 3.1. A tentative conceptual framework for the treatment of ADHD.

The framework shows that treatment should start with establishing a well-structured environment, which should be maintained for a long period. The next step to be considered is the addition of behaviour therapy in order to diminish disruptive behaviour and to establish new, more adaptive behaviour. The third step to take into consideration is cognitive–behavioural therapy. This treatment mode is aimed at increasing self-control, whereas structuring the environment and behaviour therapy can be seen as external means of controlling the behaviour of the child.

Each of the three treatment modes mentioned above can be complemented with *medication*. Gunning (1996) found that methylphenidate is less effective when the child is not offered enough external control. He suggests one should first provide sufficient structure in the home and classroom, and then evaluate whether behaviour therapy is possible without medication. If not, medication should be attempted. If medication is offered from the start, subsequent behaviour improvement may discourage children (and their caretakers) from taking an active part in the treatment. Thus, they may learn to depend on pills rather than on their own efforts. If medication appears to be helpful, it places the child in a relatively better starting position to profit from behaviour therapy (Gunning, 1994). During behaviour therapy, the application of medication should continue since such behaviour therapy alone is often insufficient (Gunning, 1994). Another reason not to refrain from medication is that it affects symptoms other than those influenced by behaviour therapy (Gunning, 1996). Research findings also suggest that the simultaneous administration of medication and behaviour therapy is more effective than each of these modes separately (Pelham *et al.*, 1980). This applies to both short-term and long-term effects (Satterfield, Satterfield & Shell, 1987).

Again, it should be noted that the treatment modes presented in Figure 3.1 supplement each other. They are needed in the handling of a vast variety of problems throughout treatment. In the course of treatment, however, the intensity of a particular treatment mode may be increased or decreased.

Apart from the selection of treatment modes, a distinction can be made between the contexts within which the treatment is carried out. It is usually not enough to restrict the treatment to one context (for example exclusively at school, at home, or in a residential group), since for children with ADHD, transfer of training is poor (Braswell & Bloomquist, 1991). Further, certain problems are context specific. Sleeping problems, for example, cannot be treated at school. These are important reasons for children's parents and teachers to be actively involved with the therapy.

Parent mediation programmes are gaining popularity in clinical practice. In this type of therapy, systematically parents are provided with information on the problem behaviour of their child and are subsequently taught ways to modify it. Most parent training programmes are based on behaviour management principles and rely strongly on operant conditioning techniques (e.g. Barkley, 1987). Programmes which apply CBT principles have been presented by Braswell and Bloomquist (1991) and Koning *et al.* (1993b). Braswell and Bloomquist teach parents how to prompt and reinforce their children in their use of cognitive strategies for different sorts of problems. Koning *et al.* (1993b) instruct parents how to teach their children to stop-think-and-do. This programme is directed at cognitive tasks, practical skills (like laying the table and tidying up one's room), and social skills. More information about this programme is given in the next section. Based on his review of the literature, Barkley (1990) concluded that parent training in the context of ADHD could be therapeutically beneficial, although more research is necessary before final conclusions can be drawn.

Concerning the effects of treatment in general, Barkley (1994) points out that only temporary effects can be expected. For example, once medication is withdrawn or the environment becomes less structured, behaviour reverts to its formerly impaired range. Barkley believes that the core feature of ADHD consists of a fundamental impairment in delayed responding, which occurs outside conscious or voluntary control. He asserts that the deficit of children with ADHD is not as much in thinking as in waiting long enough to give thinking a chance to occur and then to affect responding. Barkley points out that neither CBT nor other psychosocial therapies address the fundamental impairment in the relatively automatic delay or inhibition process in children with ADHD. This implies that at present ADHD cannot be cured. However, by treatment, the children may be able to bring conscious and effortful control to improve their response inhibition, provided they are prompted and reinforced for doing so. Barkley supports treating these children in their natural settings for a considerable period of time.

More intensive treatment is possible if a residential or day-care facility is available. The Nijmegen Paedological Institute (in which the authors work) is a centre for child care, special education and applied research, providing residential and day-care treatment for children of primary school age with serious developmental, emotional and behavioural disorders. The children attend a special school that is linked to the institute. When receiving residential care, they spend every other weekend, and all school holidays, at home. Approximately a quarter to one third of the centre's population suffers from ADHD.

Until the early 1980s, treatment consisted primarily of a structured environment in the group and at school, supplemented with behaviour modification for disruptive behaviour. Medication was only applied in extreme cases. At the end of the 1980s, an individual cognitive training programme was developed by the staff, based on the programme 'Think Aloud' (Camp & Bash, 1981). By means of this programme, children are taught a problem-solving strategy. The programme utilises a number of cognitive–behavioural training techniques, which have been put forward by Meichenbaum (1977). Specifically, children are to pose to themselves, the following four questions when confronted with a problem or task:

1. What is the problem? (Problem exploration.)
2. What is my plan? (Generating possible strategies to tackle the problem.)
3. Do I use my plan? (Self-monitoring and self-guidance while executing the plan.)
4. How did I do? (Self-evaluation of solution.)

This is accomplished by using a cognitive modelling technique. To start with, the *adult* goes through all the steps while constantly verbalising what he or she is thinking and doing, and monitoring and instructing himself or herself aloud. Subsequently, the *child* imitates the adult's behaviour, talking out loud as well. In the next stage the child is instructed to whisper instead of talk out loud. Finally, the child guides his or her own behaviour by silent, inner speech.

In a training programme, individually administered by a remedial teacher, children are taught to apply this stop-think-and-do approach while performing school tasks (like mathematical problems), practical tasks (like handicraft), and social activities (like negotiating with another child about what game to play). Residential group workers and teachers are informed about the nature and application of the training principles, thus enabling the extension of the training to both the live-in group and classroom settings. Parents are involved in the treatment of their child, in order to accomplish an around-the-clock programme. Based on the 'Think Aloud' training of Camp and Bash (1981) and also drawing upon the programmes by Barkley (1987, 1990), Braswell and Bloomquist (1991), and Shure and Spivack (1978), an experimental cognitive–behavioural parent training programme is applied (Koning *et al.*, 1993b; Van der Vlugt *et al.*, 1995).

The present version of the programme consists of eight sessions, once every fortnight. The sessions are led by a professional trainer with a group of up to five couples. The parents learn how to teach their children cognitive–behavioural skills at home. Sessions comprise theoretical introductions and practical (role-playing) exercises. After each session, homework tasks are performed by parents and children at a specific time of the day. In addition, parents are stimulated to practise stop-think-and-do principles throughout the day whenever a suitable situation arises.

A token reward and response–cost system is applied: children receive a sticker of a smiling face on properly completing a task, and a sticker of a sad face if they fail a task. At the end of the session, one smile sticker is removed for each sad sticker. The remaining smile stickers can be exchanged for tangible rewards.

In the *first two sessions* the child is taught to stop-look-and-listen. These are considered basic prerequisite skills on the way to self-control. Before children can think about and make a suitable plan to deal with a problem, they must learn to pace down and stop their activities, examine their environment, and subtract relevant information from it. Stopping, looking and listening are taught by means of visual and verbal cues. For example, each time the child is about to rush into things, the parent raises a stop signal and says 'stop'. Eventually stopping should become an automatic act. Looking and listening intently are taught by means of imitation (copying movements, mimicking facial expressions, and repeating words and sentences, for example) and by prompting (giving instructions such as 'Walk towards the door and knock three times').

Once these prerequisite stop-look-and-listen skills have been acquired, the children must learn to think out loud while performing simple skills like drawing, lacing their shoes, and getting dressed. It is assumed that verbalisation and (in a later stage of development) internalisation of speech diminish impulsive behaviour and promote self-control. Children with ADHD, however, do not utilise speech while monitoring and controlling their behaviour. Initially, the children are prompted to think out loud while performing various tasks. Later on, they should whisper these self-verbalisations. And eventually, they exert control over their behaviour by means of inner or 'silent' speech. This is addressed in the *third session*, by means of cognitive modelling: the parent performs a task while thinking out loud, and subsequently the child performs the same task, while thinking out loud as well.

In the *fourth session*, children learn to recognise problems and to apply strategies to deal with them. Before getting started with a task or problem, they should ask themselves what exactly is its nature and decide on the best way to tackle it. The programme emphasises the process of planning as such rather than the merits of the proposed solution for a specific problem. While talking out loud, children pose and answer the following questions: 'Stop: what is my problem?' and 'What is my plan?'. After a couple of trials, the children start to whisper instead of talk aloud. Finally, whispering is faded out and replaced by inner speech. The latter transition should not take place too soon, since inner speech makes it impossible for the adult to monitor and correct the child's thinking process.

In the *fifth session* children learn self-monitoring, self-guidance and self-evaluation. While executing their plan, they pose to themselves questions like 'Do I use my plan?' and 'How did I do?'.

An example of such self-instructions is given in the following. John has to set the table for dinner. Before doing so he asks himself aloud: 'Stop! What is my problem?'. He replies: 'I have to set the table for five people.' Then: 'What is my plan? First I lay the tablecloth on the table. Next I fetch five plates, forks, knives, spoons and napkins from the cupboard. And next I place them all neatly on the table'. While doing so: 'Am I using my plan? I first place the tablecloth on the table properly . . . Now I fetch the plates, knives, spoons and forks from the cupboard, five of each. Oops, I almost forgot the napkins! Now I lay them all down in groups for each person. . .' And finally: 'How did I do? I've been using the four questions. . . I followed my plan. I noticed in time that I nearly missed the napkins. I did a good job!'

The *sixth* and *seventh sessions* deal with social situations. Children are trained to use the four questions in making plans for preventing as well as handling social conflicts. Apart from being instrumentally effective, plans should meet two ethical criteria: 'Is it fair to me and to the other person?' and 'Is it pleasant for me and for the other person?' For example: John's friend Peter has come to see him. John suggests they play a computer game together. Peter, however, prefers to go biking. They do not come to an agreement and start yelling at each other. John's mother intervenes by holding up a stop sign and prompting John to stop-think-and-do. John stops yelling and says aloud: 'What's my problem? I want to play a Nintendo game with Peter, but he wants to go biking . . . Now the next question is: What are we going to do about it?' Mother: 'Precisely, now go and find a way to solve this problem? Remember, the solution should be fair and pleasant for both of you.' John: 'We could play Nintendo because we're in my house!' Peter: 'If you do that I will go out biking alone'. Mother: 'Is this plan fair?' Both boys agree. Mother: 'And is it pleasant for both of you? You want to have a nice time together, don't you?' John: 'We could first play a couple of Nintendo games and then go biking.' Mother: 'What other plans could you make?' Peter: 'We could think of something we both like to do.' Eventually, John and Peter decide on an activity which they both enjoy. As the boys are playing, mother may stop them once again and remind John to pose himself the third question: 'Am I using my plan?' Finally, the fourth question will be addressed: 'How did I do?' This example illustrates that in many situations the parent keeps playing an active role in stimulating and coaching the cognitive processes of the child.

Session eight is an evaluation meeting in which benefits and problems parents have encountered during and after the programme are discussed. A date for a follow-up session is set.

Transfer of training is promoted by applying the stop-think-and-do principles in a variety of situations, including school. In school, children with ADHD typically are hindered by inattentiveness and impulsivity while performing school tasks such as arithmetic and spelling. For example, children may arrive at a wrong answer because they do not notice that the task is to subtract rather than to add two numbers.

The programme has been evaluated in a small-scale study with two main questions in mind:

1. Does a parent training programme positively affect the way parents of children with ADHD perceive and are able to handle their parenting situation?
2. Does it bring about better self-control and a decrease in behaviour problems in the children?

Other objectives of the study were to explore the strengths and weaknesses of the parent training programme and to assess the significance and practicability of a multi-modal approach.

Subjects were six children (aged 8 to 11 years) and their families. The children were diagnosed as having ADHD according to guidelines proposed by DSMIII.R. Each child was used as his or her own control, thus the study had a multiple n = 1 pre-test–post-test design. In order to assess changes in the way parents evaluated their parenting situation, they completed the Nijmegen Child-rearing Situation Questionnaire (Wels & Robbroeckx, 1989, 1991a, 1991b) before and after the training. Behavioural changes in the children were assessed in questionnaires completed by their parents, residential group workers and teachers before and after the training. These questionnaires included the Child Behavior Check List and the Teacher Report Form (Achenbach, 1991). Changes in children's self-control were assessed in different ways. For instance, teachers and residential group workers completed the Self-control Rating Scale (Kendall & Wilcox, 1979), and the children were subjected to a neuropsychological screening test battery (Van der Vlugt, 1988) before and after the training. The battery covers the following functions: general intelligence, memory, language, attention and concentration, visual–constructive skills, and fine motor skills.

Case illustration

Peter is the youngest child in a middle-class family. At the start of the training he was 9.6 years old. At that time he had been in residential care for one and a half years. Though he was of average intelligence, his educational level was one year behind that of his peers. Peter behaved in an excited, nervous and impulsive way. When interacting with others he was hasty, superficial, impertinent, obstreperous and dominant. Before and during the training period he received medication.

During the individual cognitive–behavioural training for cognitive and practical tasks, Peter regularly posed himself the four basic questions previously noted. During social tasks, however, he was less motivated. By applying a combined reward and response–cost system (gaining or losing chips for respective compliance or non-compliance to a task set out for him) behaviour was somewhat improved

Peter's parents were strongly motivated and closely involved in the training. Initially, Peter resisted the use of the four questions of the stop-think-and-do strategy in his home environment. His parents resolved this problem by asking siblings to apply the strategy as well. Rewards, such as allowing the choice of a TV programme or being read to, also motivated Peter. After some time, a signal from the parents was sufficient to prompt Peter into using the four basic questions. However, the execution of his plans was variable: Peter was often careless, heedless of time and easily distracted.

After the training, both parents experienced a clear reduction in family and rearing burdens. They claimed that the help they received benefited their own abilities and skills in handling and changing Peter's behavioural problems. Peter clearly displayed fewer behavioural problems at home after the training period. His parents found him to be quieter and more relaxed. He became angry less quickly, and admitted to faults more readily.

At school and in the residential group Peter's behavioural problems during the training programme were somewhat reduced, but after the training they again increased. No change in self-control skills was noted.

The systematic evaluation showed that a majority of the parents reported that they became more confident of their own child-rearing abilities, and more conscientious and objective in handling their children. They experienced a notable reduction in familial disruptions. Partners co-operated and understood each other better.

Furthermore, the parents experienced the training as a support of their child-rearing abilities. They felt the methods taught were useful and applicable. They found it difficult to give an initial oral demonstration of the stop-think-and-do strategy that was to serve as a model for their children. Also, operant techniques such as prompting, cueing and response–cost remained necessary to stimulate the children into using the four stop-think-and-do questions and executing their plans in an appropriate way. The co-operative approach between parents and the institute in the handling of their children was highly valued by parents. The fact that training sessions were held in the home environment was experienced as being very motivating. The limited time period for training was unsatisfactory. Too much was covered in a short time span.

Although the majority of the children achieved better self-control during the individual training, in the home situation behavioural improvements and increased self-control were only reported by a minority of the parents. In the residential situation, no behavioural changes were noted. Neuropsychological testing revealed an improved self-control in most children.

The results suggest that cognitive–behavioural parent training can have a positive impact on the way parents experience their child-rearing situation in general, and on the way they evaluate their competence to handle their children in particular. Parents appreciated the content as well as the process of the training, and they testified that the training had been valuable and helpful to them in their parental role. This was probably due to the fact that they had gained a better understanding and acceptance of their children's needs and handicaps, and had obtained more motivation and resilience in coping with the exceptional educational problems they were confronted with daily. The mere fact that parents spent more 'quality time' with their children may have contributed to the results as well.

However, even with this expensive, labour-intensive programme, the behaviour, and more specifically the amount of self-control of the children themselves, did not significantly improve. There is a variety of possible reasons for this disappointing finding.

Among them was the timing of the programme at the end of the school year, when there were many interruptions to the school routine.

Hinshaw and Melnick (1992) suggest that some disappointing results of cognitive–behavioural training may be attributed to failure to apply complementary measures such as medication, behavioural strategies, and help with school work. Thus, it still remains to be demonstrated that CBT has a clinically significant effect on the behaviour of children with ADHD.

Summary and discussion

Children with ADHD can be characterised as inattentive, impulsive and hyperactive. They show multiple problems within different environments, such as school and home. For this reason, treatment should be multi-modal and cover all the contexts of the children's daily lives. On the basis of literature and their own clinical experience, the authors suggest a multi-modal treatment approach, which is built up as follows. Treatment should always start with creating a well-structured, 'prosthetic' environment. Such an environment prevents the children from being overstimulated, and provides them with clear rules, prompts and consequences. As a second step, specific behaviour problems are addressed by clear-cut behavioural therapeutic interventions, mainly consisting of operant techniques. A third step in building up treatment can be the addition of CBT. Each of these three modes can be complemented with medication.

The effects of CBTs which are aimed at the children's lack of self-control and problem-solving abilities, have not yet been unequivocally demonstrated. Even embedding such a therapy in a multi-modal treatment context does not necessarily result in a significant improvement of the children's behaviour, as is illustrated by the study presented in this chapter. This outcome may be attributed to the relatively poor timing and rather short period of training (four months just before summer vacation).

Whatever the precise underlying deficit of ADHD may be, the syndrome is currently considered as a developmentally handicapping condition, which – at present – cannot be cured, and calls for long-term treatment and guidance. Cognitive–behavioural therapy can be a helpful therapeutic element, in that it may enhance the children's self-control and provide them with strategies to deal with everyday problems.

A multi-modal approach to ADHD will need further elaboration. Notably, attention should be paid to the development of treatment protocols which deal with issues such as the sequencing and combining of treatment modes, and the selection of contexts within which the treatment is conducted.

Acknowledgements

The authors gratefully acknowledge the assistance of Dr Huub M. Pijnenburg and Dr Mark Leiblum in preparing this chapter.

References

Abikoff, H. & Klein, R.G. (1992). Attention-deficit hyperactivity and conduct disorder: Comorbidity and implications for treatment. *Journal of Consulting and Clinical Psychology*, **60**, 881–92.

Achenbach, T.M. (1991). *Integrative guide for the 1991 CBCL/4–18,YSR, and TRF profiles*. University of Vermont, Department of Psychiatry, Burlington.

American Psychiatric Association (1995). *Diagnostic and statistical manual of mental disorders*, 4th edn. American Psychiatric Association, Washington DC.

Barkley, R.A. (1987). *Defiant children: A clinician's manual for parent training*. Guilford Press, New York.

Barkley, R.A. (1990). *Attention deficit hyperactivity disorder: A handbook for diagnosis and treatment*. Guilford Press, New York.

Barkley, R.A. (1994). Impaired delayed responding. In *Disruptive behavior disorders in childhood* (ed. D.K. Routh), pp. 11–58. Plenum Press, New York.

Braswell, L. & Bloomquist, M.L. (1991). *Cognitive behavioral therapy with ADHD children: child, family, and school interventions*. Guilford Press, New York.

Camp, B.W. & Bash, M.S. (1981). *Think aloud: Increasing social cognitive skills – A problem-solving program for children*. Research Press, Champaign, Il..

Compernolle, Th. (1996). Contextuele behandeling van aandachtsen activiteitsstoornissen. In *Kinder- en jeugdpsychiatrie III, Behandeling en begeleiding* (ed. F. Verhey & F.C. Verhulst), pp. 359–66. Van Gorcum, Assen.

Douglas, V. (1972). Stop, look and listen: The problem of sustained attention and impulse control in hyperactive and normal children. *Canadian Journal of Behavioral Science*, **4**, 259–76.

Goodman, R. & Stevenson, J. (1989). A twin study of hyperactivity: II. The aetiological role of genes, family relationships, and perinatal adversity. *Journal of Child Psychology and Psychiatry*, **30**, 691–709.

Gunning, W.B. (1994). Gedragstherapie en farmacotherapie bij ADHD: Effect en fasering. *Gedragstherapie*, **27**, 251–67.

Gunning, W.B. (1996). Medicamenteuze benadering van aandachtsen activiteitsstoornissen. In *Kinder- en jeugdpsychiatrie III, Behandeling en begeleiding* (ed. F. Verhey & F.C. Verhulst), pp. 345–52. Van Gorcum, Assen.

Hinshaw, S.P. (1994). *Attention deficits and hyperactivity in children*. Sage Publications, Thousand Oaks, Ca.

Hinshaw, S.P. & Melnick, S. (1992). Self-management therapies and attention-deficit hyperactivity disorder: Reinforced self-evaluation and anger control interventions. *Behavior Modification*, **16**, 253–73.

Kendall, P.C. (1992). *Cognitive-behavioral therapy for impulsive children, treatment manual/stop and think workbook*, 2nd edn. Temple University, Department of Psychology, Philadelphia.

Kendall, P.C. (1993). Cognitive behavioral therapies with youth: Guiding theory, current status, and emerging developments. *Journal of Consulting and Clinical Psychology*, **61**, 235–47.

Kendall, P. C., Panichelli-Mindel, S.M. & Gerow, M.A. (1995). Cognitive-behavioral therapies with children and adolescents. In *Behavioral approaches for children and adolescents, challenges for the next century* (ed. H.P.J. van Bilsen, P.C. Kendall & J.H. Slavenburg), pp. 1–18. Plenum Press, New York.

Kendall, P.C. & Wilcox, L.E. (1979). Self-control in children: Development of a rating scale. *Journal of Consulting and Clinical Psychology*, **47**, 1020–9.

Koning, A., Pijnenburg, H.M., Snijkers, A., Van der Vlugt, H. & Wels, P.M.A. (1993a). *Opvoedingsondersteuning voor ouders van kinderen met ADHD: Een oriënterend onderzoek naar de mogelijkheden voor toepassing van een gedragsmodificatieprogramma door ouders in de thuissituatie*. Paedologisch Instituut en Katholieke Universiteit, Nijmegen.

Koning, A., Pijnenburg, H.M., Snijkers, A., Van der Vlugt, H. & Wels, P.M.A. (1993b). *Trainershandboek en ouderwerkboek voor het ADHD programma: Experimentele versie*. Onderzoeksrapport. Paedologisch Instituut, Nijmegen.

Lauth, G.W. & Schlottke, P.F. (1995). *Training mit aufmerksamkeitsgestörten Kindern*. Beltz Psychologie Verlags Union, Weinheim.

Meichenbaum, D.H. (1977). *Cognitive behavior modification: An integrative approach*. Plenum Press, New York.

Pelham, W.E., Schnedler, R.W., Bologna, N. & Contreras, A.(1980). Behavioral and stimulant treatment of hyperactive children: a therapy study with methylphenidate probes in a within-subject design. *Journal of Applied Behavior Analysis*, **13**, 221–36.

Petersen, L. (1995). STOP THINK DO. In *Behavioral approaches for children and adolescents: Challenges for the next century* (ed. H.P.J.G. van Bilsen, P.C. Kendall & J.H. Slavenburg), pp. 103–11. Plenum Press, New York.

Prins, P.J.M. (1994). Gedragsstoornissen bij kinderen: conceptualisering en behandeling. *Gedragstherapie*, **3**, 27, 187–214.

Quay, H.C. (1989). The behavioral reward and inhibition systems in childhood behavior disorder. In *Attention deficit disorder III: New research in treatment, psychopharmacology, and attention* (ed. L.M. Bloomingdale), pp. 176–86. Pergamon Press, New York.

Satterfield, J.H., Satterfield, B.T. & Shell, A.M. (1987). Therapeutic interventions to prevent delinquency of hyperactive boys. *Journal of the*

American Academy of Child and Adolescent Psychiatry, **26**, 56–64.

Shure, M.B. & Spivack, G. (1978). *Problem-solving techniques in childrearing*. Jossey-Bass, San Francisco.

Van der Vlugt, H. (1988). *Handleiding bij een neuropsychologische testbatterij: Theorie en praktijk*. Interne publikatie. Tilburgs Ambulatorium voor Neuropsychologie, Katholieke Universiteit Brabant.

Van der Vlugt, H., Pijnenburg, H.M., Wels, P.M.A. & Koning, A. (1995). Cognitive behavior modification of ADHD: a family system approach. In *Behavioral approaches for children and adolescents: Challenges for the next century* (ed. H.P.J.G. Van Bilsen, P.C. Kendall & J.H. Slavenburg), pp. 65–75. Plenum Press, New York.

Wels, P.M.A. & Robbroeckx, L.M.H. (1989). *Handleiding bij de Nijmeegse Vragenlijst voor de Opvoedingssituatie (NVOS, versie 3.2)*. (Technisch Rapport November 1989, ISBN 90 5085 015 4). Instituut voor Orthopedagogiek, Katholieke Universiteit Nijmegen.

Wels, P.M.A. & Robbroeckx, L.M.H. (1991a). Gezinsbelasting en hulpverlening aan gezinnen (I). Een model voor gezinsbelasting ten gevolge van een problematische opvoedingssituatie. *Tijdschrift voor Orthopedagogiek*, **30**, 5–19.

Wels, P.M.A. & Robbroeckx, L.M.H. (1991b). Gezinsbelasting en hulpverlening aan gezinnen (II). De betrouwbaarheid en validiteit van de NVOS onderzocht. *Tijdschrift voor Orthopedagogiek*, **30**, 63–79.

4

Childhood obsessive – compulsive disorder

Roz Shafran

Introduction

Obsessive–compulsive disorder (OCD) in children is considered to be similar to the disorder in adults, and the diagnostic criteria for childhood and adult OCD are almost identical (Swedo *et al.*, 1989). According to the *Diagnostic and statistical manual of mental disorders*, 4th edition (DSM-IV; American Psychiatric Association, 1994), obsessions for both children and adults are defined as unwanted, intrusive ideas, thoughts, images or impulses that cause distress, are time consuming or interfere with functioning, and are independent of another Axis I disorder. However, for children, the criterion of insight into the disorder, i.e. that at some point during the disorder the person has recognised that the obsessions or compulsions are excessive or unreasonable, does not apply. It is clear from diagnostic criteria that the compulsions, defined as repetitive behaviour performed in response to an obsession or according to rigid rules, are meaningful; their purpose is to reduce or prevent distress, or to prevent a dreaded event or situation, but they are not realistically connected with the event they are designed to prevent, or are clearly excessive.

Throughout this chapter, OCD in children and adolescents is often compared with work on adult OCD, since that is the origin of the majority of cognitive–behavioural analyses. However, there may be important aetiological, phenomenological and therapeutic differences between OCD in children younger than 12 years of age and the disorder that begins in adolescence, i.e. 12–18 years old, and the disorder in adolescence is volatile (Rachman, personal communication; Rettew et al., 1992; Valleni-Basile *et al.*, 1994). Despite this, since the majority of work has not distinguished between childhood and adolescent OCD, and for the purposes of review, the disorder in children and adolescents (18 years or younger) is considered jointly.

The fears of death, danger and germs that characterise obsessions experienced by children and adolescents are similar in content to the obsessions in the adult population. Typical examples include a young girl's unwanted thought of her parents in a car accident, or a fear that an object is contaminated and that contact with the object could cause a disease. Often children will say that they are frightened that they are going mad because of the persistence and ego-dystonic nature of the intrusion. The literature on the epidemiology and the phenomenology of the disorder has recently been reviewed by March and Leonard (1996), and a summary of the findings from the main investigations of obsessions and compulsions in this population are summarised in Table 4.1.

As in adults with OCD, the common compulsive behaviour that children engage in to reduce the anxiety or to prevent a dreaded event includes checking, washing and repeating activities, often in a ritualised, stereotypical manner (Swedo et al., 1989; Toro et al., 1992). For example, one adolescent had to write every fifth word of a homework assignment five times before the next word could be written and she could continue. Interruption of the compulsive behaviour would result in having to start the homework assignment again. In addition to overt behaviour, children may try to ignore/suppress the intrusion, or 'cancel out' the obsession by engaging in a covert ritual which can lead to slowness and accusations of 'daydreaming'. For example, one boy was unable to engage in his schoolwork until he was no longer experiencing unwanted intrusions; as a consequence, he would spend up to one hour unsuccessfully trying to suppress his obsessions. Stimuli that trigger the obsession, such as ill-kept washrooms, will be avoided as far as possible. The actual form of childhood OCD is not static but varies over time (Rettew et al., 1992; Rapoport, Swedo & Leonard, 1992; Hanna, 1995; Thomsen & Mikkelsen, 1995). There is some evidence that symmetry and ordering symptoms appear earlier than contamination and religious themes, with the majority of children experiencing multiple obsessions and compulsions (Last & Strauss, 1989; Swedo et al., 1989; Rapoport et al., 1992). Case reports of children with fear of AIDS contamination are becoming more common (e.g. Wagner & Sullivan, 1991; Fisman & Walsh, 1994), as has been noted in adults (Faulstich, 1987).

Although the mean age of onset of OCD is in the early twenties (Rachman & Hodgson, 1980; Rasmussen & Eisen, 1992), one-half to one-third of adults with obsessive–compulsive disorder report onset during childhood (Kringlen, 1970; Black, 1974; Rachman & Hodgson, 1980). Furthermore, between 50 per cent and 70 per cent of children with OCD continue to have the disorder in adulthood (Hollingsworth et al., 1980; Leonard et al., 1993; Bolton, Luckie & Steinberg, 1995). Notable differences between childhood and adult OCD include (1) the over-involvement of the family in childhood cases, (2) males outnumber females either 3:2 or 2:1 (Last & Strauss, 1989; Swedo et al., 1989; Hanna, 1995) in children/adolescents compared with an equal gender distribution in adults (Rasmussen & Eisen, 1992); (3) there is a trend for relatively higher rates of psychiatric disturbance amongst first-degree relatives of children with OCD than in the adult population, although figures range from 1 per cent to 30 per cent (Hollingsworth et al., 1980; Lenane et al., 1990; Riddle et al., 1990; Last et al.,

Table 4.1. Summary of main findings from descriptive, epidemiological, familial and CBT studies of OCD in childhood and adolescence (excluding case studies with n < 5)

Study	Sample	Design	Main findings
Apter et al. (1996)	861 community 16 year olds	Epidemiological	2.3% met diagnostic criteria for OCD 50% of cases were male Most common symptoms: neatness, orderliness, repeating 8% of sample spent 1 hour or more per day on obsessional thoughts or compulsive behaviours OCD and subclinical OCD cases differed from non-OCD cases but not from each other
Valleni-Basile et al. (1996)	3283 community adolescents	1-year follow-up of Valleni-Basile et al. (1994)	1-year incidence of rate OCD was 0.7% Only 17% with initial diagnosis retained diagnosis at 1-year follow-up Initial diagnosis of subclinical OCD was not predictive of diagnosis of OCD at follow-up
Bolton, Luckie & Steinberg (1995)	14 clinically referred British adolescent patients	9–14 year follow-up of Bolton, Collins & Steinberg (1983)	53% of cases were male 43% still met diagnostic criteria for OCD Initial response to treatment was not predictive of long-term outcome No clear prognostic indicators were identified
Douglass et al. (1995)	930 community 18 year olds	Epidemiological	45% of cases were male 4% prevalence rate High comorbidity with depression (62%), social phobia (38%), and substance dependence (24% alcohol) 86% had either obsessions **or** compulsions (14% had both) Most common obsessions: accidental harm, immoral thoughts Most common compulsions: checking, counting, order, touching
Hanna (1995)	31 clinically referred children and adolescents	Retrospective chart review	61% male 29% of cases were onset before 7 years; 52% had onset between 8 and 12 years 55% had insidious onset; 39% had gradual onset; 6% had sudden onset 71% of cases had symptoms that changed over time 100% of cases had obsessions and compulsions Most common obsessions: contamination (87%), aggressive (81%), symmetry (64%) Most common compulsions: washing (84%), checking (64%), repeating (64%), ordering (61%), touching (58%), counting (42%) 84% had other lifetime psychiatric diagnoses

Table 4.1. (*cont.*)

Study	Sample	Design	Main findings
Thomsen (1995a)	47 clinically referred children and adolescents	6–22-year follow-up	60% of cases were male Social outcome: good – 38%, moderate – 40%, poor – 21% Childhood OCD patients were more socially isolated in adulthood than a non-OCD comparison group No prognostic indicators for social outcome were identified
Thomsen & Mikkelsen, (1995)	23 clinically referred children and adolescents	1.5–5-year follow-up	65% of cases were male 50% retained OCD diagnosis; of these, 1/3 had episodic course, 2/3 had chronic course
March, Mulle & Herbel (1994)	15 clinically referred children and adolescents	Open trial of standardised behaviour therapy	33% of cases were male 60% of patients had at least 50% improvement Gains maintained at follow-up
Thomsen (1994)	47 clinically referred children and adolescents	6–22-year follow-up	60% of cases were male 50% met diagnostic criteria for OCD; of these, 50% had chronic course, 50% had episodic course 3% were diagnosed with OCD 55% had both obsessions and compulsions Most frequent symptoms: touching (88%), checking (86%), washing (83%), counting (52%), collecting (38%)
Valleni-Basile *et al.* (1994)	3283 community adolescents	Epidemiological	43% still met diagnostic criteria for OCD
Leonard *et al.* (1993)	54 clinically referred children and adolescents	2–7-year follow-up	70% continued to take medication Initial response to CMI did not predict outcome Best predictor of outcome at follow-up was severity of symptoms at week 5 of CMI treatment Presence of Axis I psychiatric disorder predict follow-up OCD severity
DeVeaugh-Geiss *et al.* (1992)	60 clinically referred children and adolescents	Comparison of CMI versus placebo	65% of cases were male CMI was significantly more effective than placebo 37% reduction in symptoms with CMI; 8% with placebo
Rettew *et al.* (1992)	79 clinically referred children and adolescents	Case note review of NIMH children for 2–7 years	Early onset (less than 6 years) associated with compulsions not obsessions 47% of patients had both washing and checking at some time during their illness 38% of patients or relatives believed specific events triggered OCD All patients had symptoms that varied with time No age-related symptoms

Study	Sample	Study type	Findings
Last et al. (1992)	188 anxiety-disordered children and adolescents	Epidemiological	Age at onset for OCD was 10.8 years; Age at intake was 12.8 years; 53.6% of cases were male; Almost half of the children had a history of simple phobia
Toro (1992)	72 clinically referred children and adolescents	Case note review	2.2% of psychiatric cases in hospital had OCD; 65% of cases were male; Most common obsessions: death (13%), sex (6%); Most common compulsions: repeating (74%), cleaning (56%), checking (51%), ordering (42%)
Zohar et al. (1992)	562 Israeli army adolescents	Epidemiological study	94% had both obsessions and compulsions; 3.6% of sample were diagnosed with OCD; 85% of cases were male; 50% had obsessions only
Leonard et al. (1991)	26 clinically referred children and adolescents	Double-blind DMI substitution during CMI treatment	58% of cases were male; 89% of those substituted relapsed compared with 18% in the non-substituted group; OC symptomatology continued to vary while on CMI
Thomsen & Mikkelsen (1991)	61 clinically referred children and adolescents	Case review	61% of cases were male; 1.3% prevalence in the clinic; 87% discharged with a different diagnosis
Lenane et al. (1990)	145 first-degree relatives	Family study	30% of probands had a relative with OCD (25% of fathers; 9% of mothers); 45% of fathers and 65% mothers had one or more other psychiatric diagnosis (primarily affective disorder)
Riddle et al. (1990)	21 clinically referred children and adolescents	Phenomenological and family history study	43% of cases were male; 90% had obsessions and compulsions; Most common obsessions: contamination (52%), aggressive (38%), somatic (38%), religious (29%), morbid images (25%); Most common compulsions: repeating (76%), washing (67%), ordering/arranging (62%), checking (57%); 57% involved family members; 71% had parents with OCD (n = 4) or obsessive–compulsive symptoms (n = 11)

Table 4.1. (cont.)

Study	Sample	Design	Main findings
Berg et al. (1989)	66 community adolescents	Follow-up 2 years after Flament et al. (1988)	42% of cases were male Subclinical OCD did not progress to OCD at follow-up
Honjo et al. (1989)	61 clinically referred children and adolescents with obsessive–compulsive symptoms	Case note review	5% of psychiatric cases referred to clinic had OC symptoms 63% of cases were male 51% had specific (often school-related) trigger Most common obsessions: dirt (34%), death (13%), body/appearance (13%), harm (12%), disasters (10%) Most common compulsions: washing (38%), checking (23%), rituals (15%), neutralising (15%) 8% involved family members in rituals Symptoms age related
Last & Strauss (1989)	20 clinically referred children and adolescents	Descriptive	60% of cases were male 80% had both obsessions and compulsions First-degree relatives: 8% OCD, 33% any anxiety disorder, 15% depression, 51% any Axis I disorder
Leonard et al. (1989)	48 clinically referred children and adolescents	Double-blind crossover trial of CMI and DMI	63% of cases were male CMI superior to DMI
Swedo et al. (1989)	70 clinically referred children and adolescents	Descriptive study	67% of cases were male Children performing rituals for 6 months or more prior to parents becoming aware of problem Most common obsessions: fear of contamination (40%), fear of harm (24%), symmetry/exactness (17%), scrupulosity (13%) Most common compulsions: washing (85%), repeating (51%), checking (46%), touching (20%)
Apter & Tyano (1988)	496 clinically referred children and adolescents	Epidemiology	2.8% met diagnostic criteria for OCD
Flament et al. (1988)	5,596 students	Epidemiological study	1.9% lifetime prevalence rate 95% had both obsessions and compulsions Most common obsessions: fear of contamination (35%), fear of harm (30%) Most common compulsions: washing (85%), checking (40%), straightening (35%), repeating (15%) Poor outcome (see Berg et al., 1989)
Flament et al. (1985)	19 clinically referred children and adolescents	Double-blind placebo controlled cross-over	74% of cases were male CMI superior to placebo No predictors of drug response No evidence that responders had better long-term outcome than non-responders (Flament et al., 1990)

Study	Sample	Type	Findings
Apter, Bernhaut & Tyano (1984)	8 in-patient adolescents	Outcome trial	63% of cases were male 7/8 improved with combination therapy (medications and behaviour therapy)
Bolton, Collins & Steinberg (1983)	15 clinically referred adolescents	Outcome trial	53% of cases were male 80% improved with cognitive–behavioural and family therapy 50% maintained improvement following discharge
Rapoport et al. (1981)	9 clinically referred adolescents	Descriptive	OCD is a valid syndrome in children All cases had a history of major depressive disorder
Hollingsworth et al. (1980)	10 clinically referred children and adolescents	1.5–14-year follow-up	76% of the initial 17 subjects were male 70% had obsessive–compulsive symptoms 82% parents had psychiatric problems Elevation of medical problems in the sample
Adams (1973)	49 clinical cases	Descriptive	Male preponderance Early age of onset
Judd (1965)	405 children referred to psychiatric clinic	Descriptive	1.2% met criteria for OCD 60% of cases were male All cases had sudden onset, both obsessions and compulsions, symptoms interfered with functioning, persistent guilt, strong moral code, no evidence of psychosis History of psychopathology in the parents was common
Despert (1955)	68 paediatric cases	Case note review	Children often hide symptoms, and present requesting help for depression or anxiety; children are aware of abnormality of symptoms

CMI, clomipramine; DMI, desipramine.

1991; Thomsen, 1995b) – despite this, it is important to bear in mind that the vast majority of adults with OCD do not have children with the disorder (Rachman & Hodgson, 1980; Sawyer *et al.*, 1992); (4) pure obsessions-only are rarely found in the childhood population and compulsions without obsessional content are more common in children than in adults; and (5) tics, neurological and neuroendocrine abnormalities are more common in the childhood population than in the adult population (see Swedo & Leonard (1994) for a review).

Obsessive–compulsive disorder in children has traditionally been considered to be rare and clinicians-in-training, at least in the UK, have been told not to expect to treat such an uncommon disorder during their years of practice (Tallis, personal communication). This assertion is based on studies such as the comprehensive Isle of Wight survey in which no cases of OCD were found in an unselected sample of 2000 children aged 10–11 years, and the prevalence rate of mixed anxiety/obsessional disorders was 0.3 per cent (Rutter, Tizard & Whitmore, 1970). Within child psychiatric clinics, early prevalence estimates of OCD ranged from 0.2 per cent to 1.2 per cent (Berman, 1942; Judd, 1965; Hollingsworth *et al.*, 1980).

However, in a widely cited two-stage community study of 5596 *adolescents* in New Jersey, Flament and colleagues (1988) found point-prevalence rates of 1 per cent and lifetime prevalence rates of 1.9 per cent. The adolescents in the community sample were similar to clinical cases of National Institute of Mental Health (NIMH) in the types of obsessions experienced (fear of contamination, fear of harm) and compulsions performed (washing, checking, symmetry), with the majority of subjects experiencing multiple obsessions and compulsions. Subsequent community-based studies in Israel and the USA have indicated prevalence rates of up to 4 per cent (e.g. Zohar *et al.*, 1992; Nestadt *et al.*, 1994; Valleni-Basile *et al.*, 1994; Douglass *et al.*, 1995), but approximately half (or more) of the identified 'cases' had either obsessions *or* compulsions but not both. This indicates that these cases are not similar to those seen in a clinical setting, where 80–100 per cent have both obsessions and compulsions (Last & Strauss, 1989; Hanna, 1995). Furthermore, the male : female ratio of OCD in childhood is approximately 3 : 2 or 2 : 1 (Swedo *et al.*, 1989; Last & Strauss, 1989; Hanna, 1995), whereas the ratio in community-based studies is either equivalent (Valleni-Basile *et al.*, 1994) or else females far outnumber males (Douglass et al., 1995). Given these differences, care must be taken when generalising from community studies (e.g. Valleni-Basile *et al.*'s (1996) one-year follow-up in which only 17 per cent of cases retained their diagnosis of OCD) to the clinic.

One possible reason for the surprisingly high prevalence rates in community studies could be the confusion between the purposeful compulsions that characterise OCD and the 'empty' stereotypies seen in autism and tics (see Shapiro & Shapiro, 1992). Despite surface similarities, motor tics and stereotypies differ from compulsions in a number of ways, including intent, form and resultant distress (e.g. George *et al.*, 1993; Holzer *et al.*, 1994). Although minor tics have been noted in the childhood population, Tourette's syndrome is far less common in children with a primary diagnosis of OCD than checking behaviours in a population of children with Tourette's syndrome (Pauls *et al.*, 1986, 1995; Pitman *et al.*, 1987; George *et al.*, 1993; Holzer *et al.*, 1994). Far more frequent than comorbid Tourette's disorder are affective and anxiety disorders. In the NIMH sample of 70 children, only 18 (26 per cent) had OCD as their only diagnosis, with 35 per cent receiving a comorbid diagnosis of depression, and 40 per cent having a comorbid anxiety disorder (Swedo *et al.*, 1989). In other clinical studies of children and adolescents, a similar proportion (60–80 per cent) had other lifetime diagnoses apart from OCD (Last & Strauss, 1989; Hanna, 1995). In community studies, depression is commonly associated with obsessional symptoms (e.g. Valleni-Basile *et al.*, 1996), and it is possible that the episodic course of a substantial number of patients with childhood OCD can be attributed to variability in depression (Thomsen and Mikkelsen, 1995). Investigations of the comorbidity between OCD, depression and anxiety are summarised in Table 4.2.

A second possible reason for the discrepancy between clinical prevalence estimates and community estimates is the confusion between normal childhood rituals and compulsive behaviour. At first glance, childhood OCD can appear as a normal developmental phenomenon in that superstitions are part of many children's games, and repetitions, perseverations and rhythmic behaviour are a normal part of childhood (Leonard, 1990). However, the content, intensity and distribution of superstitious behaviour are distinct from those in OCD. Compulsions in childhood and adult OCD are characterised by checking, washing and repeating rituals, and are driven by ego-dystonic fears of contamination and danger whereas superstitions are concerned with good and bad luck, are not ego-dystonic or resisted, and do not cause distress (Leonard, 1990). Furthermore, superstitions are commonly shared beliefs, whereas obsessions tend to be personal and partly idiosyncratic in content.

Rationale for using cognitive – behaviour therapy

Behaviour therapy (BT) for OCD is based upon traditional behavioural theories such as the two-stage model of anxiety formation and persistence (Mowrer, 1939, 1960). The cornerstone of the behavioural theory is that anxiety is elicited by exposure to the feared stimulus and that compulsions serve to reduce anxiety (Rachman and Hodgson, 1980, p. 167). Central to the model is the suggestion that the same normal learning mechanisms produce normal and abnormal intrusions (Rachman & deSilva, 1978; Salkovskis & Harrison, 1984). A wide variety of evidence supports the model, including the results of psychometric studies (Hodgson & Rachman, 1977; Goodman & Price, 1990; van Oppen, 1992), experimental manipulations (Rachman & Hodgson, 1980), genetic research (Rasmussen, 1993) and the outcome of behavioural therapy (Abel, 1993; van Balkom *et al.*, 1994). The cognitive–behavioural analysis of OCD arose directly from behaviour theory and therapy.

Table 4.2. Comorbidity between OCD and other psychiatric disorders (from 1988 onwards)

Study	Sample	Measure	Percentage with OCD + current major depressive disorder	Percentage with OCD + current anxiety	Percentage with OCD + any psychiatric disorder
Hanna (1995)	n = 31 patients Mean age = 13.5 years 61% male	DICA	32	26	84
Douglass et al. (1995)	n = 37 community adolescents Age range 11–18 years 41% male	DIS, DISC-C (Adapted)	62	38 social phobia 19 simple phobia 16 agoraphobia	84
Valleni-Basile et al. (1994)	n = 26 community adolescents Mean age = 13 years 35% male	K-SADS	45	34 separation anxiety 29 phobia	Not stated
Johnson (1993)	n = 100 patients with obsessions Mean age = 12.8 years (boys), 12.4 years (girls) 60% male	Retrospective controlled comparison case note review	26	23 anxiety or fear	Not stated
Toro et al. (1992)	n = 72 patients Mean age = 12 years 65% male	Case note review	22	41.6	72.8
Riddle et al. (1990)	n = 21 patients Mean age = 12.2 years 43% male	Clinical interview	10	38	62
Last & Strauss (1989)	n = 20 patients Mean age = 12.7 years 60% male	K-SADS	10	60	70
Swedo et al. (1989)	n = 70 patients Mean age = 13.7 years 67%	DICA	26	7 separation anxiety 16 over-anxious 17 simple phobia 36 school refusal	74
Honjo et al. (1989)	n = 61 clinically referred Mean age = 13.4 years 63%	Case note review	8		Not stated
Flament et al. (1988)	n = 20 identified cases Mean age = 16.2 years 55% male	DICA	25	20	75

Behaviour therapy primarily comprises *graded exposure to the feared stimulus with prevention of the typical response* (exposure with response prevention, ERP). The traditional behavioural model is based upon the premise that anxiety is reduced by a process of habituation, and that habituation is facilitated by both (1) exposing the patient to the feared stimulus, and (2) preventing the compulsions (Meyer, 1966). ERP is also believed to be therapeutic by enabling patients to test personal beliefs. For example, some patients believe that if they do not engage in compulsive behaviour, their anxiety levels will rise exponentially and they will 'crack up'. ERP allows patients to test this belief in a relatively safe environment by monitoring what happens if compulsive urges are resisted. In the majority of cases, the anxiety resulting from ERP declines within an hour (Rachman & Hodgson, 1980) and the feared consequence ('cracking up') never occurs. Hence behavioural tests can facilitate cognitive change, can emphasise that obsessions are harmless, and that it is not necessary to respond to them as if they were important or meaningful. These important cognitive components were incorporated into theoretical models during the 'cognitive revolution' of the mid-1980s.

Obsessive–compulsive disorder was a prime candidate for a cognitive re-analysis, given that phenomenology of the disorder incorporates obvious cognitive distortions concerning risk appraisal and responsibility (Carr, 1974; McFall & Wollersheim, 1979; Rachman, 1993). Salkovskis (1985) conceptualised obsessions within the hypothesised framework of cognitive phenomena proposed by Beck (Beck, Emery & Greenberg, 1985). The essence of the cognitive–behavioural model is that there is 'an inflated belief in the probability of being the cause of serious harm to others or self, or failing to avert harm where this may have been possible' (Salkovskis, 1985, p. 575). Responsibility has been defined as 'the belief that one has power which is pivotal to bring about or prevent subjectively crucial negative outcomes' (Salkovskis *et al.*, 1992). According to the theory, appraisal of an intrusion in terms of responsibility for harm leads to the need for action. The person will therefore attempt to suppress the thought, image or impulse or else to 'neutralise' it. Neutralising takes the form of overt or covert compulsions that are designed to reduce distress and/or the probability of the feared event occurring. Recently, cognitive distortions other than responsibility are being considered as important in OCD, such as the over-interpretation of intrusive thoughts (including the belief that thought is similar to action), the need to control intrusive thoughts, intolerance for uncertainty/ambiguity and the overestimation of danger (Freeston, Rheaume & Ladouceur, 1996; Shafran, Thordarson & Rachman, 1996; Rachman, 1997). These cognitive distortions are often considered within the context of an inflated sense of responsibility for harm, although the most recent cognitive theory of obsessions is broader. Specifically, it is proposed that 'obsessions are caused by catastrophic misinterpretations of the significance of one's thoughts (images, impulses). The obsessions persist as long as these misinterpretations continue and diminish when the misinterpretations are weakened' (Rachman, 1997).

A wide variety of evidence supports the addition of the cognitive component to the behavioural model and the role of responsibility in adults. For example, manipulating responsibility results in a corresponding change in anxiety, estimates of the probability of harm and the urge to perform neutralising behaviours (Lopata & Rachman, 1995; Ladouceur et al., 1995; Shafran, 1997). Empirical and psychometric data support the model (Freeston et al., 1992a; 1992b), and the thought-suppression literature is also consistent with the model (Muris et al., 1992; Salkovskis & Campbell, 1994). However, outcome data comparing behaviour therapy with CBT in adults are equivocal (see later).

The cognitive–behavioural model was developed to explain adult OCD, and the experimental and psychometric data are almost exclusively based on the adult population. Although CBT has become the psychotherapeutic treatment of choice for adults with OCD (March, 1995), Salkovskis's cognitive model is not mentioned in the literature for the younger population, and the work conducted is primarily behavioural, with the notable exception of March's work (March, Mulle & Herbel, 1994; March, 1995) and some case reports (e.g. Piacentini et al., 1994). In the work on children, it has been difficult to disentangle CBT from BT, and there is a lack of consensus in the childhood literature as to the cognitive component of treatment. A recent review (March, 1995) describes CBT in terms of three-stages – information gathering, ERP and homework assignments – all of which may be considered primarily behavioural. In the majority of the studies, the emphasis has clearly been on the behavioural component of treatment (ERP and extinction), with any cognitive component largely comprising cognitive self-statements which are seen to 'boss back' the OCD (March et al., 1994) or as a coping strategy (Bolton, Collins & Steinberg, 1983; Francis, 1988; Rapoport et al., 1993; March et al., 1994; Piancinti et al., 1994). The statements could be construed as challenging negative automatic thoughts but do not explicitly address the issue of appraisal of intrusive thoughts in terms of responsibility for harm (Salkovskis, 1985, 1996), despite the clinical salience of inflated responsibility among the younger population. Details of the therapeutic procedures are given later in this chapter.

Techniques of assessment for childhood obsessive–compulsive disorder

Although there are many assessment measures available to ascertain the content and severity of the obsessive–compulsive problem, accurate assessment may be impeded since the obsessions are often considered shameful and the patient is secretive about the nature and extent of the problem. It is reported that compulsions without obsessions are more common in childhood than in the adult population (Rapoport et al., 1992) but this may be attributable to the inability to assess the obsessional component in children, for whom it can be difficult to articulate the obsession. It may therefore appear that the problem is primarily one of empty compulsive behaviour since patients may report not knowing why they have to engage in rituals, but thorough assessment may reveal the driving force behind the activity. Assessment may be a lengthy and ongoing process, involving several different techniques.

Interviews

Diagnostic interviews

Standardised structured and semi-structured interviews can be used for diagnostic purposes (see Wolff & Wolff, 1991; deHaan & Hoogduin, 1992), although there is a lack of data on the reliability and validity of the OCD subsections (Hodges, 1993). When using the standardised structured and semi-structured interviews, care must be taken to clarify the meaning of the terms 'obsessions' and 'compulsions'. The interviewer must be trained in the use of the specific interview schedule, and also be knowledgeable about OCD in order to be able to distinguish between behaviour which does not cause distress, is not time consuming and is not driven by an obsession (for example having a bedtime routine, not stepping on pavement cracks, checking or arranging for no reason) and behaviour that is a manifestation of OCD.

Results from studies of the reliability and validity of the different assessment tools are inconsistent and often contradictory (see Hodges (1993) for a review). As a consequence, there is no current 'gold standard' on which to base reliable and valid diagnostic procedures, resulting in difficulties in establishing accurate diagnosis of OCD in the younger population (Dulcan, 1996). Currently, the most common diagnostic interviews used are the Diagnostic Interview for Children and Adolescents – Revised (DICA-R; Herjanic *et al.*, 1975; Reich & Welner, 1988), the Schedule for Affective Disorders and Schizophrenia for School Aged Children (K-SADS; Puig-Antich & Chambers, 1978) and the Diagnostic Interview Schedule - Child Version Revised (DISC-R; Costello, Edelbrook, & Costello, 1985; Shaffer *et al.*, 1988; Piacentini *et al.*, 1993). The DISC-R has itself been revised and the resultant DISC-2.3 has good reliability for the parent version, but is less satisfactory for the child version (Shaffer *et al.*, 1996). A new assessment tool for children, the Anxiety Disorders Interview Schedule – Revised, looks promising but further psychometric data are required (ADIS-R; Silverman, 1991; Silverman & Eisen, 1992).

Specific interviews

The most specific interview for OCD in children is the Children's Yale–Brown Obsessive Compulsive Scale (CY-BOCS; Goodman *et al.*, 1989a, 1989b.). The scale is based on the well-established adult version, and has a similar format and items with minor word modifications, e.g. in the definition of obsessions. The CY-BOCs comprises ten questions and yields separate scores for obsessions and compulsions. The questions are based on symptoms that are elicited during the course of the semi-structured interview and cover obsessions and compulsions separately. The semi-structured interview starts by defining obsessions and compulsions, and then inquires about a range of obsessions, including those concerned with aggression (e.g. the fear of harming someone), contamination (e.g. concerns with bodily waste and secretions), sexual matters (e.g. forbidden sexual images), hoarding/collecting, religion (e.g. blasphemy), symmetry/arranging (accompanied by magical thinking or not), miscellaneous obsessions such as a 'need to know' and somatic obsessions. The compulsions are then assessed separately (e.g. cleaning behaviour, counting, checking, repeating, ordering/arranging, hoarding, and miscellaneous compulsions such as touching or mental rituals). After eliciting the primary or 'target' obsessions and compulsions, five questions are asked about obsessions (e.g. time taken up by obsessions, interference caused by the obsessions, associated distress, degree of resistance and degree of control), followed by five similar questions on compulsions. The scores on the obsessions and compulsions subscales are added together to form the total CY-BOCs score. Additional questions are asked about insight, avoidance, indecisiveness, responsibility, slowness and doubting, and the clinician then makes a judgement of the global severity of the patient's illness, global improvement (if applicable) and reliability of the rating scores obtained.

The adult Y-BOCS has good reliability and validity (e.g. Goodman *et al.*, 1989a, 1989b; Woody, Steketee & Chambless, 1995; Taylor, 1995), and some early work on the child version indicates that it too has good psychometric properties (deHaan & Hoogduin, 1992; Hanna, 1995; Scahill et al., 1997). The adult version has been adapted to a self-report inventory (Steketee *et al.*, 1996) and it is possible that a self-report child/adolescent version for older children may do equally well in this format.

Self-report inventories

Leyton Obsessional Inventory, Child Version
The most commonly used self-report instrument is the child version of the Leyton Obsessional Inventory (LOI-CV; Berg, Rapoport & Flament, 1986; Berg *et al.*, 1988), although the Leyton is rarely used by modern researchers in the adult field owing to confusion as to whether it is measuring OCD symptoms or personality traits (see Taylor (1995) for a review). The Leyton began as a study of houseproud housewives (Cooper 1970) and took the form of a card-sorting test. The measure was adapted to a pencil-and-paper test (Snowdon, 1980), and child versions of the card-sort (Berg *et al.*, 1986) and questionnaire (Berg *et al.*, 1988) have been developed. A 20-item survey form of the inventory has been widely used in screening studies in order to identify children in the community who may have OCD (Flament *et al.*, 1988; Thomsen, 1993). The 20-item self-report instrument has good norms, and has been shown to have a low false-negative rate but a high false-positive rate (see Wolff & Wolff, 1991). Recently, the test–retest reliability of this survey form of the LOI-CV has been shown to vary as a function of age, with adequate reliability in the 14–16-year-old age range, but poor reliability for 8–10 year olds (King *et al.*., 1995). Interestingly, the subjects with high scores on the LOI-CV in the large screening study of Flament and colleagues (1988), but with no diagnosis of OCD, were not more likely to have developed the disorder at two-year follow-up than subjects with low scores on the LOI-CV (Berg *et al.*, 1989), indicating that it is not a good measure for identifying 'at-risk' subjects.

Maudsley Obsessional Compulsive Inventory

The Maudsley Obsessional Compulsive Inventory (MOCI; Hodgson & Rachman, 1977) is widely used in adult research and has good reliability and validity (Hodgson

& Rachman, 1977; Rachman & Hodgson, 1980; see Taylor (1995) for a review). This inventory is a 30-item True/False inventory with subscales of washing, checking, doubting and slowness/consciousness, and has been used to assess obsessionality in adolescents (Allsopp & Willliams, 1991). In adults, modest correlations have been found between the Y-BOCS, LOI and MOCI (Richter, Cox & Direnfeld, 1994). The MOCI has been substantially revised and combined with selected questions from the CY-BOCS to form the Childhood Obsessional Compulsive Inventory (COCI; Shafran *et al.*, 1997). The self-report instrument comprises 19 items to assess compulsions and 13 to assess obsessions, and each item is rated on a three-point frequency scale. The main obsessions and compulsions are listed separately and rated in terms of time/frequency, interference, distress, resistance and controllability. An investigation of this scale's psychometric properties is currently underway (copies are available on request).

Clinician-rated scales

A variety of clinician-rated scales is used to provide information independently from the child's reporting. The Children's Global Assessment Scale (CGAS; Shaffer *et al.*, 1983) is a measure of global impairment rated by the clinician on a scale from 1 (not at all ill) to 6 (severely ill). The NIMH global scale has a childhood OCD subsection (Murphy, Pickar & Alterman, 1982) which is easy to complete and is commonly used, as is the four-item Obsessive Compulsive Rating Scale (OCR; Rapoport, Elkins & Mikkelson, 1980) . These scales can be easily used to monitor progress throughout therapy, and there is adequate interrater reliability (see Wolff & Wolff, 1991). However, the clinician often cannot provide an objective measure of improvement and there is little information on the validity of the measures.

Observational measures

Self-monitoring, direct observation by family members, and direct observation by the therapist and staff can all be useful assessment techniques (e.g. Ownby, 1983; Francis, 1988), especially if conducted in a systematic and organised manner. Recording frequency, duration and distress caused by obsessions and compulsions can be beneficial, providing that the recording does not itself become ritualised. Behavioural avoidance tasks, similar to those used in the treatment of phobias, can be extremely valuable in order to determine long-term and short-term treatment gains (Turner & Beidel, 1988; Steketee *et al.*, 1996; Rachman, personal communication). In these tests, children are asked (a) to get as close to a feared object as they can manage comfortably in the clinic test room, and (b) to report their fear level at this closest point. Hence, two recordings are made: the closest approach point and their fear at the closest approach point (Rachman personal communication). An example would be the following: if the child is afraid to touch a contaminated object, he or she is asked to get as close to the object (e.g. doorknob) as can be comfortably managed. The distance away from the object (e.g. hand 6 inches (about 15 cm) from the doorknob) and fear (using a 1–10-point 'fear thermometer') are recorded. This is repeated for a series of three tasks at different points on the child's fear hierarchy. A variation on the behavioural avoidance task is to fix the distance from the object (e.g. 4 inches (about 10 cm) from the doorknob) and assess fear levels at this point before and after treatment. If the behavioural avoidance task is to be used as an objective assessment measure, care must be taken not to confuse the task with an exposure exercise. The task must be carried out quickly in order to prevent habituation, and cognitive techniques (e.g. eliciting beliefs associated with the exposure) should be kept to a minimum. The behavioural avoidance task yields important clinical information, has good reliability and validity, but must be standardised in order to have utility in larger research trials (Turner & Beidel, 1988; Steketee *et al.*, 1996).

Techniques of treatment

Accurate assessment is important for many reasons, but primarily because it will expedite appropriate treatment. Treatment of childhood OCD is derived from CBT with adults, with some modifications. The emphasis of CBT in children is clearly in the behavioural domain, with little work on cognitive aspects, and no therapy on the cognitive components suggested by Salkovskis or Rachman (Salkovskis, 1985, 1996; Rachman, 1997). In the younger population, exposure with response prevention is the mainstay of CBT with some important adaptations. Exposure consists of 'facing the fear' so, for example, the child is asked to touch the sole of a shoe which he or she fears is dirty or contaminated and has been actively avoiding. The response prevention consists of not engaging in rituals to reduce anxiety, e.g. washing the hand that touched the shoe. It may be that the response is prevented for 5 minutes, then 15 minutes and then half an hour. The child is asked to monitor his or her anxiety throughout and to notice that anxiety does come down, even if the compulsion is not performed.

A 'fear ladder' is built in which the most frightening exposures are at the top of the ladder (e.g. touching the toilet bowl) and the least frightening are at the bottom (e.g. touching the bedroom door). A fear thermometer can be used to assess the degree of fear or anxiety associated with the exposure in order to build the ladder. The exposure exercises are chosen by the child and are linked to the child's homework and progress. To facilitate exposure, the therapist can model exposure to behaviour therapy to convey the information that the action is 'safe' and can be taken without any disastrous consequences (e.g. by demonstrating touching a toilet seat, shoe etc.).

For children, the family is involved in the behavioural programme and given advice on how not to comply with rituals, for example ignoring requests for reassurance (Francis and Pinto, 1993). Often the normal behavioural principle of reward can be applied in order to increase compliance with the behavioural programme (deHaan & Hoogduin, 1992). Reward may take the form of soda, points, money, cassettes or magazine or, ultimately, the improvement in obsessional symptoms. For example, one client received one pound for every occasion that she managed to shower for less than 30 minutes; another was told that if he managed to go for a week without repeatedly checking that the drawers in his bedroom were shut, he would receive tickets to a football match. The therapist and parents decide jointly on a suitable incentive. In addition to rewards, some clinicians have utilised response–cost procedures such as writing a letter to a grandparent (e.g. Apter, Bernhout & Tyano, 1984).

The C in CBT for children, derives from work primarily conducted by March, who has published a standardised CBT manual (March et al., 1994). The manual does not incorporate Salkovskis's (1985) ideas on responsibility or Rachman's (1997) proposal concerning the personal significance of intrusions. Instead, the cognitive component comprises monitoring within story metaphors (the child can be instructed to create a new story, 'authoring out' the OCD from his or her life), anxiety management training and 'constructive self-talk' in order to 'boss back' the OCD (March et al., 1994, p.335).

Other cognitive techniques can be usefully employed for children, particularly the use of behavioural tests to collect evidence to challenge dysfunctional beliefs. For example, if patients report a belief that they will become intensely anxious and remain anxious for 'hours' if they do not wash their hands after touching a contaminant, they are asked to (a) predict the anxiety, (b) touch the contaminant without washing, (c) report immediate anxiety, (d) report anxiety after a delay of 5, 10 and 30 minutes. In the majority of cases, the anxiety will decline significantly with the delay period (30 minutes), and the patients are asked what they have learned about their anxiety and their belief that they will experience intense anxiety for 'hours' if they do not wash their hands upon exposure. This integration of cognitive and behavioural techniques can be used for children, and two case illustrations are given below. The first case primarily comprised exposure with response prevention, whereas the second required more extensive cognitive work to challenge the meaning of the patient's intrusions.

Case illustrations
Case 1
Simon, a 12-year-old boy, presented with a seven-month history of 'contamination' fears and compulsive washing behaviour. He had been to a summer camp where he had experienced intense anxiety; thereafter, anything associated with the camp was 'contaminated' and elicited anxiety accompanied by the fear that he would be forced to return to camp. The 'contamination' spread upon Simon touching objects. For example, if he touched the hairbrush that had been to camp with him and then touched the cupboard, the cupboard was also considered as 'contaminated'. On touching a contaminated object, Simon would wash his hands excessively. He engaged in extensive avoidance and refused to touch objects for fear that he would spread 'contamination'; if forced to touch objects, he would cover his hands with his sleeves.

At the time of assessment, he was taking 30 mg paroxetine and was within the severe clinical range on the CY-BOCS. Therapy began by building a graded hierarchy, with 'touching the door handle with my sleeve over my hand but not washing' at the bottom and 'returning to camp and not washing my hands' at the top. Simon underwent graded exposure with response-prevention and used relaxation to help him resist the urge to wash his hands. He overpredicted the degree of anxiety he would feel if he touched 'contaminated' objects, and was surprised to learn that his anxiety rapidly dissipated with relaxation and distraction. Within four sessions of hour-long therapy, he had completed all steps of the hierarchy, had been able to return to camp with minimal anxiety, and his score on the CY-BOCS was within the normal range.

Case 2

Mary, a 15-year-old girl, presented with a history of obsessive–compulsive problems that had considerably worsened in the past three months after learning that her mother had narrowly escaped being seriously injured in a work-related accident. At assessment, she reported intrusive images that she would be responsible for harm coming to others (e.g. that they would be in a car accident that would be her fault), and violent intrusive images of other children in school. She reported that she believed the thoughts indicated that she was going crazy, that she was a 'bad kid' for having the thoughts and that she would grow up to be 'bad'. On the occurrence of an intrusive image, she felt driven to repeat whatever action she had been carrying out (e.g. repeatedly pulling up her socks, packing her schoolbags, standing up/sitting down, washing her hands). Mary scored within the clinical range on the CY-BOCS but did not report experiencing symptoms of depression.

Therapy focused on building a 'fear ladder'. At the bottom of the hierarchy was 'experience an intrusive image whilst putting down an object and not repeating the action'; at the top of the hierarchy was 'experience an intrusive image whilst reading and not re-read the sentence'. Mary underwent graded exposure with response-prevention and, after each exposure, reported on her anxiety and urge to repeat the behaviour. Other behavioural tasks were conducted to test the belief that she would be unable to complete her schoolwork if she continued to work whilst experiencing the images. She was asked to continue to work despite having the images and anxiety. The urge to repeat the work was monitored throughout the exposure and response-prevention and, to her surprise, Mary was able to experience the image and continue to work despite her anxiety.

The belief that the images meant that Mary was going crazy was challenged by providing Mary with a more benign explanation for her intrusions, namely that it was because she was trying to suppress the images that they recurred so often. The proposal that suppression of images leads to their recurrence was examined by asking Mary to suppress her images and rate their frequency and intensity. This was compared to an exercise in which she was asked to expose herself to the images and deliberately concentrate upon them. She discovered that the intensity of images decreased with exposure and response-prevention, but increased with suppression. She was asked to monitor the intensity of her images for one week, during which she deliberately focused on them, and she discovered that they decreased in intensity.

To counter the cognition that the thoughts indicated that she was going crazy, Mary was asked to 'go crazy' and 'lose control' deliberately. She reported that she did not know how to go crazy, and concluded that it was unlikely that she was at risk of doing so. To challenge the belief that she was 'bad' for having the images, the work on normal/abnormal obsessions was presented (Rachman & deSilva, 1978) and she reported that she considered the 'normal' obsessions, experienced by 90 per cent of the population, to be as bad as her own. She was also asked to place herself on a continuum of 'worst person in the world' (e.g. Clifford Olson, the notorious serial killer) and 'best person in the world' (e.g. Mother Teresa) and concluded that she had a long way to go before becoming 'bad'. At the end of six sessions, Mary reported significant improvement in her obsessions and compulsions.

It is important to note that CBT has a sound rationale based on theory-driven, empirical and outcome data that places OCD within normal learning theory (e.g. Rachman & deSilva, 1978; Salkovskis & Harrison, 1984). It is helpful to provide children and adolescents with a rationale for their therapy, and there is no need to give a rationale for CBT which 'places OCD securely within a medical model' (March *et al.*, 1994, p. 334). Similarly, although it may sometimes be helpful for children to externalise the OCD and view it as the enemy that must be defeated, this does not necessitate a description of the disorder as 'a prototypic neurobehavioural condition' (March, Leonard & Swedo, 1995, p. 507), with compulsions construed as hiccups of the central nervous system that are devoid of intrinsic meaning' (March *et al.*, 1994).

Given the lack of data on CBT in children, it is not clear which children are likely to benefit from this technique, and which are not. It is likely that prognostic indicators are similar for children and adults, i.e. that lack of insight, comorbid severe depression, and lack of motivation/compliance will be poor prognostic indicators (Steketee & Shapiro 1995; Rachman & Shafran, in press). Again similar to the adults, at present there is no way of determining which children (if any) are better suited to one type of treatment (e.g. CBT) than to another (e.g. medication) and when multiple treatments may be required.

Use of multi-component therapy

Cognitive–behavioural therapy for children and adolescents has usually incorporated a family component, with 'an emphasis on simplicity, clarity and correct identification of feelings' (Adams, 1973, p.459; 1985). Behaviour therapy and family therapy have been combined since the earliest reports (e.g. Adams, 1973; Fine, 1973; Friedmann & Silvers, 1977; Bolton *et al.*, 1983) and this combined approach remains strong in both theory and practice (Piacentini *et al.*, 1993; March *et al.*, 1994; Bolton, 1996). The most experienced clinicians in the field suggest that drug treatment, behaviour therapy and family counselling are all needed to improve long-term outcome (Rapoport *et al.*, 1993). In a recent study of CBT, parents and family members had weekly family meetings over the course of therapy, with the goals of providing education about OCD and helping the family develop more normalised patterns of family functioning (Piancentini *et al.*, 1994). March's standardised protocol (March *et al.*, 1994) explicitly incorporates two family sessions, primarily psychoeducational. The parents are actively involved in response-prevention or extinction and are given a 'self-help' booklet on how to manage themselves with respect to their child's OCD. The booklet is linked to the child's home-work, the parents are encouraged to stop giving advice, and parents are invited to comment on the progress of treatment at the beginning of each session. Anxiety management training is an important adjunct to CBT and is given in the form of relaxation training, breathing techniques, humorous visualisations and positive coping strategies

(March *et al.*, 1994; Piacentini *et al.*, 1994). CBT has not yet been dismantled and it is difficult to know the separate contributions of each component of treatment.

However, it is notable that all but one of the children in March's study were receiving concurrent treatment with a serotonin re-uptake inhibitor for at least a portion of the study interval, thus making it impossible to determine the effects of CBT independent of medication. A large treatment trial of children and adolescents found that use of clomipramine hydrochloride treatment for eight weeks was superior to placebo, and gains were maintained providing that the subjects continued on the medication (DeVeaugh-Geiss *et al.*, 1992). However, in the childhood population, outcome with medication alone is 'surprisingly poor' (Swedo and Rapoport, 1993, p. 214) and a 20-week double-blind, crossover trial with 14 patients showed minimal differences between fluoxetine and placebo (Riddle *et al.*, 1992). There has been no controlled treatment trial comparing CBT with medication either alone or in combination, although it is possible that behaviour therapy may prevent relapse when medications are discontinued (March *et al.*, 1994), as is the case with adults (see Abel (1993) for a review; Steketee, 1993).

The school psychologist has an important role in the identification, assessment and treatment of OCD in children (Adams *et al.*, 1994), and a 'behavioural consolidation approach' is suggested (e.g. Bergan & Kratochwill, 1990). In this approach, the problem is identified, with the parents, child and teacher working together. The teacher may be included in a behavioural programme, for example by being instructed not to provide reassurance when requested repeatedly. Depending on the nature of the obsessions and compulsions, it may be necessary to conduct ERP within the school setting, in which cases collaboration with teachers is essential to completing these tasks successfully. Finally, children who have difficulty with reading or writing compulsions may need to be given special consideration, e.g. tolerance of messy notebooks.

Existing evidence for the effectiveness of cognitive–behavioural therapy in obsessive–compulsive disorder

Cognitive–behavioural therapy is considered the treatment of choice for adults with OCD (Salkovskis, 1996), given that it is at least as effective as medication, if not more so, and has a far lower relapse rate (Abel, 1993; Steketee, 1993; van Balkom *et al.*, 1994). However, work on CBT in children has been hindered by the lack of clear cognitive theories for the development and maintenance of childhood OCD, and there is no clear definition of the cognitive component of treatment (see earlier). The majority of studies are case reports (e.g. Fine, 1973; Willmuth, 1988; Zikis, 1983; Giedd *et al.*, 1996) or single-case designs using behaviour therapy (e.g. Francis, 1988; Harris and Wiebe, 1992). There have been no group comparisons, systematically controlled treatment trials, or replication studies.

In March's (1995) review of 32 articles of treatment of childhood OCD, 17 studies included formal exposure, applied according to a graded hierarchy, and there was a reduction in symptoms in the majority of cases (e.g. Bolton *et al.*, 1983). Twenty-six of the 32 studies successfully used response prevention; in the remainder of the studies, response prevention was not a viable option owing to the particular subtype of OCD (e.g. obsessional slowness; Clark, 1982). ERP was used to tackle covert compulsions in some cases, with patients repeating their obsessions vocally or in writing. Defining extinction as the elimination of OCD-related behaviour through removal of positive reinforcement, especially from parents, some therapists (e.g. Francis, 1988) successfully used 'ignoring' and other extinction methods to reduce compulsions. Two studies have used thought-stopping to interrupt rather than challenge the obsessions – with a good outcome (Campbell, 1973; Kellerman, 1981) – and it is suggested that thought-stopping may facilitate ERP in some patients (March *et al.*, 1994; see March and Leonard (1996) for a review).

Cognitive therapy in the form of rational emotive therapy was used in only one study (Kearney & Silverman, 1990); exposure was considered to reduce the compulsions, with the rational emotive therapy reducing the obsessions. The effects of cognitive therapy alone, derived from formal cognitive models (e.g. Salkovskis, 1985), has not been investigated, although early indications from the adult population indicate that CBT is not significantly superior to BT alone (van Oppen *et al.*, 1995). However, CBT may be more effective than BT in treating children with obsessions only, as is the indication from the adult literature (Salkovskis & Westbrook, 1989; Ladouceur *et al.*., 1993).

In the long-term, the outcome of CBT appears to be poor (Hollingsworth *et al.*, 1980; Leonard *et al.*, 1993; Bolton *et al.*, 1995). In Bolton *et al.*'s 9–14-year follow-up of 14 adolescents treated mainly with BT and family therapy, 8 of the patients recovered (i.e. no longer met diagnostic criteria for OCD, were not currently taking medication, and had good social adjustment) and 6 still met diagnostic criteria for OCD (Bolton *et al.*, 1995). Importantly, there was no association between response to treatment in adolescence and a long-term outcome; there was also no association between long-term outcome and premorbid social adjustment, onset before 12 years or symptom severity at referral. The 57 per cent recovery rate is better than that of Flament *et al.*, (1990), in which 68 per cent still had OCD following medication, and the rate is similar to that of the large prospective long-term follow-up of the NIMH children treated with pharmacotherapy (combined with behaviour therapy in a third of cases; Leonard *et al.*, 1993). In this 2–7-year follow-up study, the outcomes were poor: 43 per cent still met diagnostic criteria for OCD; 70 per cent continued to take medication; and only 11 per cent were totally asymptomatic (Leonard *et al.*, 1993). Poor prognostic indicators included more severe OCD symptoms after five weeks of clomipramine, lifetime history of a tic disorder, and presence of parental Axis 1 psychiatric diagnosis. In a Danish 6–22-year long-term outcome study after treatment using medications, family therapy and behaviour therapy (for in-patients), approximately 25 per cent of the 47 patients were recovered; 25 per cent were subclinical; 25 per cent had episodic OCD; and the remaining quarter had chronic OCD (Thomsen, 1994). It was not possible to disentangle the effects of the different therapies in this study or in the subsequent prospective study in which 50 per cent of the 26 children retained a diagnosis of OCD at follow-up (1.5–5 years; Thomsen & Mikkelsen, 1995).

In the conclusion of his review, March states that 'Abundant clinical and emerging empirical evidence suggests that CBT, alone or in combination with pharmacotherapy, is an effective treatment for OCD in children and adolescents' (p. 15). The long-term value remains to be established. It must be conceded that empirical investigations of CBT with a sound methodological basis are scarce, especially when compared with the vast literature on pharmacotherapy (e.g. Flament *et al.*, 1985; Liebowitz *et al.*, 1990; Riddle *et al.*, 1992; DeVeaugh-Geiss *et al.*, 1992). Sound research studies investigating the effects of CBT in this population are needed as a matter of some urgency, given the suffering caused by OCD.

Relevant research issues

There are three main research issues to be addressed in investigating childhood OCD. The first is an increased integration between theoretical approaches to CBT in childhood and adult populations; the second is better theories of childhood OCD; and the third is improved methodology and controlled treatment outcome trials to test the theories and therapies.

As is evident from March's recent review (March, 1995), despite the consensus as to behaviour therapy (i.e. primarily, but not exclusively, exposure with response prevention), there is little agreement about the cognitive component of CBT. Closer integration with theoretical approaches in the adult population may provide a useful starting point for improving the consistency of definitions, and in facilitating comparisons across child and adult populations. For example, in adults, an international group of collaborators agrees that the cognitive component involves challenging beliefs about responsibility, the over-interpretation of intrusions, the need to control intrusions, and the overestimation of threat and intolerance for uncertainty/ambiguity. These beliefs could usefully be investigated in the younger population.

There is also a need for better theories to account for childhood OCD. At present, neurological deficit theories conceptualise OCD as a 'brain hiccup', involving structural, functional or chemical abnormalities, whereas cognitive–behaviour theories regard OCD as a psychological disorder based on normal learning processes (see Bolton, 1996 for a review). The neurological deficit theories do not appear to make easily testable predictions (e.g. Rapoport & Wise, 1988), and attempts at integrating the different theoretical approaches have proven difficult (Tallis, 1995; Bolton, 1996), despite the assertion that 'it is now clear that OCD is a neurobehavioral disorder' (March *et al.*, 1995, p. 507). It is important to improve the aetiological models to enable research studies to test competing predictions and advance theory and therapy.

The third need is for improved methodology in the research on childhood OCD, including using reliable and valid assessment and outcome measures. Only one group has published a standardised treatment manual; this is an excellent and essential first step towards establishing treatment protocols and conducting controlled outcome studies (March *et al.*, 1994). However, as yet, there have been no controlled studies into the effects of behaviour therapy with medication-free children/adolescents, and there have been no controlled trials comparing the effectiveness of behaviour therapy with other therapies such as pharamacotherapy, CBT or family therapy. There have been no published controlled trials comparing individual CBT plus family therapy with group CBT plus family therapy. Although long-term outcome studies have been published (e.g. Flament *et al.*, 1990; Leonard *et al.*, 1993; Thomsen, 1994; Bolton *et al.*, 1995), it is difficult to make sense of the data considering that a variety of treatment interventions were used during therapy and the follow-up period.

It is difficult to balance the clinical needs of the patients with the need for a pure methodologically sound research-based therapy. However, as it stands, we have medications that are 'surprisingly poor' (Swedo & Rapoport, 1993, p.216), and a lack of integration between the childhood and adult research, despite the continuity of the disorder in a substantial number of cases. On a more optimistic note, we have indicators that behaviour therapy with medications is effective (March *et al.*, 1994); there is a strong interest in the field; and assessment and treatment techniques for adults are advancing at a remarkable pace (Salkovskis, 1996). It is hoped that similar advances can be made in the theoretical and therapeutic approaches to childhood OCD.

Acknowledgements

The author is grateful to Professor S. Rachman and Dr B. Lask for their helpful comments on an earlier draft, and to the Izaak Walton Killam Memorial Foundation for financial support.

References

Abel, J. (1993). Exposure with response prevention and serotonergic antidepressants in the treatment of obsessive-compulsive disorder: A review and implications for inter-disciplinary treatment. *Behaviour Research and Therapy*, **31** (5), 463–78.

Adams, G.B., Waas, G.A., March, J.S. & Smith, M.C. (1994). Obsessive compulsive disorder in children and adolescents: the role of the school psychologist in identification, assessment, and treatment. *School Psychology Quarterly*, **9**, 274–94.

Adams, P.L. (1973). *Obsessive children: a sociopsychiatric study*. Brunner Mazel, New York.

Adams, P.L. (1985). The obsessive child: a therapy update. *American Journal of Psychotherapy*, **39**, 301–13.

Allsopp, M. & Williams, T. (1991). Self-report measures of obsessionality in a school population of adolescents. *Journal of Adolescence*, **14**, 49–56.

American Psychiatric Association (1994). *Diagnostic and statistical manual of mental disorders*, 4th ed., American Psychiatric Association, Washington, DC.

Apter, A., Bernhout, E. & Tyano, S. (1984). Severe obsessive–compulsive disorder in adolescence: a report of eight cases. *Journal of Adolescence*, **7**, 349–58.

Apter, A., Fallon, T., King, R.A., Ratzoni, G. Zohar, A., Binder, M., Weizman, A., Leckman, J.F., Pauls, D.L., Kron, S. & Cohen, D.J. (1996). Obsessive–compulsive characteristics: from symptoms to syndrome. *Journal of the American*

Academy of Child and Adolescent Psychiatry, **35**, 907–12.

Apter, A. & Tyano, S. (1988). Obsessive–compulsive disorders in adolescence. *Journal of Adolescence*, **11**, 183–94.

Beck, A.T., Emery, G. & Greenberg, R.L. (1985). *Anxiety disorders and phobias: a cognitive perspective*. Basic Books, New York.

Berg, C.Z., Rapoport, J.L. & Flament, M. (1986). The Leyton Obsessional Inventory – Child Version. *Journal of the American Academy of Child and Adolescent Psychiatry*, **25**, 84–91.

Berg, C.Z., Rapoport, J.L., Whitaker, A., Davies, M., Leonard, H., Swedo, S.E., Braiman, S. & Lenane, M. (1989). Childhood obsessive–compulsive disorder: a two year prospective follow-up of a community sample. *Journal of the American Academy of Child and Adolescent Psychiatry*, **28**, 528–33.

Berg, C.Z., Whitaker, A., Davies, M., Flament, M.F. & Rapoport, J.L. (1988). The survey form of the Leyton Obsessional Inventory – Child Version. Norms from an epidemiological study. *Journal of the American Academy of Child and Adolescent Psychiatry*, **27**, 759–63.

Bergan, J.R. & Kratochwill, T.R. (1990). *Behavioral consultation and therapy*. Plenum Press, New York.

Berman, L. (1942). Obsessive–compulsive neurosis in children. *Journal of Nervous and Mental Disease*, **95**, 26–39.

Black, A. (1974). The natural history of obsessional neurosis. In *Obsessional states* (ed. H.R. Beech). Methuen, London

Bolton D. (1996). Annotation: developmental issues in obsessive–compulsive disorder. *Journal of Child Psychology and Psychiatry*, **37**, 131–7.

Bolton, D., Collins, S. & Steinberg, D. (1983). The treatment of obsessive–compulsive disorder in adolescence: a report of fifteen cases. *British Journal of Psychiatry*, **142**, 456–64.

Bolton, D., Luckie, M. & Steinberg, D. (1995). Long-term course of obsessive–compulsive disorder treated in adolescence. *Journal of the American Academy of Child and Adolescent Psychiatry*, **34**(11), 1441–50.

Campbell, L. (1973). A variation of thought stopping in a twelve-year-old boy: a case report. *Journal of Behaviour Therapy and Experimental Psychiatry*, **4**, 69–70.

Carr, A.T. (1974). Compulsive neurosis: A review of the literature. *Psychological Bulletin*, **81**, 311–18.

Clark, D. (1982). Primary obsessional slowness: a nursing treatment programme with a 13 year old male adolescent. *Behaviour Research and Therapy*, **20**, 289–92.

Cooper, J. (1970). The Leyton Obsessional Inventory. *Psychological Medicine*, **1**, 48–64.

Costello, A.J., Edelbrook, C. & Costello, A.J. (1985). Validity of the NIMH diagnostic interview schedule for children: a comparison between psychiatric and pediatric referrals. *Journal of Abnormal Child Psychology*, **13**, 579–95.

Cottraux, J., Mollard, E., Bouvard, M. & Marks, I. (1993). Exposure therapy, fluvoxamine, or combination treatment in obsessive–compulsive disorder: one-year followup. *Psychiatry Research*, **49**(1), 63–75.

deHaan, E. & Hoogduin, C.A. (1992). The treatment of children with obsessive–compulsive disorder. *Acta Paedopsychiatrica*, **55**(2), 93–7.

Despert, L. (1955). Differential diagnosis between obsessive–compulsive neurosis and schizophrenia in children. In *Psychopathology of childhood* (ed. P.H Hoch & J. Zubin), pp. 240–53. Grune and Stratton, New York.

DeVeaugh-Geiss, J., Moroz, G., Biederman, J., Cantwell, D., Fontraine, E., Greist, J.H., Reichler, R., Katz, R. & Landau, P. (1992). Clomipramine hydrochloride in childhood and adolescent obsessive–compulsive disorder – a multicenter trial. *Journal of the American Academy of Child and Adolescent Psychiatry*, **31**, 45–9.

Douglass, H.M., Moffitt, T.E., Dar, R., McGee, R. & Silva, P. (1995). Obsessive–compulsive disorder in a birth cohort of 18-year-olds: prevalence and predictors. *Journal of the American Academy of Child and Adolescent Psychiatry*, **34**(11), 1424–31.

Dulcan, M.K. (1996). Epidemiology of child and adolescent mental disorders. *Journal of the American Academy of Child and Adolescent Psychiatry*, **35**, 852–4.

Faulstich, M.E. (1987). Psychiatric aspects of AIDS. *American Journal of Psychiatry*, **144**, 551–6.

Fine, S. (1973). Family therapy and a behavioral approach to childhood obsessive–compulsive neurosis. *Archives of General Psychiatry*, **28**, 695–7.

Fisman, S.N. & Walsh, L. (1994). Obsessive–compulsive disorder and fear of AIDS contamination in childhood. *Journal of the American Academy of Child and Adolescent Psychiatry*, **33**(3), 349–53.

Flament, M.F., Koby, E., Rapoport, J., Berg, C.J., Zahn, T., Cox, C., Denckla, M. & Lenane, M. (1990). Childhood obsessive–compulsive disorder: a prospective follow-up study. *Journal of Child Psychology and Psychiatry*, **31**, 363–80.

Flament, M.F., Rapoport, J., Berg, C.J., Sceery, W., Kilts, C., Mellstrom, B. & Linnoila, M. (1985). Clomipramine treatment of childhood obsessive-compulsive disorder. *Archives of General Psychiatry*, **42**, 977–83.

Flament, M.F., Whitaker, A., Rapoport, J.L., Davies, M., Berg, C.Z., Kalikow, K., Sceery, W. & Shaffer, D. (1988). Obsessive–compulsive disorder in adolescents: an epidemiological study. *Journal of the American Academy of Child and Adolescent Psychiatry*, **27**, 764–71.

Francis, G. (1988). Childhood obsessive–compulsive disorder: extinction of compulsive reassurance-seeking. *Journal of Anxiety Disorders*, **2**, 361–6.

Francis, G. & Pinto, A. (1993). Obsessive–compulsive disorder. In *Handbook of prescriptive treatments for children and adolescents* (ed. R.T. Ammerman, C.G. Last & M. Hersen), pp. 198–213. Allyn & Bacon, Boston.

Freeston, M.H., Ladouceur R., Thibodeau, N. & Gagnon, F. (1992a). Cognitive intrusions in a non-clinical population I. response style, subjective experience and appraisal. *Behaviour Research and Therapy*, **29**(6), 585–97.

Freeston, M.H., Ladouceur, R., Thibodeau, N. & Gagnon, F. (1992b). Cognitive intrusions in a non-clinical population. II. Associations with depressive, anxious and compulsive symptoms. *Behaviour Research and Therapy*, **30**, 263–71.

Freeston, M.H., Rheaume, J. & Ladouceur, R. (1996). Correcting faulty appraisals of obsessional thoughts. *Behaviour Research and Therapy*, **34**, 433–46.

Friedmann, C. & Silvers, F. (1977). A multimodality approach to inpatient treatment of obsessive–compulsive disorder. *American Journal of Psychotherapy*, **31**, 456–65.

George, M.S., Trimble, M.R., Ring, H.A., Sallee, F.R. & Robertson, M.M. (1993). Obsessions in obsessive–compulsive disorder with and without Gilles de la Tourette's syndrome. *American Journal of Psychiatry*, **150**, 93–7

Giedd, J.N., Rapoport, J.L., Leonard, H.L., Richter, D. & Swedo, S.E. (1996). Case study: acute basal ganglia enlargement and obsessive–compulsive symptoms in an adolescent boy. *Journal of the American Academy of Child and Adolescent Psychiatry*, **35**, 913–15.

Goodman, W.K. & Price, L.H. (1990). Rating scales for obsessive–compulsive disorder. In *Obsessive–compulsive disorders: theory and management*, 2nd edn. (ed. M.A. Jenike, L. Baer & W.E. Minichiello). Year Book Medical Publishers, Boston.

Goodman, W.K., Price, L.H., Rasmussen, S.A., Mazure, C., Fleischmann, R., Hill, C.L., Heninger, G.R. & Charney, D.S. (1989a). The Yale–Brown obsessive compulsive scale (Y-BOCS): Part I. Development, use, and reliability. *Archives of General Psychiatry*, **46**, 1006–11.

Goodman, W.K., Price, L.H., Rasmussen, S.A., Mazure, C., Fleischmann, R., Hill, C.L., Heninger, G.R. & Charney, D.S. (1989b). The Yale–Brown obsessive compulsive scale (Y-BOCS): Part II. Validity. *Archives of General Psychiatry*, **46**, 1012–16.

Hanna, G.L. (1995). Demographic and clinical features of obsessive–compulsive disorder in children and adolescents. *Journal of the American Academy of Child and Adolescent Psychiatry*, **34**(1), 19–27.

Harris, C. & Wiebe, D. (1992). An analysis of response prevention and flooding procedures in the treatment of adolescent obsessive compulsive disorder. *Journal of Behaviour Therapy and Experimental Psychiatry*, **23**, 107–15.

Herjanic, B., Herjanic, D., Brown, F. & Wheatt, T. (1975). Are children reliable reporters? *Journal of Abnormal Child Psychology*, **3**, 41–8.

Hodges, K. (1993). Structured interviews for assessing children. *Journal of Child Psychology and Psychiatry*, **34**, 49–68.

Hodgson, R. & Rachman, S. (1977). Obsessional compulsive complaints. *Behaviour Research and Therapy*, **15**, 389–95.

Hollingsworth, C.E., Tanguay, P.E., Grossman, L. & Pabst, P. (1980). Long-term outcome of obsessive–compulsive disorder in childhood. *Journal of the American Academy of Child and Adolescent Psychiatry*, **19**, 134–44.

Holzer, J.C., Goodman, W.K., McDougle, C.J., Baer, L., Boyarsky, B.K., Leckman, J.F. & Price, L.H. (1994). Obsessive–compulsive disorder with and without a chronic tic disorder: a comparison of symptoms in 70 patients. *British Journal of Psychiatry*, **164**, 469–73.

Honjo, S., Hirano, C., Murase, S., Kaneko, T., Sugiyama, T., Ohtaka, K., Aoyama, T., Takei, Y., Inoko, K. and Wakabayashi, S. (1989). Obsessive–compulsive symptoms in childhood and adolescence. *Acta Psychiatrica Scandinavica*, **80**, 83–91.

Johnson, B.A. (1993). The Maudsley's obsessional children: phenomenology, classification and associated neurobiological and co-morbid features. *European Child and Adolescent Psychiatry*, **2**, 192–202.

Judd, L. (1965). Obsessive–compulsive neurosis in children. *Archives of General Psychiatry*, **12**, 136–43.

Kearney, C.A. & Silverman, W.K. (1990). Treatment of an adolescent with obsessive–compulsive disorder by alternating response prevention and cognitive therapy: an empirical analysis. *Journal of Behaviour Therapy and Experimental Psychiatry*, **21**, 39–47.

Kellerman, J. (1981). Hypnosis as an adjunct to thought stopping and covert reinforcement in the treatment of homicidal obsession in a twelve-year-old boy. *International Journal of Clinical and Experimental Hypnosis*, **29**, 129–35.

King, N., Inglis, S., Jenkins, M., Myerson, N. & Ollendick, T. (1995). Test–retest reliability of the survey form of the Leyton Obsessional Inventory–Child Version. *Perceptual and Motor Skills*, **80**(3 Pt 2), 1200–2.

Kringlen, E. (1970). Natural history of obsessional neurosis. *Seminars in Psychiatry*, **2**, 403–19.

Ladouceur, R., Freeston, M.H., Gagnon, F., Thibodeau, N. & Dumont, J. (1993). Cognitive-behavioural treatment of obsessional ruminators. *Behavioural Modification*, **19**, 247–57.

Ladouceur, R., Rheaume, J., Freeston, M.H., Aublet, F., Jean, K., Lachance, S., Langlois, F.

& de Pokomandy-Morin, K. (1995). Experimental manipulations of responsibility: an analogue test for models of obsessive–compulsive disorder. *Behaviour Research and Therapy*, **33**, 937–46.

Last, C.G., Hersen, M., Kazdin, A., Orvaschel, H. & Perrin, S. (1991). Anxiety disorders in children and their features. *Archives of General Psychiatry*, **48**, 928–34.

Last, C.G., Perrin, S., Hersen, M. & Kazdin, A.E. (1992). DSMIII-R anxiety disorders in children: sociodemographic and clinical characteristics. *Journal of the American Academy of Child and Adolescent Psychiatry*, **31**(6), 1070–6.

Last, C.G. & Strauss, C.C. (1989). Obsessive-compulsive disorder in childhood. *Journal of Anxiety Disorders*, **3**, 295–302.

Lenane, M.C., Swedo, S.E., Leonard, H., Pauls, D.L., Screery, L. & Rapoport, J.L. (1990). Psychiatric disorders in first-degree relatives of children and adolescents with obsessive–compulsive disorder. *Journal of the American Academy of Child and Adolescent Psychiatry*, **29**, 407–12.

Leonard, H.J. (1990). Childhood rituals and superstitions: developmental and cultural perspective. In *Obsessions and compulsions in children and adolescents* (ed. J.S. Rapoport). American Psychiatric Press, Washington, DC.

Leonard, H.L., Swedo, S.E., Lenane, M.C., Rettew, D.C., Cheslow, D.L., Hamburger, S.D. & Rapoport, J.L. (1991). A double-blind desipramine substitution during long-term clomipramine treatment in children and adolescents with obsessive–compulsive disorder. *Archives of General Psychiatry*, **48**, 922–7.

Leonard, H.L., Swedo, S.E., Lenane, M.C., Rettew, D.C., Hamburger, S.D., Bartko, J.J. & Rapoport, J.L. (1993). A 2- to 7-year follow-up study of 54 obsessive–compulsive children and adolescents. *Archives of General Psychiatry*, **50**(6), 429–439.

Leonard, H.L., Swedo, S.E., Rapoport, J.L., Koby, E.V., Lenane, M.C., Cheslow, D.L. & Hamburger, S.D. (1989). Treatment of obsessive compulsive disorder with clomipramine and desipramine in children and adolescents. *Archives of General Psychiatry*, **46**, 1088–92.

Liebowitz, M.R., Hollander, E., Fairbanks, J. & Campeas, R. (1990). Fluoextine for adolescents with obsessive–compulsive disorder. *American Journal of Psychiatry*, **143**, 370–1.

Lopata, C. & Rachman, S. (1995). Perceived responsibility and compulsive checking. *Behaviour Research and Therapy*, **33**, 673–84.

March, J.S. (1995). Cognitive–behavioral psychotherapy for children and adolescents with OCD: a review and recommendations for treatment. *Journal of the American Academy of Child and Adolescent Psychiatry*, **34**(1), 7–18.

March, J.S. & Leonard, H.L. (1996). Obsessive–compulsive disorder in children and adolescents: a review of the past 10 years. *Journal of the American Academy of Child and Adolescent Psychiatry*, **34**(10), 1265–73.

March, J.S., Leonard, H.L. & Swedo, S.E. (1995). Neuropsychiatry of obsessive–compulsive disorder in children and adolescents. *Comprehensive Therapy*, **21**, 507–12.

March, J.S., Mulle, K. & Herbel, B. (1994). Behavioral psychotherapy for children and adolescents with obsessive–compulsive disorder: an open trial of a new protocol-driven treatment package. *Journal of the American Academy of Child and Adolescent Psychiatry*, **33**(3), 333–41.

McFall, M. & Wollersheim, J.P. (1979). Obsessive–compulsive neurosis: a cognitive–behavioural formulation and approach to treatment. *Cognitive Therapy and Research*, **3**(4), 333–48.

Meyer, V. (1966). Modification of expectations in cases with obsessional rituals. *Behaviour Research and Therapy*, **4**, 273–80.

Mowrer, O.H. (1939). A stimulus–response theory of anxiety. *Psychological Review*, **46**, 553–65.

Mowrer, O.H. (1960). *Learning theory and behaviour.* Wiley, New York.

Muris, P., Merckelbach, H., Van Den Hout, M. & De Jong, P. (1992). Suppression of emotional and neutral material. *Behaviour Research and Therapy*, **30**(6), 639–42.

Murphy, D.L., Pickar, D. & Alterman, I.S. (1982). Methods for the quantitative assessment of depressive and manic behaviour. In: *The behaviour of psychiatric patients* (ed. E.L. Burdock, A. Sudilvsky & S. Gershon), pp. 355–92. Marcel Dekker, New York.

Nestadt, G., Samuels, J.F., Romanoski, A.J., Folstein, M.F. & McHugh, P.R. (1994). Obsessions and compulsions in the community. *Acta Psychiatrica Scandinavica*, **89**(4), 219–24.

Ownby, R.L. (1983). A cognitive behavioural intervention for compulsive handwashing with a thirteen-year old boy. *Psychology in the Schools*, **20**, 219–222.

Pauls, D.L., Alsobrook, J.P., Goodman, W., Rasmussen, S. & Leckman, J.F. (1995). A family study of obsessive–compulsive disorder. *American Journal of Psychiatry*, **152**(1), 76–84.

Pauls, D.L., Towbin, K.E., Leckman, J.F., Zahner, G.E.P. & Cohen, D.J. (1986). Gilles de la Tourette's syndrome and obsessive–compulsive disorder. *Archives of General Psychiatry*, **43**, 1180–82.

Piacentini, J., Gitow, A., Jaffer, M., Graae, F. & Whitaker, A. (1994). Outpatient behavioral treatment of child and adolescent obsessive compulsive disorder. *Journal of Anxiety Disorders*, **8**, 277–89.

Piacentini, J.C., Shaffer, D., Fisher, P., Schwab-Stone, M., Davies, M. & Gioia, P. (1993). The diagnostic interview schedule for children – Revised Version (DISC-R): III. Criterion validity. *Journal of the American Academy of Child and Adolescent Psychiatry*, **32**, 658–65.

Pitman, R.K., Green, R.C., Jenicke, M.A. & Mesullam, M.M. (1987). Clinical comparison of Tourettes syndrome and obsessive compulsive disorder. *American Journal of Psychiatry*, **144**, 1166–71.

Puig-Antich, J. & Chambers, W. (1978). *The schedule for affective disorders and schizophrenia for school-age children (Kiddie-SADS)*. New York State Psychiatric Institute, New York.

Rachman, S. (1993). Obsessions, responsibility, and guilt. *Behaviour Research and Therapy*, **31**, 149–54.

Rachman, S. (1997). A cognitive theory of obsessions. *Behaviour Research and Therapy*, **35**, 793–802.

Rachman, S. & deSilva, P. (1978). Abnormal and normal Obsessions. *Behaviour Research and Therapy*, **16**, 233–8.

Rachman, S. & Hodgson, R. (1980). *Obsessions and compulsions*. Prentice-Hall, New Jersey.

Rachman, S. & Shafran, R. (in press). *The mechanisms of behavioral treatment and the problem of therapeutic failures*. In Maser J. (ed). NIMH conference on OCD.

Rapoport, J., Elkins, R., Langer, D.H., Screery, W., Buchsbaum, M.S., Gillin, J.C., Murphy, D.L., Zahn, T.P., Lake, R., Ludlow, C. & Mendelson, W. (1981). Childhood obsessive–compulsive disorder. *American Journal of Psychiatry*, **12**, 1545–54.

Rapoport, J.L., Elkins, R. & Mikkelson, E. (1980). A clinical controlled trial of cholorimipramine in adolescents with obsessive–compulsive disorder. *Psychopharmacology Bulletin*, **16**, 62–3.

Rapoport, J.L., Leonard, H.L., Swedo, S.E. & Lenane, M.C. (1993). Obsessive compulsive disorder in children and adolescents: issues in management. *Journal of Clinical Psychiatry*, **54** Suppl., 27–32.

Rapoport, J.L., Swedo, S.E. & Leonard, H.L. (1992) Childhood obsessive compulsive disorder. *Journal of Clinical Psychiatry*, **53** Suppl., 11–16.

Rapoport, J.L. & Wise, S.P. (1988). Obsessive–compulsive disorder: evidence for a basal ganglia dysfunction. *Psychopharmacology Bulletin*, **24**, 380–4.

Rasmussen, S.A. (1993). Genetic studies of obsessive compulsive disorder. *Annals of Clinical Psychiatry*, **5**, 241–8.

Rasmussen, S. & Eisen, J.L. (1992). The epidemiology and clinical features of obsessive compulsive disorder. *The Psychiatric Clinics of North America*, **15**, 743–58.

Reich, W. & Welner, Z. (1988). *Revised version of the Diagnostic Interview for Children and Adolescents (DICA-R)*. Department of Psychiatry, Washington University School of Medicine, St Louis, MO.

Rettew, D.C., Swedo, S.E., Leonard, H.L., Lenane, M.C. & Rapoport, J.L. (1992). Obsessions and compulsions across time in 79 children and adolescents with obsessive–compulsive disorder.

Journal of the American Academy of Child and Adolescent Psychiatry, **31**(6), 1050–6.

Richter, M.A., Cox, B.J. & Direnfeld, D.M. (1994). A comparison of three assessment instruments for obsessive–compulsive symptoms. *Journal of Behaviour Therapy and Experimental Psychiatry*, **25**, 143–7.

Riddle, M.A., Scahill, L., King, R.A., Hardin, M.T., Anderson, G.M., Ort, S.I., Smith, J.C., Leckman, J.F. & Cohen, D.J. (1992). Double-blind, cross-over trial of fluoxetine and placebo in children and adolescents with obsessive–compulsive disorder. *Journal of the American Academy of Child and Adolescent Psychiatry*, **31**, 1062–9.

Riddle, M.A., Scahill, L., King, R., Hardin, M.T., Towbin, K.E., Ort, S.I., Leckman, J.F. & Cohen, D.J. (1990). Obsessive–compulsive disorder in children and adolescents: phenomenology and family history. *Journal of the American Academy of Child and Adolescent Psychiatry*, **29**, 766–72.

Rutter, M., Tizard, J. & Whitmore, S. (1970). *Education, health & behaviour*. Longman, London

Salkovskis, P.M. (1985). Obsessional–compulsive problems: a cognitive–behavioural analysis. *Behaviour Research and Therapy*, **23**(5), 571–83.

Salkovskis, P.M. (1996). Cognitive–behavioural approaches to the understanding of obsessional problems. In *Current controversies in anxiety disorders* (ed. R. Rapee). Guilford Press, New York.

Salkovskis, P.M. & Campbell, P. (1994). Thought suppression induces intrusion in naturally occurring negative intrusive thoughts. *Behaviour Research and Therapy*, **32**, 1–8.

Salkovskis, P.M. & Harrison, J. (1984). Abnormal and Normal Obsessions: a replication. *Behaviour Research and Therapy*, **22**, 549–52.

Salkovskis, P.M., Rachman, S.J., Ladouceur, R. & Freeston, M. (1992). The definition of 'responsibility'. *World Congress of Behavioural and Cognitive Psychotherapies*, Toronto, Canada.

Salkovskis, P.M. & Westbrook, D. (1989). Behaviour therapy and obsessional ruminations: can failure be turned into success? *Behaviour Research and Therapy*, **27**, 149–60.

Sawyer, M.G., Slocombe, C., Kosky, R., Clark, J., Mathias, J., Burfield, S., Faranda, I., Hambly, H., Mahar, A., Tang, B.N. *et al.* (1992). The psychological adjustment of offspring of adults with obsessive–compulsive disorder: a brief report. *Australian and New Zealand Journal of Psychiatry*, **26**, 479–84.

Scahill, L., Riddle, M.A., McSwiggin-Hardin, M., Ort, S.I., King, A., Goodman, W.K., Cicchetti, D. & Leckman, J.F. (1997). Children's Yale–Brown Obsession–Compulsion Scale: reliability and validity. *Journal of the American Academy of Child and Adolescent Psychiatry*, **36**, 844–52.

Shaffer, D., Fisher, P., Dulcan, M.K., Davies, M., Piacentini, J., Schwab-Stone, M., Lahey, B.B., Bourdon, K., Jensen, P., Bird, H.R., Canino, G.

& Regier, D.A. (1996). The NIMH Diagnostic Interview Schedule for Children Version 2.3 (DISC-2.3): description, acceptability, prevalence rates, and performance in the MECA study. *Journal of the American Academy of Child and Adolescent Psychiatry*, **35**, 865–77.

Shaffer, D., Gould, M.S., Brasic, J., Ambrosini, P., Fisher, P., Bird, H. & Alawahlia, S.A. (1983). Children's global assessment scale (CGAS). *Archives of General Psychiatry*, **40**, 1228–31.

Shaffer, D., Schwab-Stone, M., Fisher, P., Davies, M., Piacentini, J. & Gioia, P. (1988). *Results of a field trial and proposals for a new instrument (DISC-R)*. National Institute of Mental Health, Washington, DC.

Shafran, R. (1997). The manipulation of responsibility in obsessive–compulsive disorder. *British Journal of Clinical Psychology*, **36**, 397–408.

Shafran, R., Teachman, B., Lilley, C. & Rachman, S. (1997). The assessment and development of childhood obsessive–compulsive disorder. *27th European Congress of Behaviour and Cognitive Therapy*. Venice, Italy.

Shafran, R., Thordarson, D.S. & Rachman, S. (1996). Thought–action fusion in obsessive–compulsive disorder. *Journal of Anxiety Disorders*, **10**, 379–91.

Shapiro, A.K. & Shapiro, E. (1992). Evaluation of the reported association of obsessive–compulsive symptoms or disorder with Tourette's disorder. *Comprehensive Psychiatry*, **33**, 152–65.

Silverman, W.K. (1991). *Anxiety Disorders Interview Schedule for Children*. Graywind Publications, Albany, NY.

Silverman, W.K. & Eisen, A.R. (1992). Age difference in the reliability of parent and child reports of child anxious symptomatology using a structured interview. *Journal of the American Academy of Child and Adolescent Psychiatry*, **31**, 117–24.

Snowdon, J. (1980). A comparison of the Written and Postbox forms of the Leyton Obsessional Inventory. *Psychological Medicine*, **10**, 165–70.

Steketee, G. (1993). *Treatment of obsessive–compulsive disorder*. Guilford Press, New York.

Steketee, G., Chambless, D.L., Tran, G.Q., Worden, H. & Gillis, M.M. (1996). Behavioral avoidance test for obsessive compulsive disorder. *Behaviour Research and Therapy*, **34**(1), 73–83.

Steketee, G.S. & Shapiro, L.J. (1995). Predicting behavioral treatment outcome for agoraphobia and obsessive–compulsive diosrder. *Clinical Psychology Review*, **15**, 317–46.

Swedo, S.E. & Leonard, H.L. (1994). Childhood movement disorders and obsessive compulsive disorder. *Journal of Clinical Psychiatry*, **55** Suppl., 32–7.

Swedo, S.E. & Rapoport, J.L. (1993). Obsessive compulsive disorder in childhood. *Handbook of prescriptive treatments for children and adolescents*

(ed. R.T. Ammerman, C.G. Last & M. Hersen), pp. 211–19. Allyn and Bacon, Boston.

Swedo, S.E., Rapoport, J.L., Leonard, H., Lenane, M. & Cheslow, D. (1989). Obsessive–compulsive disorder in children and adolescents. *Archives of General Psychiatry*, **46**, 335–41.

Tallis, F. (1995). *Obsessive compulsive disorder: a cognitive and neuropsychological perspective*. John Wiley & Sons, Chichester.

Taylor, S. (1995). Assessment of obsessions and compulsions: reliability, validity and sensitivity to treatment effects. *Clinical Psychology Review*, **15**, 261–296.

Thomsen, P.H. (1993). Obsessive–compulsive disorder in children and adolescents: self-reported obsessive-compulsive behaviour in pupils in Denmark. *Acta Psychiatrica Scandinavica*, **88**, 212–17.

Thomsen, P.H. (1994). Obsessive–compulsive disorder in children and adolescents: A 6-22 year follow-up study. Clinical descriptions of obsessive-compulsive phenomenology and continuity. *European Child and Adolescent Psychiatry*, **3**, 82–96.

Thomsen, P.H. (1995a). Obsessive–compulsive disorder in children and adolescents: A 6–22 year follow-up study of social outcome. *European Child and Adolescent Psychiatry*, **4**, 112–22.

Thomsen, P.H. (1995b). Obsessive–compulsive disorder in children and adolescents: a study of parental psychopathology and precipitating events in 20 consecutive Danish cases. *Psychopathology*, **28**, 161–7.

Thomsen, P.H. & Mikkelsen, H.U. (1991). Children and adolescents with obsessive–compulsive disorder: the demographic and diagnostic characteristics of 61 Danish patients. *Acta Psychiatrica Scandinavica*, **83**, 262–6.

Thomsen, P.H. & Mikkelsen, H.U. (1995). Course of obsessive–compulsive disorder in children and adolescents: a prospective follow-up study of 23 Danish cases. *Journal of the American Academy of Child and Adolescent Psychiatry*, **34**, 1432–40.

Toro, J., Cervera, M., Osejo, E. & Salamero, M. (1992). Obsessive–compulsive disorder in childhood and adolescence: a clinical study. *Journal of Child Psychology and Psychiatry and Allied Disciplines*, **33**, 1025–37.

Turner, S. & Beidel, D.C. (1988). *Treating obsessive–compulsive disorder*. Pergamon Press, New York.

Valleni-Basile, L.A., Garrison, C.Z., Jackson, K.L., Waller, J.L., McKeown, R.E., Addy. C,L. & Cuffe, S.P. (1994). Frequency of obsessive–compulsive disorder in a community sample of young adolescents. *Journal of the American Academy of Child and Adolescent Psychiatry*, **33**, 898–906.

Valleni-Basile, L.A., Garrison, C.Z., Waller, J.L., Addy, C.L., McKeown, R.E., Jackson, K.L. & Cuffe, S.P. (1996). Incidence of obsessive–compulsive disorder in a community sample of young adolescents. *Journal of the American Academy of Child and Adolescent Psychiatry*, **35**, 782–91.

van Balkom, A.J.L.M., van Oppen, P., Vermeulen, A.W.A., van Dyck, R., Nauta, M.C.E. & Vorst, H.C.M. (1994). A meta-analysis on the treatment of obsessive compulsive disorder: a comparison of antidepressants, behavior and cognitive therapy. *Clinical Psychology Review*, **14**, 359–382.

van Oppen, P. (1992). Obsessions and compulsions: dimensional structure, reliability, convergent and divergent validity of the Padua Inventory. *Behaviour Research and Therapy*, **30**(6), 631–7.

van Oppen, P., deHaan, E., van Balkom, A.J.L.M., Spinhoven, P., Hoogduin, K. & van Dyck, R. (1995). Cognitive therapy and exposure in vivo in the treatment of obsessive compulsive disorder. *Behaviour Research and Therapy*, **33**, 379–90.

Wagner, K.D. & Sullivan, M.A. (1991). Fear of AIDS related to development of obsessive–compulsive disorder in a child. Special section: Impact of HIV on child and adolescent psychiatry. *Journal of the American Academy of Child and Adolescent Psychiatry*, **30**, 740–2.

Willmuth, M.E. (1988). Cognitive–behavioral and insight-oriented psychotherapy of an eleven-year old boy with obsessive–compulsive disorder. *American Journal of Psychotherapy*, **42**, 472–8.

Wolff, R.D. & Wolff, R. (1991). Assessment and treatment of obsessive–compulsive disorder in children. *Behavior Modification*, **15**, 372–93.

Woody, S.R., Steketee, G. & Chambless, D.L. (1995). Reliability and validity of the Yale–Brown Obsessive Compulsive Scale. *Behaviour Research and Therapy*, **33**, 597–605.

Zikis, P. (1983). Treatment of an 11-year-old obsessive–compulsive ritualizer and tiquer girl with in vivo exposure and response prevention. *Behavioural Psychotherapy*, **11**, 75–81.

Zohar, A.H., Ratzoni, G., Pauls, D., Apter, A., Bleich, A., Kron, S., Rappaport, M., Weizman, A. & Cohen, D.J. (1992). An epidemiological study of obsessive–compulsive disorder and related disorders in Israeli adolescents. *Journal of the American Academy of Child and Adolescent Psychiatry*, **31**, 1057–61.

5
Anxiety disorders

Kevin R. Ronan and Frank P. Deane

Fears and anxieties in children are a normal part of growing up. Seen from an etho-logical perspective, fears and anxieties help children adapt to the world in which they live (Kendall *et al.*, 1992; Ronan, 1996a). Infants' reactions to loud noises and strangers are examples of fear-based arousal promoting increased survival. Such reactions alert caregivers that danger is imminent and protection may be required. As children get older, a primary developmental task facing them is socially based. Anxiety, in its adaptive form, helps children begin to assimilate within a world of others. Moderate levels of anxiety can serve a regulatory function, helping children monitor behaviour in accordance with social, academic and cultural expectations. On the other hand, too little or too much anxiety can be maladaptive. Those who are most often found to exhibit antisocial and conduct-related functioning are also those who tend more often to be relatively bereft of anxious arousal (e.g. Kendall & Hammen, 1995). Persistent, excessive anxiety is also maladaptive, leads to distress, and begins to interfere with a child's development.

Normative data and individual variation

If anxiety is a normal feature of development, how then do we determine what is 'too much' and maladaptive? First, we must be clear about definitions. Fear and anxiety are both related to the theme of increased threat. Fear is generally thought of as a discrete reaction to circumscribed stimuli; anxiety is a more diffuse and internalised response. Second, to understand maladaption, we must first define the upper and lower limits of normal functioning (Kendall & Ronan, 1990). Familiarity with research on develop-mental changes in the content of fears and anxieties, prevalence, and related normative data is essential when making determinations about diagnosis and the need for treatment. Owing to space considerations, these will be briefly summarised (more information is available in Kendall & Ronan, 1990; Ronan, 1996b). The frequency of childhood fears and anxieties appears to peak early (around ages two to four) and decreases somewhat thereafter. The early fears of infants and younger children tend to be related to more discrete danger cues (e.g. animals, strangers, nightmares). As children get older, fears do diminish but by no means disappear. For example, Ollendick, Matson & Helsel (1985) found 7–9 year olds reported just over 14 separate fears; 16–18 year olds reported over 11 fears. With age, the content of fears and anxieties also changes. In accordance with cognitive and developmental tasks, fears and anxieties become increasingly more anticipatory, internalised and focused on social, school, physical and health concerns. Consequently, a fear (separation from caregiver) normal for one age group (up to four to five years of age) may not be for another (e.g. adolescents). In addition to developmental changes, gender differences have also been found. Self-report and maternal report have both suggested that girls have more fears and anxieties than boys (Ollendick *et al.*, 1985). Although actual differences may exist, it is also important to note that sociocultural factors (e.g. sex role expectations) may, in some cases, lead to a 'reporting bias' that may then be reflected in observed gender differences (Kendall & Ronan, 1990).

In addition to normative features, another determinant of maladaptive anxiety lies in a consideration of individual differences (Kendall *et al.*, 1991). Children's reactions to anxiety-provoking stimuli are necessarily based on factors including temperament, past experience and context (Campbell, 1986). Based on differences in these factors, fear reactions to developmentally appropriate stimuli may be associated with excessive forms of behaviour (e.g. withdrawal, temper tantrums, clingy behaviour, peer problems). Thus, although a particular fear or anxiety may fit the developmental pattern, this does not necessarily mean it is transitory, is not problematic, or does not require treatment. Normative data provide a reference point for making clinical judgements about diagnosis and the need for treatment within the context of specific information regarding intensity, persistence and maladaptiveness for each individual.

With sufficient information concerning norm-referenced, developmentally sensitive data, assessment can begin to look at the effect of anxiety on each individual child. The question to be asked is 'Does anxiety consistently inhibit functioning to an extent that the child is overly distressed and/or experiences significant impairments in daily functioning?' If the answer is negative, parents will be relieved to learn that their child's fears are age appropriate and are likely to diminish in number and intensity with time. In these cases, advice on how to cope with normal fears is also recommended. However, in those cases where anxiety interferes with daily functioning, additional assessment and intervention are warranted. The following section briefly reviews diagnostic manifestations and prognosis for childhood anxiety disorders.

Diagnosis, incidence and prognosis

The recent revision of the *Diagnostic and statistical manual* (DSM-IV; American Psychiatric Association, 1994) has changed the way childhood anxiety is diagnosed. Avoidant and overanxious disorders have now been reclassified within the more general class of anxiety disorders. What was formerly known as avoidant disorder is now social phobia; overanxious disorder, is now generalised anxiety disorder. Although these disorders are now in a category that is not childhood specific, each does contain specific features relating to childhood manifestations of symptoms (e.g., more peer-focused, reduced number of symptoms required). Only separation anxiety has been retained as an anxiety disorder specific to disorders of childhood. Apart from these core diagnostic categories, the other disorders within the anxiety disorders class can also be applied to children and adolescents. This includes panic disorder and agoraphobia, specific phobias, obsessive–compulsive disorder, post-traumatic stress disorder (PTSD), and acute stress disorder. This last-mentioned disorder is newly included in DSM-IV and is organised around PTSD symptoms (especially dissociative) that occur in the one-month period following a trauma.

Recent reviews have suggested anxiety disorders in children to be more common than was once thought (Anderson, 1994) with more recent prevalence estimates as high as 17 per cent (Silverman, Ginsburg & Kurtines, 1995). A significant problem in establishing prevalence involves the issue of comorbidity. When children present in clinical settings with anxiety-related problems, they more often present with comorbid symptoms (e.g. depression, ADHD; Ollendick & King, 1994). Developmental factors appear to have an additional influence on clinical presentation. Younger children have been found more often to manifest separation anxiety and simple phobia (and some with comorbid ADHD); older children are more often found with social phobia and generalised anxiety disorder (and comorbid depression or dysthymia; Ollendick & King, 1994). Many symptoms can remit with time. On the other hand, prospective research has also confirmed the persistence of anxiety-related problems and diagnoses in some children over a five-year period (Cantwell & Baker, 1989). The prognosis is better for acute and early onset problems such as school phobia, particularly when effort is mobilised to help the child quickly.

Rationale for treatment; targets for assessment

When clinicians and researchers conceptualise anxiety, they often focus on the relationships between three principal response determinants of anxiety: behavioural avoidance, physiological alerting and arousal, negative cognitive appraisal (Kendall *et al.*, 1991). In short, when a person is anxious or fearful, it is generally associated with arousal and avoidance as a result of a perceived threat and uncertainty. Within the cognitive–behavioural model of childhood anxiety, the perception of threat and uncertainty is a central principle around which other symptoms are organised. That is, cognitive appraisal processes help children make sense of environmental and internal stimuli. When cognitive processing is dominated by a pervasive sense of threat in the face of such stimuli, fear or anxiety can result.

Maladaptive anxiety implicates *distorted*, as opposed to *deficient*, cognitive processing (Kendall, 1985). Deficiencies refer to a relative inability to engage in planning and problem solving, particularly in situations where such processing would be beneficial (e.g. academic, social). Deficient processing is a primary issue in interventions aimed at disorders of self-control including ADHD and conduct disorder (Ronan & Kendall, 1991). On the other hand, distortions refer to active processing that does not accurately reflect the reality of a given situation. In the anxiety disorders, children will engage in distorted thinking, often being overly self-focused, hypercritical, overly concerned about evaluation (both self- and other-) and biased towards 'picking out' threat in ambiguous situations (e.g. Kendall *et al.*, 1992). Physiological arousal may be unnecessarily attributed to anxiety-related factors. For example, anxious older children and adolescents may experience a physiologically based hyperventilation syndrome and overly catastrophise this event (e.g. 'I must be going crazy', 'I am going to die'; Nelles & Barlow, 1988). When distorted processing becomes pervasive, associated other symptoms (increased stress, avoidance and physical symptoms) can begin to create significant daily interference of functioning. Thus, in the typology proposed by Kendall (1985), anxious children are not deficient in their processing of situations; on the contrary, they often actively engage in evaluating situations. Unfortunately, this active engagement has a tendency to be characterised by self-statements focused on uncertainty and threat. The expectancy is that 'bad things will happen' (Ronan, 1996a).

Owing to the tendency to be overly focused on threat and uncertainty, anxious children may not be able to mobilise effective coping strategies. However, this is not to say that anxious children will not have any idea how to cope. In fact, some research supports the notion that many anxious children are able to generate coping strategies (Kendall & Chansky, 1991). Their problem is more one of translating these ideas and strategies into the effective behavioural management of anxiety. Consequently, treatment is first designed to help children learn coping strategies that may, in some form, already be within their repertoire, then to assist them in translating coping plans into behavioural action. Our cognitive–behavioural treatment model of childhood anxiety helps children practise these coping plans in increasingly stressful real-life situations. Thus, while our model emphasises the role of distorted processing interfering with active coping, it also integrates the role of behaviours and the impact of the environment as functionally related to cognitive processing factors. Thus, antecedents and consequences of anxious arousal are very much a focus of both assessment and treatment. We turn now to a consideration of these issues within a functional assessment framework.

Assessment

Assessment serves several functions including research, diagnosis and establishing which factors lead to the development and maintenance of fear behaviours, ongoing treatment response monitoring and, ultimately, treatment effectiveness or outcome. Assessment is important in our programme as it is the logical first step in the development of an individualised treatment plan. A functional assessment framework is recommended (see also King, Hamilton & Ollendick, 1988; Ronan, 1996b; Silverman & Kurtines, 1996). The value of using functional assessment is that it has potential in eliciting comprehensive information within an efficient timeframe. With some planning, such a framework makes maximal use of information derived from standardised assessment methods (Table 5.1).

The focus in functional assessment is on the antecedents and consequences of responses in each of the three response domains described earlier. Thus, the aim is to identify those factors that elicit and maintain unwanted anxious arousal as reflected in distorted cognitive processing, excessive physiological arousal, and maladaptive behavioural avoidance. This includes establishing relationships between environmental factors (e.g. classical and operant conditioning) and internal features (e.g. baseline arousal, skill deficits, physical health, self-talk). Information gathered is integrated within various contexts, including developmental, family, social and academic. For example, external events can initiate anxious processing and arousal. Other children, including adolescents, may become overly anxious as a result of more internally-based factors (e.g. self-focused criticism and scrutiny). Yet others may simply have age-appropriate fears and overly concerned parents.

As a brief example highlighting the relationships between these factors, school phobia and avoidance are problems for some children. However, the factors that elicit and maintain these problems can be quite different (Ronan, 1996a). School avoidance for some children is a result of separation anxiety and negative reinforcement (parents quelling tantrums by acquiescing to school absence). For others, normal arousal occurring at school may be misinterpreted as resulting from anxiety-based, rather than physiologically based, factors. Another child may interpret neutral responses from teachers as signs of disapproval, leading to increased fear and avoidance. Other children manifest school phobia in relation to a combination of factors: school issues (e.g. peer rejection and teasing, academic worries), skill deficits (e.g. social, academic skills), positive reinforcement (fear reactions lead to attempts at reassurance). In all cases of school avoidance, treatment would almost invariably include getting the child back to school quickly (Blagg & Yule, 1994). However, functional assessment helps determine those specific factors that will help intervention proceed efficiently (Ronan, 1996b).

To elicit relevant information, three areas of focus that supplement a more traditional testing battery and help plan for treatment include the following (King et al., 1988; Ronan, 1996b): (a) precise information about the problem (identification of the problem, antecedents, consequences, child's pattern of arousal, developmental enquiries, prior help-seeking attempts); (b) clarifying expectations (research-based

Table 5.1. Comprehensive childhood anxiety assessment battery

---

Structured interview: Anxiety Disorders Interview Schedule for Children (Silverman & Nelles, 1988)
General features/specific fears
   Revised Children's Manifest Anxiety Scale (RCMAS; Reynolds & Richmond, 1978)
   State-Trait Anxiety Inventory for Children (STAIC; Spielberger, 1973)
   Fear Survey Schedule for Children – Revised (FSSC-R; Ollendick, 1983)
   Youth Self-Report (YSR; Achenbach, 1991)
Cognitive features/coping strategies:
   Negative Affect Self-Statement Questionnaire (NASSQ; Ronan et al., 1994)
   Thought-listing (Kendall et al., 1992)
   Kidcope (Spirito et al., 1988)
Coping ability
   Coping Questionnaire (CQ) (see Assessment section)
Depressive features
   Child Depression Inventory (CDI; Kovacs, 1981)
Direct behaviour observation
   Behavioural task ('Tell Me About Yourself': see Assessment section)
Parent ratings
   Child Behaviour Checklist (CBCL; Achenbach & Edelbrock, 1983; Achenbach, 1991)
   Parent-State-Trait Anxiety Inventory for Children-Trait (P-STAIC-T; Strauss, 1987)
   Coping Questionnaire: Parent Version (see Assessment section)
Family and school assessment
   Observational methodology (coding interactions; see Dadds et al., 1994)
   Parent self-report (e.g. anxiety and depression)
   Teacher's CBCL (Achenbach, 1991)

From Ronan (1996b). Reprinted with the permission of the Association for the Advancement of Behavior Therapy (AABT).

information provision, agreement on active participation and goal setting); (c) assigning out-of-session activities (homework aimed at more precise monitoring and observation to gather specific baseline data). In asking for specific information, it is vital that the practitioner uses precise language. Starting with the general problem and moving to specific situations requires exploration of patterns of anxious arousal (e.g. 'When your tummy hurts, what thoughts pop into your head?'), antecedents ('What happened just before?'), consequences ('Then what happens?' 'What do you do to help yourself feel less scared?'). Helping the child begin to establish the relationship between response channels and causes and effects through the use of education, examples and modelling often helps elicit useful information for treatment purposes. Additionally, asking the child to 'walk' the practitioner slowly through a typical (or stressful) day is a helpful technique with some children. Finally, asking the child to do an impromptu speech 'Tell me about yourself' followed by a brief physical symptom-listing and thought-listing exercise (Kendall et al., 1992) can be instructive (e.g. 'What thoughts popped into your head? Did any thoughts make you more or less anxious? What was your body saying?').

Information gained from other assessment methods (e.g. structured interview, self-report, rating scales) can be integrated within a functional framework (Ronan, 1996b). Typically, in our practice, prior to seeing a child and family, we like to have some structured measures filled out. Parents and teachers are asked to fill out rating scales to be sent back prior to the first session. Children fill out self-report at the beginning of the first session while the parents are interviewed. For example, cognitive assessment measures can help identify negative self-statements and establish a baseline that can be used to assess the effectiveness of treatment in this domain. This not only includes changes in the frequency and intensity of negative self-statements but can also include assessment of the child's baseline 'state of mind' (ratio of positive to positive plus negative thinking; Treadwell & Kendall, 1996; Ronan & Kendall, 1997). Children can also fill out selected measures following a 'Tell me about yourself' behavioural exercise described previously. For example, on the Coping Questionnaire (Kendall *et al.*, 1992), they would rate how able they were to help themselves feel less upset on a seven-point scale. Table 5.1 presents multi-trait/multi-method assessment measures most often used to assess for features related to childhood anxiety. Where possible, comprehensive assessment is recommended. However, recent findings have established that many practitioners tend to use more general and established testing batteries which are available in their practice settings (Watkins *et al.*, 1995). Thus, some practitioners will be unwilling or unable to do all of the assessments listed in Table 5.1. Some of these measures, however, can have pragmatic value and be used to meet specific needs. Table 5.2 presents the same measures, although they are presented within a more goal-oriented, functional assessment framework (Ronan, 1996b). All measures listed have some established reliability and validity and most have been shown to be sensitive to the effects of the intervention to be described in the rest of this chapter.

When assessment determines that a child does require help, relevant information is then provided to the parents and the child. We have already described how normative data and developmental information can be provided. In addition, information provided to parents and children concerning research related to the effectiveness of child- and family-focused intervention is recommended. Providing accurate information about the efficacy or success rate of the intervention often helps create an expectation of ultimate treatment success. As many clinicians are aware, research is supportive of the idea that positive prognostic expectations contribute to the effect size of an intervention (Bergin & Garfield, 1994). Thus, if the children and their parents expect success, it may then become more likely to occur as a result of that expectation (Ronan, 1996b). Fortunately, as will be described later, the actual intervention itself has been shown to demonstrate efficacy across different populations and over time. We now turn our attention to that programme.

Treatment

The main goals of cognitive–behavioural intervention with anxious children and families are (a) management of anxiety, (b) reduction of personal distress, and (c) increasing mastery and coping skills (Kendall *et al.*, 1990, 1992). Children learn and begin to recognise early signs and triggers for anxious arousal and use these early cues

Table 5.2. Specific assessment goals, methods and measures

Goal	Method/measure
Is this fear normal for this child?	Normative/developmental data familiarity; FSSC-R, STAIC, RCMAS
Screening	Self-report and other ratings (specific and global)
Social desirability	RCMAS (Lie Scale)
Differential diagnosis	Structured interview
Identifying/quantifying features	Self- and other ratings
Cognitive features	NASSQ, thought-listing
Behavioural observation	Brief Behavioural Observation Task
Coping issues	CQ/NASSQ/self-report
Quantifying comorbid features	CDI, CBCL/YSR, structured interview
Parent report	CBCL-P; P-STAIC-T, CQ-P
School issues	CBCL-Teacher
Parent's anxiety depression	Adult anxiety and depression self-report
Family context	Family observation (Dadds *et al.*, 1994)
Treatment planning	Self-report, cognitive measure, parent/teacher CBCL followed by focused functional assessment/structured interview
Ongoing treatment assessment	STAIC-T, P-STAIC-T, CQ, NASSQ-derived thought-listing ratings, homework ratings, in-vivo ratings (e.g. Behavioural Observation Tasks), daily diary
Treatment outcome	Battery of measures (see Table 5.1)

From Ronan (1996b). Reprinted with the permission of the Association for the Advancement of Behavior Therapy (AABT).

as signals for the initiation of active cognitive and behavioural coping strategies. These skills are learned in a sequence designed to promote skill building upon skill. The overall theme is helping the child combine these individual skills within an integrated 'coping template' – known in our programme as the FEAR plan. Once learned, these skills are then applied in the second half of the programme – in increasingly anxiety-provoking, real-life situations. A parent or family component is designed to enhance gains made in individual treatment and help generalise across time and settings. First, we look at the children and their families components and general strategies used over the course of individual treatment sessions. Following this description, an integrated 16-session programme is described (Kendall *et al.*, 1990, 1992). This programme is well structured, and our experience as well as outcome studies support its effectiveness. However, various considerations (e.g. resource problems, individual child needs) mean that application of the programme needs to be flexible. Nevertheless, it is important to bear in mind the principles and structure of the programme first before proceeding to flexible applications.

Treatment components and strategies

A number of cognitive, behavioural, and affectively-based techniques are learned by the child in the first half of treatment (sessions 1–8). These include the following: (a) identification of cues to anxious arousal, (b) relaxation, (c) imagery, (d) addressing distorted self-talk, (e) problem solving, and (f) helping the child cope with both increased success (self-reinforcement) and failure through realistic self-evaluation. These major concepts are then integrated within the child's own four-step coping, or FEAR, plan. The acronym FEAR stands for:

Feeling frightened? (awareness of bodily cues and identifying anxiety)

Expecting bad things to happen? (identifying and correcting maladaptive self-talk)

Attitudes and actions that can help (coping and problem-solving strategies)

Results and rewards (Self-evaluation and reward/coping with failure).

The treatment strategies used to help the child learn these techniques in graduated sequence include (a) coping modelling, (b) role-play (c) social and tangible reward, (d) homework (Show That I Can, STIC, tasks) and, importantly, (e) a collaborative therapeutic alliance. Once learned, the FEAR plan is then practised during the second half of treatment (sessions 9–16) using both imaginal and in-vivo exposure. During exposure, children begin to practise these newly acquired skills – their own FEAR plan – in increasingly anxiety-provoking situations. As 'skill builds upon skill' during the first half of the programme, 'mastery (at coping) builds upon mastery' during the exposure phase. We turn our attention now to the integration of techniques and treatment strategies within and across treatment sessions.

Session structure

Session structure is similar within each half of treatment. During the learning phase (sessions 1–8), the beginning of each session starts with a review of homework (STIC task) that incorporates previous skills learned. Stickers or points (STIC points) are given for homework completion. These points may then be turned in after sessions 4, 8, 12 and 16 for tangible (small games, toys) or social rewards (e.g., doing something enjoyable with the therapist). Next, the new skill to be learned is introduced. Strategies used to help the child learn include the therapist modelling the use of the skill in such a way that demonstrates imperfect, but ultimately successful, coping – or, coping modelling versus mastery modelling. During coping modelling, the therapist models behaviours, thoughts and feelings in situations that demonstrate that failure is sometimes to be expected, can be planned for, and ultimately assists learning. Additionally, coping with success is also modelled. Anxious children may have as much difficulty accepting success as they have coping with failure.

Rehearsal and role play are also used to afford the child additional opportunities for learning and practice. While many children enjoy doing role-plays, some children may be more reluctant. In these cases, the therapist can take the lead with the child 'tagging along' (Ollendick, 1983). This involves the therapist role playing and the child following along enacting similar behaviours. The therapist also talks aloud thoughts and feelings, and the child is asked if he or she feels the same or different. Gradually, therapist prompting is faded, and the child is asked to do role-play with increasingly fewer instances of this form of assistance. In addition, switching roles (e.g. the therapist playing the child) often increases enjoyment and learning for the child. As with other skills and strategies, role-plays done in individual sessions should start out easy and get more difficult. In pre-session planning for role-plays, the idea is to plan for success and mastery.

Towards the close of each session, the STIC task is discussed, and the child writes it down in his or her personal journal (see session 1 below). Brief discussion links the STIC task with the focus of the current and next session. Finally, it is important to remember to allow for less-structured time with the child. It is recommended that some brief time at the beginning and at the end of each session be freed to play a game or some other activities the child enjoys (see below for more information).

The second half of treatment has a similar structure to the first half. However, the emphasis is on helping the child get ready to practise the entire FEAR plan in increasingly stressful situations. The first half of treatment will have generated a hierarchy of anxiety-provoking situations that are arranged from least to most stressful. Consequently, in the second half of treatment, imaginal, in-office exposure to lesser anxiety-provoking stimuli is used first. Thus, during these earlier sessions, the structure of the session can remain the same as during the first half of treatment.

On the other hand, later in the second half of the programme, some in-vivo practice is conducted outside of the office setting. Owing to setting demands, slight modification to session structure may sometimes be warranted. For example, planning and more elaborate modelling and role-plays may have to be conducted in an earlier session. A brief discussion or role-play in the natural setting can then be used to review the coping plan, that includes how to deal with all conceivable contingencies including perceived failure. Following in-vivo exposure, the act of coping and mastery is often naturally reinforcing for the child and should comprise the focus of discussion and feedback. STIC tasks continue to be assigned and reviewed.

Integrated treatment

As mentioned earlier, the first half of treatment is devoted to learning a systematic approach to coping with unwanted anxious arousal – the FEAR plan. The second half of the treatment applies the strategies in the FEAR plan to imaginal and real-life anxiety-provoking situations. Skills are learned in graduated sequence. Similarly, exposure is carried out, moving from less to more stressful situations. The final session is devoted to consolidation of gains through the making of a 'commercial' that advertises the child's success in treatment.

Learning the skills: sessions 1–8

The first session is illustrated at some length in order to give an idea of initial activities as well as to give a clearer picture of the structure of individual sessions. Session 1 is designed for rapport building, information gathering, and explaining basics regarding treatment. Developing a therapeutic relationship with the child is important. First, therapeutic alliance is an important factor for many children in our programme (e.g. at long-term follow-up, Kendall & Southam-Gerow, 1996). In addition, anxious children can take some time to 'warm up' to a new situation. Taking the time necessary to help the child feel more comfortable is crucial to the success of the programme. Focusing on non-threatening materials (e.g. games, toys, fun activities) can be helpful at the outset of initial sessions. In addition, leaving some time at the end of each session for a child-chosen fun activity can increase the child's motivation to do the 'work' (e.g. 'As soon as we are done with . . . we can play . . .'). In addition, consistent follow-through on such arrangements is an important part of building a trusting and collaborative relationship. Gathering information can also be introduced within a rapport-building and 'fun' framework – laying a personal facts game is one method. Child and therapist alternate answering the same question (e.g. middle name, how many siblings, favourite TV show).

Basic orientation to the programme provides an overview and emphasises 'working together'. Part of this orientation includes gaining an initial understanding of goals from the child's perspective. Linking the idea of increased coping ability with goal attainment is emphasised – for example highlighting the goal of being able to have more fun in different situations. Brief information concerning treatment effectiveness (e.g. 'This programme has worked for many children') is designed to increase prognostic expectations and encourage active involvement in treatment. Finally, within the context of the first homework (STIC) task, a personal journal is introduced. The child is asked to bring the journal to the next session and to write down details about one time during the week that he or she felt 'great' – not anxious or upset. To introduce coping modelling and role-play, the therapist should first provide examples and demonstrate how behaviours, thoughts and feelings are connected. The child is then encouraged to provide an example. The children are told they can earn stickers (younger children) or points (older children) for completed STIC tasks that can then be exchanged for rewards following sessions 4, 8, 12 and 16. Initial rewards are more tangible (toys, small games); later rewards are more socially based (e.g. time spent with the therapist doing something fun). This progression is designed to enhance generalisation and maintenance of between-session activities to naturally occurring reinforcers in the child's environment.

Session 2 (and all subsequent sessions) then begins with a review of homework and reward for completion. Session 2 also begins to help children identify anxious (and other) feelings and, in session 3, their relation to somatic arousal (**Feeling frightened?**). STIC tasks in these sessions introduce the use of the personal journal to begin identifying patterns of arousal in anxiety-producing situations. These situations are subsequently arranged hierarchically and serve as the basis for exposure during the second half of treatment. Session 4 introduces relaxation training – both cue-controlled and progressive muscle relaxation. A relaxation tape can be made for the child during the session for later practice and use.

Sessions 5 and 6 introduce anxious self-talk and problem solving and their role in anxious arousal and coping. The primary goals in these sessions, are helping the child learn to identify unrealistic thinking and modify this anxious self-talk into coping self-talk. Cartoons are used in these sessions depicting children with empty thought bubbles engaged in ambiguous or anxiety-provoking situations. First, thought bubbles are filled in with automatic thoughts related to anxiety (**E**xpecting bad things to happen?). Second, coping thoughts replace dysfunctional self-talk. In addition to cognitive restructuring, these sessions also explore the value of behavioural problem-solving strategies in anxiety management (**A**ttitudes and actions that help).

Session 7 focuses on self-evaluation and self-reinforcement for successful coping (**R**esults and rewards). This session also helps the child develop strategies for coping with failure. This includes reminding the child of a theme developed through coping modelling and earlier role-plays – that is, the idea that failure is often a necessary part of courage, bravery, genuine learning and eventual mastery.

Session 8 reviews skills learned and integrates them within the individualised FEAR acronym. The FEAR plan is written down on an index card to assist in learning and for the child to check during stressful periods when memory may be compromised. The STIC task for this session involves practice with the FEAR acronym by explaining the acronym to others and making up a story involving teaching it to a younger child. At this point the child is also reminded of the switch in focus to skill application, beginning with the next session.

Applying the skills: sessions 9–16

Planning and flexibility are important features of the exposure phase of treatment. In selecting several situations that provoke low to high anxiety, the therapist needs to plan ahead. For example, objects needed for in-office exposure (e.g. a speech to be read) and any other persons involved (e.g. an audience) need to be anticipated and prepared in advance of the actual session. Flexibility is required as each child will progress at different rates, dependent on the specific problem content, complexity, initial severity, or number of fears. The point here is not to cover every fear and anxiety the child manifests but, rather, to ensure that each child experiences mastery in coping effectively in salient anxiety-producing situations. Some children will require more initial time in imaginal exposure prior to proceeding to in-vivo exposure. Other children will be able to begin out-of-office in-vivo practice rather quickly. If the child experiences difficulty in a situation, remind him or her to self-reward for even partial success. If the child is not able to proceed at all, the therapist encourages rehearsal and role-play, coping modelling, and the use of the FEAR index card as a prompt. In other situations, the therapist may initially have to join in (tag along) to ensure some success. As the child achieves more success, he or she is then encouraged to begin using the skills more independently. We stress again to be aware of individual child needs and move exposure along at the individual child's pace.

In session 9, reorientation from learning to application continues to be emphasised, with practice of the FEAR plan in increasingly realistic life situations (both in and out of the office setting). The first step involves imaginal exposure in a low anxiety-provoking situation. The child will have had some familiarity with this form of exposure already from earlier role-plays and this provides a logical transition to in-vivo exposure. Following success with the imaginal practice, in-vivo exposure to low anxiety-provoking stimuli is next, and is generally carried out in the office. Again, this may involve prior planning, for example the child making a request to the office secretary, with the secretary fully 'briefed' about the impending request to ensure success. Session 10 follows the same sequence – low anxiety-provoking situations imaginally followed by in-vivo exposure.

Sessions 11 and 12 focus on moderately anxious situations. Session 11 uses both imaginal and in-vivo exposure. Session 12 uses only in-vivo exposure. Sessions 13 through 15 focus on real situations – generally out of the office – that provoke moderate to high levels of anxiety. Session 16 summarises and reviews the coping skills and treatment successes. At the Child and Adolescent Anxiety Disorders Clinic at Temple University, children also make a videotaped commercial that 'advertises' their successes during this session (see Kendall *et al.*, 1992). Review with the child and parents also focuses on maintenance and continued generalisation of the FEAR plan (e.g. need for continuing practice). Saying goodbye includes expressions of feelings by the child and the therapist and provisions for 'booster' sessions if required. Therapist telephone follow-up (e.g. at three months) is recommended.

Treatment outcome

The programme described has been subject to controlled, randomised clinical trials (Kendall *et al.*, 1992; Kendall, 1994). Findings have supported the benefits of the programme across gender and racial groups and parent and child measures compared with a wait-list control condition. Clinical significance has been demonstrated. Approximately two-thirds of the anxiety-disordered children participating in treatment were diagnosis free following treatment. By contrast, only 5 per cent (1/20) of the children randomly assigned to the wait-list condition were similarly diagnosis free following the wait-list control period (Kendall, 1994). One-year (Kendall, 1994) and over three-year (Kendall & Southam-Gerow, 1996) follow-up supports the maintenance of treatment effects. Another related study (Treadwell & Kendall, 1996) found beneficial changes in treated children's states-of-mind ratios (balance of positive to negative thinking, see Assessment section) compared to a wait-list control group. Despite the obvious success of the programme as rated by parents and children, it is important to point out that differences between treated and wait-list conditions were not shown on teacher ratings at post-treatment. However, it is also the case that teachers often did not view these children as having significant problems initially. Since many of the symptoms in anxiety-disordered children are 'internalised', they may go relatively unnoticed in school settings compared to 'externalising' symptoms (e.g. acting out). Teacher ratings are often primary outcome indicators of externalising conditions like ADHD and conduct disorder but they may be less sensitive for anxiety disorders. Additional research is needed to address this issue.

Parents and families in treatment

What about the additional benefits of including parents in the treatment? Generally, parent involvement is recommended. First, anxious children have decision-making styles (e.g. choosing avoidant solutions) that can sometimes be reinforced within families (Dadds *et al.*, in press). Consequently, gains made in treatment may not be maintained or generalised in the absence of appropriate parental monitoring. Second, recent outcome data are supportive of the inclusion of a family-based component as a supplement to the programme just described, particularly for younger children and girls (Barrett, Dadds & Rapee, 1996).

Inclusion of parents can take the form of parent education or a family-based intervention (Kendall *et al.*, 1992). In the treatment just described, a separate parent session is included following session 3 to explain more fully the programme and the value of the parents' involvement. More comprehensive family-based approaches have also been examined. Barrett et al. (1996) used what they referred to as a Family Anxiety Management (FAM) programme.

In FAM, following 30 minutes of individual therapy as described above, the therapist meets with the parents and child together for 30–40 minutes. The theme here is of the parents and child working together as an 'expert team' to solve anxiety-producing problems. Process and content strategies are used to empower the family towards becoming problem-solving experts. Process methods include an open sharing of information, emphasis on joint collaboration, and reinforcing the family for already existing expertise (Sanders & Dadds, 1993). Content aims are threefold: (a) helping parents learn how to reward courageous acts while extinguishing maladaptive levels of anxiety – social (e.g. descriptive praise) and tangible rewards for taking healthy risks are combined with planned ignoring of excessive anxiety; prompting the child to use coping strategies is also emphasised; (b) teaching parents management of their own anxiety; and (c) communication and family problem solving – this also includes planning daily and regular family-based problem-solving discussions designed to encourage maintenance and generalisation of gains. This treatment was carried out in 12 sessions with four sessions devoted to each content area (contingency management, coping with anxiety, parent communication).

In a controlled clinical trial, Barrett et al. (1996) found the inclusion of FAM added to the effectiveness of the individual programme for anxiety disordered children. Importantly, at 12-month follow-up, 70 per cent of the children in the individual treatment condition were diagnosis free, whereas 96 per cent of the children in the individual plus FAM condition no longer met diagnostic criteria. Given these encouraging results, the inclusion of parents in the anxiety management programme is recommended.

Case illustrations

The following vignettes are based on cases seen by the first author in an outpatient clinic, private practice (as part of a paediatric outpatient practice) and an inpatient setting.

Case 1: broad-based assessment and treatment

Jason, a 13-year-old adolescent from the inner city of a large urban area, was initially seen in an outpatient clinic and, later, at his school. He was referred by his grandmother (and school) for problems related to avoidance of activities outside home (school, peers, public places). He was assessed using broad-based assessment (see Table 5.1). He met the criteria for an anxiety disorder diagnosis (overanxious, prominent features of separation anxiety) and had multiple fears (from FSSC-R, see Table 5.1) concerning evaluation, peer relations (especially with girls), physical safety, going out in public, and separation from his grandmother (primary caregiver). Jason rated himself as being unable to cope effectively (1 or 2 out of 7 on a seven-point rating scale) in these situations. Thinking was dominated by distorted processing: on a self-statement questionnaire (Ronan, Kendall & Rowe, 1994), Jason endorsed items that included perceiving others to be 'looking at me and laughing', 'I am going to make a fool of myself', 'when I took my test, I thought I would fail', 'I usually mess things up', and 'I don't deserve to have good things happen to me'. Other self-report items noted a particular pattern of physical arousal associated with anxious self-talk (e.g. stomachaches, sweaty palms).

Initial sessions were geared towards developing a relationship that included immediate school re-entry. School attendance was increased by working with both his grandmother and with the school (e.g. not allowing him to 'play sick', social reward for attendance). Additionally, owing to school support, some treatment sessions were able to be carried out in the school setting. This encouraged attendance at school and also set the stage for the development of in-vivo practice in a naturalistic setting. The 16-session protocol was followed but was adjusted to account for individual needs. For example, specific relaxation strategies (e.g. tensing and releasing stomach muscles combined with controlled breathing) were emphasised throughout treatment as they appeared to be very beneficial for the physiological symptoms Jason experienced. Additionally, in the latter phase of the first half of treatment, and more characteristic of an adolescent, Jason wanted to take more of a lead in treatment sessions.

Following the learning of the FEAR acronym, Jason came to the eighth session and announced that he had developed a story relating to the FEAR acronym. The session structure for that day was modified slightly to account for his enthusiasm – he took the lead in helping the therapist learn more about how a basketball player (Michael Jordan) might be able to use the FEAR plan to play basketball, and how he too could use it to overcome his fears. The use of metaphor – superheroes, admired figures, even 'FEAR force battalions' – has been effective in our programme (see also Kendall et al., 1991, 1992) and was likewise effective in helping Jason learn and be more willing to practice the FEAR plan.

In-vivo work included giving a speech, initially to the therapist and subsequently in class, talking to girls, taking a bus with the therapist, going to a shopping mall. These and other exposure sessions required planning and flexibility. For example, taking the bus required a number of sessions and, during the course of this assignment, Jason missed a session due to 'sickness'. This was a signal to the therapist to be sensitive to the potential of moving too quickly. However, with exposure geared towards working at the pace of this adolescent, by the end of therapy Jason was able to take a bus with a friend to the shopping mall and to the movies. Although he did continue to get anxious in a number of situations, he felt more confident – with his own superhero by his side – in his increasing ability to manage anxiety, take healthy risks, and have more fun in his life. These changes were reflected by both parent and self-report measures (e.g. fewer endorsed negative self-talk items).

Case 2

Steven was an 8-year-old boy referred by a paediatrician and his parents for problems reported at school. One question raised by the paediatrician was whether or not some of his problems (e.g. distractable, fidgety, problems listening and following instructions) were related to ADHD. Prior to seeing the family, rating scales (e.g. CBCL; specific ADHD rating scales) were completed by Steven's parents and teacher. Distractability and other problems were noted but, according to both the parent and teacher reports, were related to anxious functioning (overanxious disorder) and not to ADHD. For example, the teacher noted that Steven often cried in class because of 'worries (relating to) "not understanding anything", forgetting assignments, or doing them incorrectly'. Further, these worries appeared to be without a realistic basis, and the teacher noted that 'When we do discuss directions and assignments one on one, he usually does understand'.

The first session with Steven and his parents was geared towards functional assessment. This assessment revealed some ongoing concerns but also identified relatively acute exacerbation of anxiety one month earlier that appeared to be related to anticipating the receipt of a report card. Fears about evaluation appeared to be a dominant theme in Steven's self-talk. These fears and self-talk also related to a specific pattern of physiological arousal (e.g. 'freezing up') and other symptoms (excessive crying). Parental expectations improved with information from assessment provided within a framework of normative data and treatment efficacy (i.e. good prognosis). Treatment was geared towards helping Steven 'have more fun in his life' through the learning of anxiety-management strategies. Steven himself was skeptical about ever feeling 'normal like other kids'. Some time was spent normalising anxiety as well as providing him with information concerning the value of the programme for other children who had similar worries. Realistic goals were set. For example, Steven currently rated his baseline level of anxiety at school as 4 out of 5. When asked about a realistic goal (in the context of normalised anxiety), he said he thought being at 2 out of 5 would be 'great'.

Steven and his parents were seen for a total of 10 sessions. The 16-session protocol was condensed within this timeframe due to limitations imposed by the managed care insurance coverage. Additionally, and at the beginning of each session, Steven provided four ratings of his level of anxiety – 'now, before school, at school today, at school this week'. The therapist (author) coping modelled how to fill out self-ratings. Of interest in this case was the consistent rating of 4 out of 5 by Steven at the beginning of sessions 1 through 7. This rating was accompanied by a pessimistic tone that 'this will never work for me'. The therapist, on the other hand, noted the value of persistence and that Steven's willingness to try new things (e.g. role-play) was already an indicator of eventual success. Following the seventh session and immediately prior to more in-vivo exposure, Steven was given a STIC task to 'write a story about a boy who uses bravery and the FEAR plan to be less nervous and have more fun at school'. The emphasis on this task was on the 'attitudes and actions' component of the FEAR plan. At the beginning of the eighth session, Steven reported his anxiety at school to have been fluctuating between a 2 and 3 out of 5 over the week. In reviewing his STIC task, it was clear that he enjoyed creating a number of different coping-related stories on the family home computer, complete with graphics and computer-generated pictures. He had stressed that his characters were 'being brave and just doing it'. Other coping thoughts and actions included 'It's okay to be nervous', 'I have always got good grades even when I am nervous', 'if I just do my work, I'll feel better'. Also included in the stories was the idea of increased coping as a means to having more fun, self-reinforcement, and the anticipation of the boy's parents being proud of his efforts.

Initially, in-vivo exposure was conducted in the office (e.g. speech, doing a 'pop' quiz). It was then completed in the school setting. Planning was necessary in order to use naturally occurring situations and ensure initial and ongoing success. Steven's parents were taught the FEAR plan and asked to participate in helping Steven prepare for in-vivo practice. His teacher was also prompted to provide positive feedback even in the event of minor successes. Role-plays, supplemented by coping modelling, were conducted in-session to help Steven anticipate coping in the real situation. As a result of this planning, Steven's parents and his teacher noted Steven's growing mastery of anxiety-producing situations. By the tenth session, Steven himself noted his anxiety level to be consistently 2 out of 5. His teacher's global rating of anxiety went from 6.5 to 2 or 3 out of 7 and she stated that she thought Steven was 'doing much better'. Three months following the last session, a brief phone call to Steven's mother noted that he was doing 'terrifically'. She noted that although he still occasionally tended to become overly anxious, he was likewise able – with parental assistance and support – to 'just do it' and cope effectively.

Case 3: comorbidity

Alex, a 13-year-old boy, was a client in an inpatient setting with both externalising problems (ADHD/oppositional defiant disorder/features of conduct disorder) and overanxious disorder. Additionally, Alex was diagnosed with a learning disability. It appeared that some of his acting out was related to increased anxiety. For example, in the school section of the treatment centre, Alex was observed to act out (e.g. turning over desks) when it was understood that academic evaluation was part of the daily plan (e.g. test, oral report). Functional assessment suggested that acting out appeared to help him avoid a number of anxiety-provoking situations. With peers, increased anxiety appeared largely related to fears about being rejected and teased. He would often isolate himself in his room during free time on the unit. At other times he appeared to act out in order to be taken out (e.g. timed out) of anxiety-provoking social situations. When approached to do formal assessment, he refused. Assessment then proceeded within a more functionally based framework. More structured direct observation was carried out in school and on the unit. Teachers and direct care staff filled out rating forms. The staff psychologist also began to drop by for informal chats with the youngster. After forming a relationship, the psychologist was able to gather some information, though Alex still refused to engage in 'all that testing'. With time, however, the psychologist was able to weave some items from self-reports within these chats. It was established that a functional relationship existed between anxiety and reactive aggression with this youngster.

Alex was then seen in individual therapy. The first part of therapy included a focus on the anxiety-management programme to help him stay in school. Alex was slow to 'warm up' to the programme – again, extra time was needed to develop a collaborative relationship. Also, the therapist took more initial time using coping modelling before asking Alex to try out rehearsal and role-play. Once Alex became more convinced that he could trust the therapist not to 'leak' information to others, he somewhat reluctantly began to engage in the programme. One tactic that appeared to encourage more active involvement was using humour and role-plays that were characterised by exaggerated behaviours on the part of the therapist. This modelling appeared to increase Alex's willingness to take some healthy risks himself such that, by the last session of the learning phase, Alex had developed a rap song to help remember the FEAR plan.

Exposure focused on situations in academic and social contexts. Alex refused to allow any others to participate with regard to early in-vivo practice. However, giving an oral report to the therapist only was sufficient to provoke a severe anxiety response characterised by 'freezing up' and followed by avoidance through an escalating pattern of acting out. As in the first half of treatment, extra time was required to move at Alex's pace to ensure mastery. To get through the oral report successfully took almost three full sessions. In-vivo practice included helping Alex get ready for naturally occurring situations in school (tests, oral reports). Regarding peer-related functioning (e.g. how to deal with bullying, self-consciousness, fears of being rejected), imaginal exposure took some additional time as additional issues (e.g. social skills deficits) also had to be addressed. With time, Alex gained some competency in being able to walk up to an admired peer and initiate a conversation with him that did not culminate in rejection by the peer or acting out on the part of Alex. By the end of treatment, Alex was able to remain in school more consistently without avoiding stressful situations. He was also more able to remain on the unit for longer periods with other peers without isolating himself in his room. Direct observation data revealed a reduction in behaviours which had previously required Alex to be placed in time-out.

However, Alex continued to experience difficulties. It became apparent that some of his acting out was not entirely secondary to anxiety. For example, he explained that acting out was the only way that he knew to get any attention from an absent father. Typically, when Alex got in trouble, his father would come over to Alex's home (paternal grandmother's) to give him a punishment (beating). Other instances of proactive aggression also had instrumental value for Alex (e.g. intimidating younger kids for money, perceived status).

The cognitive–behavioural programme was helpful for Alex in reducing his anxiety and the frequency of some of his reactive aggression. However, owing to the severity and multiplicity of his problems, only partial success was achieved. A focus on anxiety was one part of a more comprehensive inpatient-based intervention (behavioural programming, group treatment, etc.) This included many of the elements of other manualised treatment approaches including problem-solving skills training (Kendall & Braswell, 1993) and multisystemic therapy for delinquent youth (Hengeller & Borduin, 1990). Alex also received extra assistance in school owing to ADHD and his learning disability. With continued work on multiple fronts, Alex was eventually able to be discharged. At a three-month follow-up, Alex did report that the anxiety-management skills were helpful for him, particularly in school. Teacher reports confirmed that he was better able to work on difficult academic topics, take tests and so forth without 'too much' acting out. He was also reported to be getting along better with his peers. In this case, the anxiety-management programme was helpful for some of Alex's concerns but was clearly not sufficient. The case does highlight, however, that practitioners should remain mindful of the potential of increased relationship between anxiety and disruptive behaviours for some children and adolescents.

Closing comments

Anxiety is a normal, and adaptive, part of every child's functioning. Consequently, our treatment programme is not designed as a 'cure' for anxiety (Kendall *et al.*, 1992). Rather, it is designed to help children and their families reduce unwanted anxiety to more manageable levels and is an approach which has some demonstrated efficacy. Other questions are as yet unanswered. For example, what particular interventions are most helpful for children who are anxious and show a comorbid externalising disorder? Is there a sequence of various treatment interventions – or, alternatively, an integrated treatment approach – that would be most helpful for these children? In the instance of anxious children who are also conduct-disordered, intervention may necessarily have to begin by focusing on safety-related issues related to dangerous behaviours (i.e., ensuring safety of others) followed by other components including anxiety management. Related to the issue of comorbidity is the issue of research looking at the 'transportability' of 'lab-based' treatments into 'real-world' clinical settings (Ronan, 1996). As highlighted in Case 2, can briefer forms of this intervention demonstrate consistent effectiveness? Are some components of the treatment package more 'active' than others (e.g. cognitive restructuring versus exposure)? Can this programme be conducted in group formats? For younger children, is parent education alone (training parents to apply the programme) sufficient to bring about wanted change? For older children, is individual intervention, without a parent or family component, more desirable? The next generation of research in this area should be designed to assess the advantages of the programme that take into account such real-world and other considerations.

References

Achenbach, T.M. (1991). *Integrative guide for the 1991 CBCL/4–18, YSR, and TRF profiles.* Department of Psychiatry, University of Vermont, Burlington.

Achenbach, T.M. & Edelbrock, C. (1983). *Manual for the child behavior checklist and revised child behavior profile.* Department of Psychiatry, University of Vermont, Burlington.

American Psychiatric Association (1994). *Diagnostic and statistical manual of mental disorders*, 4th edn. American Psychiatric Association, Washington, DC.

Anderson, J.C. (1994). Epidemiological issues. In *International handbook of phobic and anxiety disorders in children and adolescents* (ed. T.H. Ollendick, N.J. King & W. Yule), pp. 43–66. Plenum Press, New York.

Barrett, P.M., Dadds, M.R. & Rapee, R.M. (1996). Family treatment of childhood anxiety: A controlled trial. *Journal of Consulting and Clinical Psychology*, **64**, 333–42.

Bergin, A.E. & Garfield, S.L. (1994). *Handbook of psychotherapy and behavior change*, 4th edn. John Wiley, New York.

Blagg, N. & Yule, W. (1994). School refusal. In *International handbook of phobic and anxiety disorders in children and adolescents* (ed. T.H. Ollendick, N.J.King & W. Yule), Plenum Press, New York.

Campbell, S.B. (1986). Developmental issues. In *Anxiety disorders of childhood (ed. R. Gittelman), pp. 24–57. Guilford Press, New York.*

Cantwell, D.P. & Baker, L. (1989). Stability and natural history of DSM-III childhood diagnoses. *Journal of the American Academy of Child and Adolescent Psychiatry*, **28**, 691–700.

Dadds, M.R., Barrett, P.M., Rapee, R.M. & Ryan, S. M. (in press). Family process and child psychopathology: An observational analysis of the FEAR effect. *Journal of Abnormal Child Psychology.*

Dadds, M.R., Rapee, R.M. & Barrett, P.M. (1994). Behavioral observation. In *International handbook of phobic and anxiety disorders in children and adolescents* (ed. T.H. Olllendick, N.J. King & W. Yule), pp. 349–64. Plenum Press, New York.

Hengeller, S.W. & Borduin, C.M. (1990). *Family therapy and beyond: A multisystemic approach to treating the behavior problems of children and adolescents.* Brooks/Cole, Pacific Grove, Calif.

Kendall, P.C. (1985). Toward a cognitive-behavioral model of child psychopathology and a critique of related interventions. *Journal of Abnormal Child Psychology*, **13**, 357–72.

Kendall, P.C. (1994). Treating anxiety disorders in children: Results of randomized clinical trial. *Journal of Consulting and Clinical Psychology*, **62**, 100–10.

Kendall, P.C. & Braswell, L. (1993). *Cognitive-behavioral therapy for impulsive children*, 2nd edn. Guilford Press, New York.

Kendall, P.C. & Chansky, T.E. (1991). Considering cognition in anxiety disordered youth. *Journal of Anxiety Disorders*, **5**, 167–85.

Kendall, P.C., Chansky, T.E., Friedman, M., Kim, R., Kortlander, E., Sessa, F.M. & Siqueland, L. (1991). Treating anxiety disorders in children and adolescents. In *Child and adolescent therapy: Cognitive-behavioral procedures* (ed. P.C. Kendall), pp. 131–64. Guilford Press, New York.

Kendall, P.C., Chansky, T.E., Kane, M.T., Kim, R. S., Kortlander, E. Conan, K.R., Sessa, F.M. & Siqueland, L. (1992). *Anxiety disorders in youth: Cognitive behavioral interventions.* Allyn & Bacon, Needham Heights, Mass.

Kendall, P. C. & Hammen, C. (1995). *Abnormal psychology.* Houghton Mifflin, New York.

Kendall, P.C., Kane, M., Howard, B. & Siqueland, L. (1990). *Cognitive-behavioral therapy for anxious children: Treatment manual.* (Available from Philip C. Kendall, Department of Psychology, Temple University, Philadelphia, PA 19122).

Kendall, P.C. & Ronan, K.R. (1990). Assessment of children's anxieties, fears, and phobias: Cognitive-behavioral models and methods. In *Handbook of psychological and educational assessment of children* (ed. C.R. Reynolds & R.W. Kamphaus), pp. 223–244. Guilford Press, New York.

Kendall, P.C. & Southam-Gerow, M.A. (1996). Long-term follow-up of a cognitive-behavioral therapy for anxiety-disordered youths. *Journal of Consulting and Clinical Psychology*, **64**, 724–30.

King, N.J., Hamilton, D.I. & Ollendick, T.H. (1988). *Children's phobias: A behavioural perspective.* Wiley, Chichester.

Kovacs, M. (1981). Rating scales to assess depression in school aged children. *Acta Paedopsychiatria*, **46**, 305–15.

Morris, R.J. & Kratochwill, T.R. (1985). Behavioral treatment of children's fears and phobias: A review. *School Psychology Review*, **14**, 84–93.

Nelles, W.B. & Barlow, D. (1988). Do children panic? *Clinical Psychology Review*, **8**, 359–72.

Ollendick, T.H. (1983). Reliability and validity of the Revised Fear Survey Schedule for Children (FSSC-R). *Behaviour Research and Therapy*, **21**, 685–92.

Ollendick, T.H. & King, N.J. (1994). Diagnosis, assessment, and treatment of internalizing problems in children: The role of longitudinal data. *Journal of Consulting and Clinical Psychology*, **62**, 918–27.

Ollendick, T.H., King, N.J. & Yule, W. (1994). *International handbook of phobic and anxiety disorders in children and adolescents.* Plenum Press, New York.

Ollendick, T.H., Matson, J.L. & Helsel, W.J. (1985). Fears in children and adolescents: Normative data. *Behaviour Research and Therapy*, **23**, 465–7.

Reynolds, C.R. & Richmond, B.O. (1978). 'What I Think and Feel': A revised measure of children's manifest anxiety. *Journal of Abnormal Child Psychology*, **6**, 271–280.

Ronan, K.R. (1996a). Cognitive-behavioral practice in pediatric primary care. *The Behavior Therapist*, **18**, 44–5.

Ronan, K.R. (1996b). Bridging the gap in childhood anxiety assessment: A practitioner's resource guide. *Cognitive and Behavioral Practice*, **3**, 63–90.

Ronan, K.R. & Kendall, P.C. (1991). Non-self-controlled adolescents: Applications of cognitive-behavioral therapy. In *Adolescent psychiatry: Developmental and clinical studies* (ed. S.C. Feinstein), pp. 479–505. University of Chicago Press, Chicago.

Ronan, K.R. & Kendall, P.C. (1997). Self-talk in distressed youth: states of mind and content specificity. *Journal of Clinical Child Psychology*, **26**, 330–7.

Ronan, K.R., Kendall, P.C. & Rowe, M. (1994). Negative affectivity in children: Development and validation of a self-statement questionnaire. *Cognitive Therapy and Research*, **18**, 509–28.

Sanders, M.R. & Dadds, M.R. (1993). *Behavioral family intervention.* Pergamon Press, New York.

Silverman, W.K., Ginsburg, G.S. & Kurtines, W.M. (1995). Clinical issues in treating children with anxiety and phobic disorders. *Cognitive and Behavioral Practice*, **2**, 93–117.

Silverman, W. K., & Kurtines, W. M. (1996). *Anxiety and phobic disorders: A pragmatic approach.* New York: Plenum Press.

Silverman, W.K. & Nelles, W.B. (1988). The Anxiety Disorders Interview Schedule for Children. *Journal of the American Academy of Child and Adolescent Psychiatry*, **27**, 772–8.

Spielberger, C. (1973). *Manual for the State–Trait Anxiety Inventory for Children.* Consulting Psychologists Press, Palo Alto, California.

Spirito, A., Stark, L.J. & Williams, C. (1988). Development of a brief coping checklist for use with pediatric populations. *Journal of Pediatric Psychology*, **13**, 555–74.

Strauss, C. (1987). Modification of trait portion of State-Trait Anxiety Inventory for Children – parent form. (Available from the author, Western Psychiatric Institute and Clinic, 3811 O'Hara Street, Pittsburgh, PA 15213.)

Treadwell, K.R.H. & Kendall, P.C. (1996). Self-talk in anxiety-disordered youth: States-of-mind, content specificity, and treatment outcome. *Journal of Consulting and Clinical Psychology*, **64**, 941–50.

Watkins, C.E., Campbell, V.L., Nieberding, R. & Hallmark, R. (1995). Contemporary practice of psychological assessment by clinical psychologists. *Professional Psychology: Research and Practice*, **26**, 54–60.

6
Conduct disorders in young children

Veira Bailey

Conduct disorder in childhood includes excessive levels of fighting or bullying; cruelty to animals or other people; severe destructiveness to property; fire-setting, stealing, repeated lying; frequent and severe temper tantrums; defiant provocative behaviour and persistent severe disobedience; truanting from school and running away from home. As the child grows, not only do problems escalate but the response to treatment is reduced (Olweus, 1979; Patterson, 1982). Several well-conducted longitudinal studies indicate that conduct disorder is relatively stable over time and predicts anti-social behaviour in adult life. There are increased rates of delinquency and anti-social personality disorders (Farrington, 1995). Follow-up studies suggest high rates not only for alcoholism, substance abuse, physical illness, suicide and accidental death, but also for widespread social dysfunction, with poor work records and difficulties in all relationships, including marital relationships. (Robins & Rutter, 1990).

The prediction of anti-social behaviour is stronger for men than for women. For girls, conduct disorder in childhood predicts depression and anxiety disorders more strongly than anti-social behaviour and substance abuse (Robins & Price, 1991).

In addition to anti-social behaviours, there may be co-existing attention deficit and hyperactivity, frequently including cognitive deficits and academic failure (Farrington, 1995). This is associated with particularly poor outcome (Sturge, 1982; Taylor et al., 1996).

Disruptive and anti-social children are often unpopular with other children and are extruded from groups of normally functioning children, associating only with other anti-social children and becoming part of a deviant subculture (Kupersmidt, Core & Dodge, 1990). They therefore lack pro-social models and do not learn how to negotiate and fit in with the pro-social mainstream cultural group. Similarly, anti-authority attitudes and an inability to settle in class lead to a lack of satisfaction with the school and increasing alienation, disaffection and disruptive behaviour.

Parents of conduct-disordered children engage in incompetent child management practices which are associated with the inadvertent development and maintenance of aggressive and anti-social child behaviour (Patterson, 1991).

Rationale for using cognitive–behaviour therapy

Conduct-disordered children have been shown to have a range of cognitive deficits and distortions (Crick & Dodge, 1994). They recall high rates of hostile cues in social situations, attend to few cues when interpreting the meaning of others' behaviour, and attribute the behaviour of others in ambiguous situations to hostile intentions (Dodge & Newman, 1981; Dodge, 1986; Dodge *et al.*, 1990). When in conflict with others, conduct-disordered children underestimate their own level of aggression and responsibility in the early stages of a disagreement (Lochman, 1987). When problem solving, conduct-disordered children generate fewer verbal assertive solutions and many more action-oriented and aggressive solutions to interpersonal problems (Dodge & Newman, 1981).

When upset, or in situations that might cause upset feelings, conduct-disordered children show an unusual pattern of affect-labelling; they anticipate fewer feelings of fear or sadness. When highly aroused, the feeling is interpreted as anger and increasingly action-oriented responses result. However, when aggressive children are encouraged to use deliberate rather than quick automatic responses, their rates of competent and assertive solutions can increase (Lochman, White & Wayland, 1991).

A positive view of aggression and its use to solve social problems appears to be incorporated into the belief system of conduct-disordered children: they expect their aggressive actions to reduce negative consequences; they think aggressive behaviour enhances their self-esteem; and they value social goals of dominance and revenge more than affiliation (Slaby & Guerra, 1988).

Cognitive deficits in conduct-disordered children can be addressed through emotional education, self-monitoring of feelings and behaviour, self-instruction including inhibitory self-talk, self-reinforcement, social perspective-talking, and social problem solving. These are components of most problem-solving skills training (PSST) and aim to teach children how to approach interpersonal problem solving adopting a step-by-step approach.

Distorted cognitions may be dealt with in parallel with problem-solving skills training by continued reference to concepts of fairness, safety and what the other person feels. In this chapter, a cognitive–behavioural approach to conduct disorders in 6–11-year-old children is described. Management of such problems in younger children is described by Douglas (see Chapter 2) and in adolescents by Herbert (see Chapter 11).

Assessment for treatment

Assessment should be broadly based and needs not only to include the diagnosis of disorder in the child but should pay attention to an assessment of parenting competence. The possibility of child abuse, treatable mental illness in the parent, and the presence or absence of support systems for parents in the community should all be considered. An assessment also needs to be made of the child's social functioning at school with adults and with peers and of the nature and extent of academic difficulties (Moffitt, 1990a). A psychometric assessment should be made to detect any cognitive deficit.

It is important to detect comorbid hyperkinetic disorder. The presence of severe anti-social symptoms with undoubted poor parenting and possibly abuse can dominate the picture. This may lead to a classic diagnostic pitfall, as hyperkinetic disorder if untreated is associated with a high risk of persisting anti-social behaviour (Moffitt, 1990b). Cognitive–behavioural approaches to hyperkinetic disorder are described by van der Krol and colleagues (see Chapter 3).

Another diagnostic difficulty may be presented by the child who is well engaged with an experienced clinician and symptom free at interview but impulsive and distractible in other situations. The use of standardised questionnaires (Conners, 1969; Behar & Stringfield, 1974; Routh, 1978; Barkley, 1990; Goodman, 1997) may help in diagnosis. A different problem occurs when the diagnosis of hyperkinetic disorder, manifest by inattention, overactivity and impulsiveness, is made correctly but because a broad-based assessment is not carried out, conduct disorder may be missed. The presence of depression should also be considered. A social assessment may be necessary in some cases, not only to provide a child-protection risk assessment, but also to assess the need for respite provision and advice on housing and finances.

Interventions: general considerations

While research papers may focus on comparing and contrasting the efficacy of different treatment approaches, in practice, a broad-based combination of treatment procedures should be used. Combinations of approaches are likely to be complementary and maximally beneficial (Kazdin, Siegel & Bass, 1992; Earls, 1994; Kazdin, 1997), although research methodology may need to be adjusted in order to take account of the particular problems involved in evaluation (Kazdin, 1996).

A combined treatment approach will need careful orchestration of the various elements involved and should include regular networking and consultation with other agencies, such as education and social services, to avoid conflict and confusion. Occasionally, children may 'need' admission to local authority care or to an inpatient unit. Satisfactory controlled studies of inpatient versus community care are limited. A somewhat flawed comparison showed that community placement produced at least as favourable results as inpatient treatment (Wimsberg *et al.*, 1980).

In practice, it is both difficult and undesirable to separate the cognitive and behavioural elements of a treatment programme. Therapists, parents and teachers should use modelling, positive reinforcement of desired behaviour, extinction and mild negative consequences (such as loss of privileges) for undesirable behaviour in order to foster the development of pro-social behaviour.

Parent management training is essential to change the powerful modelling and negative reinforcement of anti-social behaviour which is otherwise likely to persist. This may need to involve a cognitive component to help parents whose maladaptive cognitions or negative automatic thoughts, such as 'I can't let him have the last word' or 'spare the rod . . .', interfere with their ability to carry out effective positive parenting.

Parent management training

The theoretical and practical basis for this work was developed by Patterson, Reid and colleagues at the Oregon Social Learning Center (OSLC). They describe an escalating cycle of coercive interactions between parent and child – the *coercive hypothesis*. This postulates that children learn to escape or avoid parental criticism by escalating their negative behaviours (such as temper tantrums, defiance), which leads to increasingly negative parental behaviour (such as telling the child off, yelling or hitting the child). Over time, the 'coercive training' in the family continues with an increasing rate and intensity of parent and child aggressive behaviour. Thus both parents and child are caught in the 'negative reinforcement trap' which effectively trains children to be conduct-disordered (Patterson, 1980).

In addition to the negative reinforcement, the child also experiences effective modelling of anti-social behaviours from observation of parental aggression. Furthermore, parents may also positively reinforce the child's misbehaviour, for example by paying attention to the child only when he or she is shouting or behaving badly and ignoring the child when playing quietly.

Five family management practices form the core components of the OSLC programme

1. Parents are taught how to pinpoint the problem behaviours and track them at home, e.g. recording compliance versus non-compliance.
2. Parents are taught reinforcement techniques such as praise, points systems, treats and rewards.
3. When parents see their children behaving inappropriately, they learn to apply a mild consequence or a short-term deprivation of privileges, e.g. one hour loss of television time or bike use.
4. Parents are taught to 'monitor' (or supervise) their children at all times, even when they are away from home. This involves parents knowing where their

children are at all times, what they are doing and when they will be returning home.

5. Finally, the parents are taught problem-solving and negotiating strategies. They also become increasingly responsible for designing their own programmes.

This programme typically requires 20 hours of direct contact with individual families and includes home visits in order to improve the generalisation of parenting strategies.

A parent training programme designed to treat non-compliance in young children aged 3 to 8 was developed by Forehand and McMahon (1981). This incorporated the idea of *alpha* and *beta* commands based on the observation that parents with reasonably obedient children give more so-called alpha commands and parents with conduct-disordered children give more negative beta commands. Alpha commands are characterised by being clear, specific and direct, being given one at a time and being followed by a wait of 5 seconds for compliance. Beta commands are vaguely phrased chains of instruction and comment, often delivered as a question and frequently followed by a rationalisation. An example of a beta command is 'How may times have I told you, if you don't come away from there, Darren. . .I don't know how I'm going to keep my hands off you. . .you know I've had a bad day, what with that letter from the welfare people and now the TV's on the blink. . . Darren what have I told you!' As an alternative, parents are taught to give alpha commands using clear, specific, direct instructions and waiting 5 seconds for compliance. The child is also named and eye contact is achieved. Parents are encouraged to use a firm but not a cold voice and are encouraged to refrain from telling their children what to stop doing. Parents are also taught how to play with their children in a non-directive way and how to identify and reward children's pro-social behaviours through praise and attention. Treatment is carried out in a clinic playroom, equipped with a one-way mirror, and can involve the use of an 'ear bug' through which the therapist can directly coach or prompt the parent while playing with the child. This is called the *parent–child game*.

The Group Discussion Videotape Modelling Programme (GDVM) was developed by Webster-Stratton as a parent-training programme for young conduct-disordered children. It includes components of the Forehand, McMahon and Patterson programmes as well as problem-solving and communication skills (Webster-Stratton, 1982; D'Zurilla & Nezu, 1982).

The basic parent training programme consists of a series of ten videotape programmes, modelling parenting skills. There are 250 vignettes, each of which lasts approximately 1–2 minutes. These are shown by a therapist to groups of 8 to 12 parents per group. After each vignette, the therapist leads the group discussion of the relevant interactions and encourages parents' ideas and problem solving as well as role-play and rehearsal. Parents are given homework exercises to practise a range of skills at home, but the children do not attend. Great efforts were made to use models of different sexes, ages, cultures, socio-economic backgrounds and temperament in order to enhance the power of the modelling by enabling parents to identify with the models.

The programme has also been used by parents of conduct-disordered children as a self-administered intervention, viewing the video vignettes and completing the home-work assignment without therapist feedback or group support. A recent development has been a further six videotape programmes called ADVANCE, which focus on family issues other than parenting skills, including anger management, coping with depression, marital communication skills, problem-solving strategies, and how to teach children to problem-solve and manage their anger more effectively (Webster-Stratton, 1994). Enhancing parent management training by including work on parental concerns such as job stress, family disputes and personal worries has enabled behavioural gains for children to be maintained (Dodds, Schwartz & Sanders, 1987) and has reduced attrition (Prinz & Miller, 1994). For mild behavioural problems, the provision of a brochure alone is often sufficient to produce behavioural change (Clark, Risley & Cataldo, 1976; McMahon & Forehand, 1978).

Family therapy techniques have emphasised general principles rather than the con-tingency management of antecedents and consequences of specific target behaviours. The emphasis has been on altering maladaptive patterns of interaction and commu-nication through broad principles of child management, the strengthening of genera-tional boundaries, the interpersonal interactions of family members, marital relationships and improving the self-esteem of carers.

Individual behavioural programmes for conduct-disordered children using parents as co-therapists have been shown to be most successful when attention is paid both to the antecedents and to the consequences of the desired behaviour. This makes use of the ABC model, a helpful mnemonic for parents as well as therapists (Herbert, 1987).

A stands for **a**ntecedent events – what happens immediately before the targeted behaviour.

B stands for targeted **b**ehaviour.

C stands for the **c**onsequences – what happens after the targeted behaviour.

Paying attention to the antecedents and consequences of targeted behaviours leads to intervention programmes which aim to increase pro-social behaviours by giving clearer instructions and positive reinforcement ('catch the child doing something good') for desirable behaviours.

Anti-social behaviour can be decreased by a range of techniques such as extinc-tion, over-correction, time-out from positive reinforcement and, most importantly, teaching and reinforcing pro-social behaviour that is incompatible with the anti-social behaviour.

Behavioural and cognitive techniques with the child

Social skills training approaches have been increasingly used with young conduct-disordered children. Initially, *operant techniques* were developed, rewarding pro-social behaviour and discouraging anti-social behaviours. *Modelling strategies* were also used, teaching by allowing children to observe appropriate social behaviour modelled by adult or child models. Coping modelling with a model talking through the task, including how to deal with setbacks and frustration, has been found to be more effective than a mastery model demonstrating ideal or perfect behaviour (Meichenbaum & Goodman, 1971). *Coaching* was used in which principles of competent social behaviour were taught, often using role-play of problem situations such as what to do when hit by another child or punished unfairly by a teacher. *Interpersonal cognitive problem-solving training* (ICPS) emphasised the paramount importance of interpersonal communication and negotiating skills, seeing the other person's point of view, and achieving compromise within the social situation. The training developed thinking processes: *how* to think rather than *what* to think.

The aim of therapy for these children is to remedy the deficits and distortions in behaviour and cognitions. Several programmes and models have been developed for *problem-solving skills training* (PSST) and most have several elements in common. *Emotional education* enables the child to identify and label different emotions and the situations in which they occur. The therapist may model expression of feelings and empathising with others in addition to using pictures and games to increase the repertoire. Self-monitoring of behaviour and of feelings whose intensity can be rated enables the children to feel empowered to manage their own behaviour and feelings. *Self-instruction* may use a 'Stop! Think! What can I do?' approach to inhibit or slow automatic responses; while *self-reinforcement techniques* teach the children to use *positive self-talk* – for example 'Well done, I didn't answer back' – to enhance the development of pro-social skills. *Social perspective taking* uses vignettes, modelling, role-play and feedback in order to help children become aware of the intentions of others in social situations. *Social problem solving* such as in the Think Aloud Programme uses a cartoon of Ralph the bear to teach a self-instructional approach to problem solving: 'What is the problem? What can I do about it? Is it working? How did I do?' (Camp & Bash, 1985). Cognitive strategies to control impulsivity are provided in the *Stop and think workbook* (Kendall, 1989).

An approach used by the Hahnemann Programmes (Spivack, Platt & Shure, 1976) emphasises deficits in *alternative thinking*, the ability to generate multiple solutions to interpersonal problems; *consequential thinking*, the ability to foresee the immediate and long-term consequences of the solution; and *means–end thinking*, the ability to plan a series of actions to attain the goal, devising ways around obstacles within a realistic timeframe. They use simple word concepts as a foundation for problem solving; for example *or* and *different* to help generate alternatives: 'I can hit him *or* I can tell him I am upset' – 'Hitting is *different* from telling'. *Cognitive restructuring* can be introduced in parallel where problem solving includes consideration of concepts of fairness, safety and what the other person would feel, the aim being to change basic beliefs and attitudes.

All these elements must be incorporated into a matrix of enjoyable activities in order for therapy itself to be enjoyable for the child. When working with groups, the therapist must pay attention to group composition and be able to manage and control the behaviour of the group using behavioural methods such as positive reinforcement for participation.

In order to encourage the generalisation of pro-social behaviours learned in therapy to home and to school, goal setting and operant techniques should be used. Goals should always be specific and attainable and must be carefully monitored. The contingent use of social reinforcement (e.g. praise, particularly the approval of a valued person), activity reinforcements (treats) and tangible reinforcements (rewards) can be tailored to a particular child's need. Pairing social reinforcement by parents, teachers or therapists with other reinforcements may be particularly important for conduct-disordered children as they often have poor relationships with authority figures and are minimally motivated by adults' reinforcement. Other techniques may focus particularly on anxiety (Garrison & Stolberg, 1983) or anger management (Garrison & Stolberg, 1983; Lochman et al., 1987) and may use group feedback with whiteboards, flipcharts, video feedback, role-play and group discussion. Interventions which explicitly target anger-coping skills, especially recognising the triggers (anger cue recognition), and which rehearse specific coping strategies appear to produce more positive outcomes, whether with conduct disorder or ADHD (Hinshaw, Henker & Whalen, 1984; Lochman & Curry, 1986).

Liaison with schools

Teacher liaison is necessary in order to aid generalisation by reinforcing the development of pro-social behaviours and to change inappropriate beliefs or behaviours by the teacher. Teachers may also be helped by advice on management and structuring of the classroom (Merrett & Houghton, 1989; Wheldall & Lam, 1987), in training in positive teaching methods (Wheldall & Merrett, 1991) and in teaching problem solving (Kendall & Bartel 1990). It may also be necessary to integrate specific educational remediation for a child whose educational attainments are retarded. School approaches to bullying (Olweus, 1994) are useful in reducing a school culture of anti-social behaviour.

Case illustrations
Case 1: a combined programme for a child with conduct disorder and ADHD
John, aged 11, is a child of mixed race, the older of two children living with his unmarried mother. He and his younger brother, Wayne (aged 4), have different fathers who are not in contact with

the children. Two years previously, his mother was beaten up by the man with whom she was living and the family lived in a women's refuge for a few months.

When seen initially, John was aged 10 and was in care, having been pushed downstairs by his mother following an argument. His mother complained of John's disobedience, argumentativeness, anger and violence; at school he was described as having significant behaviour problems, and being volatile and aggressive towards his peers. Because of his behavioural difficulties, it was thought unlikely that he would be able to cope in mainstream secondary school.

Work with John's mother was initially difficult because of her pessimism about the eventual outcome, which was shared by her social worker, who openly expressed the view that only residential treatment in a psychoanalytically oriented unit would be useful. John was admitted to a day unit programme, where he attended for three sessions a week in a small group of eight children aged 10 to 11 with two therapists, one of whom was a teacher. Because of the difficulties in engaging John's mother, particular care was taken at the intake meeting to describe to John and his mother the areas which John would work on in the day unit.

These were specified as: (1) to learn to be polite and friendly towards others; (2) to do as asked immediately; (3) to learn to keep calm; (4) to learn to make and keep friends; (5) to stay in his seat; (6) to get on with his work without disturbing others; (7) to talk about his worries and feelings. It was agreed that John's mother would be seen regularly by an outpatient worker for parent management training and that the day unit specialist teacher would liaise with John's school. As soon as his mother had agreed, the contract was signed by all involved, that is, John, his mother, the Day Unit staff, outpatient worker, social worker, and John's school teacher.

In the day unit programme, group rules are formulated in order to teach children the pro-social behaviours necessary for mainstream school. In John's group the rules were: (i) we will do as we are asked immediately; (ii) we look, listen and are quiet when someone else is talking; (iii) we put up our hand when we want to speak; (iv) we are polite and friendly to others; (v) we stay sitting in our seats. At the beginning of every session, the rules are rehearsed and each child's individual task is reviewed.

Initially, John found it very difficult to sit still on his chair during the group meeting that started each session. This was therefore specified as John's initial task and was soon achieved by using techniques of positive reinforcement. Whenever John was sitting still he was praised. This was linked to a points system and stars, where every fifth star was a gold star, leading to a letter home to his mother, describing John's achievement and asking her to reward him. A reward menu of small rewards had already been arranged with his mother and John frequently chose a chocolate bar from the reward box.

Modelling was also used, with children who were role models in the group; they showed John how to sit calmly. John tended to look around the room instead of maintaining eye contact. The group leaders therefore used coping modelling to demonstrate the effect of this by talking to each other when looking at the ceiling or looking out of the window. This was done in a way that was both clear and amusing.

John was an articulate boy who was well able to identify his main problems, think about alternative solutions and predict consequences. He was very aware that the consequence of his difficult behaviour at home had been admission to a children's home. *Social perspective-taking* was used to help John see his mother's point of view in a variety of situations. Role-play was used, involving all group members, and various solutions to problems were acted out.

John was also eager to remain in a mainstream school and to improve his behaviour in class. *Self-monitoring* was used in the day unit and in John's classroom. John was given a task, for example to work on an activity without disturbing others. He was able to shade a section of a chart every 10 minutes he remained on task. Feedback was then given after each 30-minute period and John was able to earn stickers for each section shaded. Over time, the shading chart and sticker system was faded out and was replaced with John's ability to use *self-instruction* and *self-talk*: 'I must finish this work by 11 o'clock, then I can go out to play and I will also get a positive comment in my home school book'.

While in the group, it quickly became apparent that restless, inattentive, fidgety behaviour, poor concentration and distractibility were major features of John's difficulties which had been obscured by the child protection issues and had not been apparent in the initial assessment interviews. An additional diagnosis of ADHD was made, which was confirmed by observation at school and by a high score on the Conners' teachers' and parents' questionnaires. Medication was added to John's treatment programme. John used self-talk to remind himself of his achievements: 'Ritalin helps a little', 'I can and do work hard to improve my behaviour'.

In order to improve the generalisation of John's coping behaviour using problem solving in the day unit to school and home, he agreed to carry a pocket book with him which his teachers, the day unit staff and John's mother filled in daily. John was rewarded with a sticker for any positive comments. Any negative comment was discussed in detail. It was stressed to his mother and to the teachers that he should not be told off but should be asked to problem solve on how he could do things differently.

John's mother was given feedback after each day unit session. She rewarded him for positive comments and gave mild negative consequences (such as missing a favourite television programme or going to bed half an hour early) for negative incidents. With John's improving behaviour, it was possible to work more co-operatively with his mother on parent management techniques and she was more compliant in carrying them out, including keeping charts. Some work was also done with her on her negative automatic thoughts which led to her feelings of anger and hopelessness. John made good use of problem solving on his return home, where there were difficulties with his mother establishing sensible routines. John was also able to contribute well to others children's problem solving, contributing alternative solutions and looking at the advantages and disadvantages in the group setting. This enhanced his self-image.

As John was particularly interested in fishing, football and gymnastics, he was motivated to earn activities and equipment related to his hobbies. John's mother was thus able to use a range of positive reinforcement for good comments from the day unit, linking praise with treats and rewards he enjoyed. When John's behaviour was disruptive in the day unit, his mother was able to implement mild negative consequences. These included: (i) John not being able to play with friends after school; (ii) John spending time in his room; and (iii) John going to bed earlier than usual.

After 3 to 4 months, the situation was much improved at home and at school. He was very responsive to positive reinforcement and his mother was consistent with behavioural management at home. His motivation to do well and his confidence in being able to cope at home and at school were markedly improved.

After the summer break, John transferred to secondary school, where his improvement was maintained. John was keen to leave the group and be at school full time, which happened after half-term. At home, his mother appeared to have difficulties in maintaining a routine and supporting him in doing his homework. John's progress will be monitored and if difficulties arise, booster sessions will be introduced.

Case 2: Problem-solving skills training for a 6 year old

Larry is a 6 year old, referred because of aggressive, angry and defiant behaviour towards other children at school and at home. Larry has two older half sisters and a baby brother, each having a different father. He was having daily tantrums and was frequently hit by his mother and her partner. Larry was admitted to a group for 5 to 7 year olds in the day unit for three sessions a week. His contract included an undertaking to work on the following areas: (1) to play with others without hitting or hurting; (2) to do as I am asked straightaway; (3) to ask when I want something; (4) to learn to express my needs and feelings; (5) to deal with my anger in an appropriate way; (6) to wait my turn.

Management training was arranged for Larry's mother and her partner, focusing in particular on increasing the positive reinforcement and reducing punishment.

Larry responded well to the structure of the group, that is, the boundaries and rules which were clearly defined with stickers awarded every 20 minutes after each activity if the rules were maintained.

He appeared as a defiant child, able only to express his needs aggressively rather than verbally. When provoked by others, he would hit out, initially needing time out of the room to calm down. He did not like time-out from positive reinforcement in the group and was therefore encouraged to express his needs and feelings verbally to avoid it. He was also encouraged to express himself verbally in the group meeting as he needed to develop his ability to help himself and help others problem solve, and to think of alternative solutions to problems at home and at school. He liked this responsibility, which enabled him to improve his self-image.

Praise for Larry was directed towards shaping his ability to develop positive self-talk. Step one in problem solving – his ability to talk about a problem – was worked on each time an opportunity arose spontaneously in the group. For example, when he wanted to use colouring pencils and not felt tips in a craft activity, his initial reaction was to sulk. (On admission he would have lashed out.) When he was asked what was wrong and was reminded that he could not be helped unless he talked about the problem, he responded and was reinforced by therapist praise and a swift solution to the problem. Talking about a problem was then generalised to home and school by discussing with Larry the probability of solving his problems at home and at school by talking. This was further reinforced by having a school/home/day unit book in which Larry's problems and his solutions were recorded.

Larry responded well to social cues and modelling, particularly when reinforced by social reinforcement (praise and non-verbal signs of approval) paired with token reinforcement for appropriate social behaviour. In his case, the tokens were friendly smiley stickers, which were put into an envelope and at the end of the week were counted and linked to a friendly award badge. This helped Larry think about his personal goals, and the goals of others in the group.

Problems naturally arising in the group were talked through using instant problem solving at the time. For example, conflicts about who lines up first at the door would be dealt with by talking through alternatives and their consequences, reaching a solution bearing in mind concepts of fairness, safety and what the other person would feel. Problem-solving techniques were also highlighted using puppets and role-playing solutions and by the use of a 'traffic lights' system, where the red light was a reminder to stop and define the problem, the amber light to think of four alternatives and their consequences, and the green light to choose the solution. Larry made very good use of problem solving, learning to remain calm and express his needs verbally. This was complemented by emotional education, talking about his feelings through art work, stories and games.

Week by week, Larry's tasks were refined, and 4 months after joining the group his main task was to stay calm at all times. This was defined in his school/home/day unit book and, after discussion with Larry, further reinforced by colouring in a picture of a dog. This was linked to attention from his mother and her partner, with the ultimate goal of them getting a dog for Larry. Larry responded very well to this co-ordinated approach, which he perceived as clear and fair. He was helped by explicit efforts to generalise his improved behaviour to home and school and to reinforce this in both situations.

Simultaneous work was carried out with his mother. Efforts were made to meet with her cohabitee, but he did not attend. However, she was increasingly able to use positive parenting techniques with Larry as his behaviour obviously improved. There was some slippage over the Christmas holidays when star charts were prematurely abandoned, and Larry reacted adversely, feeling that his mother and her partner were not keeping to their contract. His behaviour at home improved rapidly when the charts were re-established. Gradually, his mother became less defensive, and had more confidence in her ability to manage Larry. She was more able to look at her own behaviour and cognitions, not only with Larry, but also in relationship to her other children and to her partner. Further enhancement to this was offered by a place for her in the parents' group for parents of infants and primary school children attending the day unit.

Outcome

Treatment effects of cognitively based treatments have been found to significantly reduce aggressive behaviour at home, at school and in the community (Kazdin, 1997). These effects have been replicated in several controlled studies and gains have been evident up to one year later. A useful meta-analysis of relevant studies is provided by Durlak, Fuhrman & Lampman (1991).

A carefully designed, controlled study of cognitive–behavioural problem-solving skills training demonstrated a significantly greater decrease in aggressive behaviour and behaviour problems at home and at school, together with an increase in prosocial behaviours and overall adjustment. These effects were evident immediately after treatment and at a one-year follow-up (Kazdin et al., 1987). The development of CBT for the child is of particular importance when there is effectively no parent to work with. This may be due to severe family dysfunction causing removal of the child from the home (e.g. due to neglect or abuse) or when the parent is unwilling or unable to participate in parent management training. When problem-solving skills training is combined with parent management training, more marked changes in child and parent functioning occur and place a greater proportion of those treated within the normal range of functioning (Kazdin et al., 1992).

Unfortunately, the characteristics of parents which lead to parenting difficulties are those which are also associated with poorer outcomes (Webster-Stratton, 1989a;

Patterson, 1991). These factors include multiple social problems, marital problems, single parents of low socio-economic status, and a strong punishment ideology in the parents. Components can therefore be added to address these difficulties. Close liaison with social services will be helpful where there are multiple social problems, perhaps using family aide support or respite care to reduce stress, while couple therapy to address problems in the parents' relationship may reduce marital difficulties interfering with their parenting.

The underlying behaviour principles of parent management training have a face validity which parents appreciate and which may increase their compliance. Programmes generally have high parental ratings of acceptability and consumer satisfaction (Webster-Stratton, 1989b). However, while teaching parenting skills empowers parents, it also makes demands on them, with consequent difficulties in engaging in therapy and high drop-out rates (Kazdin *et al.*, 1992).

Although programmes treating conduct-disordered children are steadily developing and the therapeutic elements are being evaluated in randomised controlled trials, the central problems of working with families who are difficult to engage remain. Overall, it appears helpful to recognise that conduct disorder is a chronic condition and that 'booster sessions' may be necessary.

While public anxiety about delinquency and violence is high, it is important to emphasise the cost-benefit and potential health gain of early intervention with conduct-disordered children (Offord, 1989; Light & Bailey, 1993) as well as the opportunities for creative therapeutic interventions.

References

Barkley, R.A. (1990). Attention-deficit hyperactivity disorder. *A hand book for diagnosis and treatment*, 2nd edn. Guilford Press, New York.

Behar, L.B. & Stringfield, S. (1974). A behaviour rating scale for the preschool child. *Developmental psychology*, **10**, 601–10.

Camp, B.W. & Bash, M.A.S. (1985). *Think aloud; increasing social and cognitive skills – a problem-solving programme for children*. Research Press, Champaign, Ill.

Clark, H.B., Risley, T.R. & Cataldo, M.F. (1976). Behavioural technology for the normal middle-class family. *Behaviour modification and families* (ed. E.J. Mash, L.A. Hamerlynk & L.C. Hardy). Brummer/Mazel, New York.

Conners, C.C. (1969) A teacher rating scale for use in drug studies with children. *American Journal of Psychiatry*, **126**, 884–6.

Crick, N.R. & Dodge, K.A. (1994). A review and reformulation of social information processing mechanisms in childrens' social adjustment. *Psychological Bulletin*, **115**, 74–101.

Dodds, M.R., Schwartz, S. and Sanders, M.R. (1987). Marital discord and treatment outcome in behavioural treatment of child conduct disorders. *Journal of Consulting and Clinical Psychology.* **55**, 396–403.

Dodge, K.A. (1986). Attributional bias in aggressive children. In *Advances in Cognitive-Behavioural Research and Therapy* (ed. P.C. Kendall), pp. 71–100. Academic Press, San Diego.

Dodge, K.A. & Newman, J.P. (1981). Biased decision making processes in aggressive boys. *Journal of Abnormal Psychology*, **90**, 375–9.

Dodge, K.A., Price, J.M., Bachorowski, J. & Newman, J.P. (1990). Hostile attributional biases in severely aggressive adolescents. *Journal of Abnormal Psychology*, **99**, 385–92.

Durlak, J.A., Fuhrman, T. & Lampman, C. (1991). Effectiveness of cognitive–behaviour therapy for maladapting children: a meta-analysis. *Psychological Bulletin*, **110**, 204–14.

D'Zurilla, T.J. & Nezu, A. (1982). Social problem-solving in adults. In *Advances in Cognitive Behavioural Research and Therapy*, Vol. 1, (ed. P.C. Kendall). Academic Press, New York.

Earls, F. (1994). Oppositional and conduct disorders. In *Child and Adolescent Psychiatry* (ed. M. Rutter, E. Taylor & L. Hersov), pp. 308–29. Blackwell, Oxford.

Farrington, D.P. (1995). The development of offending and anti-social behaviours from childhood: key findings from the Cambridge Study in Delinquent Development. *Journal of Child Psychology and Psychiatry*, **36**, 929–64.

Forehand, R.L. & McMahon, R.J. (1981). *Helping the non-compliant child: a clinician's guide to parent training*. Guilford Press, New York.

Garrison, S.T. & Stolberg, A.G. (1983). Modification of anxiety in children by affective imagery training. *Child Psychology*, **11**, 115–30.

Goodman, R. (1997). The strengths and difficulties questionnaire: A research note. *Journal of Child Psychology and Psychiatry*, **38**(5), 581–6.

Herbert, M. (1987). *Behavioural treatment of children with problems: a practice manual*. Academic Press/ Harcourt Brace Jovanovich, London.

Hinshaw S.P., Henker, B. and Whalen, C.K. (1984). Cognitive behavioural and pharmacological interventions for hyperactive boys: comparative and combined effects. *Journal of Consulting and Clinical Psychology*, **52**(5), 739–49.

Kazdin, A.E. (1996). Combined and multimodal treatments in child and adolescent psychotherapy: issues, challenges and research directions. *Clinical Psychology: Science and Practice*, **3**(1), 69–100.

Kazdin, A.E. (1997). Practitioner review: psychosocial treatments for conduct disorder in children. *Journal of Child Psychology and Psychiatry*, **38**, 161–78.

Kazdin, A.E., Esveldt-Dawson, K., French, A.E., & Unis, A.S. (1987). Problem-solving skills training and relationship therapy in the treatment of antisocial child behavior. *Journal of Consulting and Clinical Psychology*, **55**, 76–85.

Kazdin, A.E., Siegel, T. & Bass, D. (1992). Cognitive problem solving skills and parent management training in the treatment of antisocial behaviours in children. *Journal of Consulting and Clinical Psychology*, **60**, 733–47.

Kendall, P.C. (1989). *Stop and think workbook*. Available from Workbooks, 238 Meeting House Lane, Merrion Station, PA 19066, USA.

Kendall, P.C. & Bartel, N.R. (1990). *Teaching problem solving for students with learning and behaviour problems: a manual for teachers*. Available from Workbooks, 238 Meeting House Lane, Merrion Station, PA 19066, USA.

Kupersmidt, J.G., Core J.D. & Dodge, K.A. (1990). The role of peer relationships in the development of disorders. *Peer rejections in childhood* (ed. G.R. Asher & J.D. Coie), pp. 274–308. Cambridge University Press, Cambridge.

Light, D. & Bailey, V. (1993). Pound foolish. *Health Service Journal*, **11**, 16–18.

Lochman, J.E. (1987). Self and peer perceptions and attributional biases of aggressive and non-aggressive boys in dyadic interactions. *Journal of Consulting and Clinical Psychology*, **55**, 404-10.

Lochman, J.E. & Curry, J.F. (1986). Effects of social problem-solving training and self-instruction with aggressive boys. *Journal of Consulting and Clinical Psychology*, **15**, 159–64.

Lochman, J.E., Lampron, L.B., Gemmer, T.C., Harris, R. & Wyckoff, G.M. (1987). Anger coping intervention with aggressive children: a guide to implementation in school settings. In *Innovations in clinical practice: a source book* (ed. P.A. Keller & S.R. Heyman), pp. 339–56. Professional Resource Exchange.

Lochman, J.E., White, K.J. & Wayland, K.K. (1991). Cognitive behavioral assessment and treatment with aggressive children. In *Child and adolescent therapy: cognitive behavioral procedures* (ed. P.C. Kendall), pp. 25–65. Guilford Press, New York.

McMahon, R.J. & Forehand, R. (1978). Non-prescriptive behavior therapy: effectiveness of a brochure in teaching mothers to correct their child's inappropriate mealtime behaviors. *Behavior Therapy*, **9**, 814–20.

Meichenbaum, D. & Goodman, J. (1971). Training impulsive children to talk to themselves: a means of developing self-control. *Journal of Abnormal Psychology*, **77**, 115–26.

Merrett, F. & Houghton, S. (1989). Does it work with the older ones? A review of behavioural studies carried out in British secondary schools since 1981. *Educational Psychology*, **9**, 287–309.

Moffitt, T.E. (1990a). The neuropsychology of delinquency: a critical review of theory and research. In *Crime and justice: an annual review of research*, Vol. 12 (ed. N. Morris & M. Tonry), pp. 99–169. University of Chicago Press, Chicago.

Moffitt, T.E. (1990b). Juvenile delinquency and attention deficit disorder: Boys' developmental trajectories from age 3 to age 15. *Child Development*, **61**, 893–910.

Moffitt, T.E. & Henry, B. (1991). Neuropsychological studies of juvenile delinquency and juvenile violence. In *Neuropsychology of aggression* (ed. J.S. Milner), pp. 67–91. Kluwer Academic Publishers, Boston.

Offord, D.R. (1989). Conduct disorders: risk factors and prevention. In *Prevention of mental disorders, alcohol and other drug use in children and adolescents* (ed. D. Shaffer, I. Philips, N.B. Enzer & M.M. Silverman), pp. 273–307. OSSAP Prevention Monograph, 2. US Department of Health and Human Services, Rockville, MD.

Olweus, D. (1979). Stability of aggressive behavior patterns in males: a review. *Psychological Bulletin*, **86**, 852–75.

Olweus, D. (1994). Bullying at school: basic facts and effects of a school based intervention programme. *Journal of Child Psychology and Psychiatry*, **35**, 1171–90.

Patterson, G.R. (1980). Mothers: the unacknowledged victims. *Monographs for the Society for Research in Child Development*, **45**(5), 1–64.

Patterson, G.R. (1982). *Coercive family process.* Castalia, Eugene, Oregon.

Patterson, G.R. (1991). Performance models for antisocial boys. *American Psychologist*, **41**, 432–44.

Prinz, R.J. & Miller, G.E. (1994). Family based treatment for childhood antisocial behaviour: experimental influence on dropout and engagement. *Journal of Consulting and Clinical Psychology*, **62**, 645–50.

Robins, L.N. & Price, R.K. (1991). Adult disorders predicted by childhood conduct problems: Results from the NMH Epidemiologic Catchment Area Project. *Psychiatry*, **54**, 116–32.

Robins, L.N. & Rutter, M. (Eds.) (1990). *Straight and devious pathways from childhood to adulthood.* Oxford University Press, Oxford.

Routh, D.K. (1978). Hyperactivity. In *Psychological management of pediatric problems*, 2 (ed. P. Magrab), University Park Press, Baltimore.

Slaby, R.G. & Guerra, N.G. (1988). Cognitive mediators of aggression in adolescent offenders: 1 Assessment. *Developmental Psychology*, **24**, 4, 580–8.

Spivack, G., Platt, J.J. & Shure, M.B. (1976). *The problem-solving approach to adjustment.* Jossey-Bass, San Francisco.

Sturge, C. (1982). Reading retardation and antisocial behaviours. *Journal of Child Psychology and Psychiatry*, **23**, 21–31.

Taylor, E., Chadwick, O., Heptinstall, E. & Danckaerts, M. (1996). Hyperactivity and conduct problems as risk factors for adolescent development. *Journal of the American Academy of Child and Adolescent Psychiatry*, **35**(9), 1213–26.

Webster-Stratton, C. (1982). Teaching mothers through video tape modelling to change their children's behaviors. *Journal of Pediatric Psychology*, **1**, 279–294.

Webster-Stratton, C. (1989a). Predictors of treatment outcome in parent training for conduct disordered children. *Behavior Therapy*, **16**, 223–43.

Webster-Stratton, C. (1989b). Systematic comparison of consumer satisfaction of three cost-effective parent training programmes for conduct problem children. *Behavior Therapy*, **20**, 103–15.

Webster-Stratton, C. (1994). Advancing videotape parent training: a comparison study. *Journal of Consulting and Clinical Psychology*, **62**(3), 583–93.

Wheldall, K. & Lam, Y.Y. (1987). Rows versus tables. II. The effects of two classroom seating arrangements on classroom disruption rate, on-task behavior and teacher behaviors in three special school classes. *Educational Psychology*, **7**, 303–12.

Wheldall, K. & Merrett, F. (1991). Effective classroom behaviour management: positive teaching. In *Discipline in schools: psychological perspectives on the Elton Report* (ed. K. Wheldall), pp. 46–65. Routledge, London.

Wimsberg, B.G., Bialer, I., Jupietz, S., Botti, E. & Balka, E. (1980). Home versus hospital care of children with behavior disorders. *Archives of General Psychiatry*, **37**, 413–18.

7
Children with learning difficulties and their parents

Jeremy Turk

The term 'learning difficulties' as used in this chapter refers to a global developmental delay leading to substantial intellectual impairment consistent with performance on a test of intellectual functioning which would give an intelligence quotient (IQ) of below 70. It is synonymous with the older terms 'mental handicap' and 'mental retardation', but must be distinguished from the North American use of the term which corresponds to what is usually described as 'specific developmental delays' (e.g. dyslexia). Having a generalised learning difficulty is associated with increased risk of emotional and behavioural disturbance for a variety of reasons (see Turk (1996a) for review). Having a child with learning difficulty also causes great problems for parents (Gath, 1977; Dupont, 1986; Romans-Clarkson *et al.*, 1986) and siblings (Gath & Gumley, 1987; Gath, 1989). The major determinant of familial adjustment is the associated behavioural disturbance rather than the level of intellectual impairment. However, there is good evidence that the likelihood of having a psychiatric disorder, and of its being severe, are associated with the degree of learning difficulty and the related central nervous system dysfunction (Rutter, Graham & Yule, 1970; Bernal & Hollins, 1995).

For a family with a learning-disabled child, CBT may be focused on the child personally. More often, other family members will be employed as co-therapists, or indeed may be the focus of therapy themselves. Work with learning-disabled individuals and their carers has confirmed just how intellectually impaired a person may be yet still have the potential to benefit from cognitively based approaches (Kuschlik, 1989). The important issue is whether the individual can entertain alternative hypotheses and appreciate that these can be evaluated practically. Earlier suspicions that such sophisticated thinking develops late during childhood have been superseded by awareness of just how young, or developmentally delayed, a person can be yet still benefit from cognitive techniques.

This chapter commences with a definition of cognitive–behavioural psychotherapy as applied to families who have a child with learning difficulties. Important components of CBT relating to this are then reviewed, followed by discussion of the relevance of distinguishing between cognitive deficiencies and cognitive distortions. The relevance of a functional analysis of behaviour and cognitions is described, with examples of common logical errors and useful cognitive techniques applicable to this client group. The chapter concludes with descriptions of areas of theory particularly relevant to this area: attributional style (Alloy *et al.*, 1984) and chronic sorrow (Wikler, Wasow & Hatfield, 1981), and three illustrative case histories.

Definition

Cognitive–behavioural psychotherapy as applied to families who have a child with learning difficulties can be defined as:

> any psychotherapeutic process addressing behaviour and/or thoughts directly as a means of producing change in the functioning of the young person with learning difficulties, parents or siblings, either individually or together.

This definition emphasises that a wide range of techniques is available and applicable to this field of work. Furthermore, the focus of psychotherapy, and desired outcomes, will vary with family, presenting problem and psychotherapist. Certain fundamental principles of cognitive approaches are particularly applicable. These are based on the tenet that in CBT the therapist does not act to persuade the child or family that their views are illogical or inconsistent with reality. The skill of the psychotherapist is to assist the children or their families in discovering this for themselves.

Important components of cognitive–behavioural psychotherapy

Cognitive–behavioural psychotherapy deals with the present ('the here and now'). This is particularly useful because of the frequently limited capacity of individuals with learning difficulties to reflect extensively and deeply on their innermost feelings in a verbally articulate way. Psychodynamically orientated approaches (Sinason, 1992) are extremely labour intensive and often continue over protracted time periods. In contrast, cognitive–behavioural approaches are brief, problem-focused, collaborative interventions involving partnership between therapist and family ('collaborative empiricism'). The priority given to clarifying and defining specific problems to be worked on, and the use of ratings of outcome, are also highly beneficial, not only in terms of confirming the nature and extent of change for therapist and family but also in justifying such approaches clinically and financially. As a means to this end, clear definitions are paramount, as are practical homework tasks whereby the 'theory' shared during psychotherapy sessions is applied back in the real world and the results analysed in sub-

Table 7.1. Important components of cognitive–behavioural psychotherapy

- Deals with the present ('here and now')
- Problem-orientated
- Objective
- Clear definitions
- Collaborative
- Practical homework tasks
- Encouragement to consider and test out alternative hypotheses in a practical fashion

sequent meetings. A main therapeutic role is to coax and encourage the children and their families to consider and test out alternative hypotheses in a practical fashion (Table 7.1).

Kendall and Lochman (1994) usefully describe the 'mental attitude' of the cognitive–behavioural therapist working with young people as one which combines the qualities of consultant (collaborating in the evaluation of ideas), diagnostician (integrating and decoding information) and educator (teaching through experience with involvement). These same attributes are relevant to the therapist when working with families and familial subunits where there is a child with learning difficulties. They complement the well-established, 'non-specific' therapeutic variables of unconditional positive regard, empathy, warmth and genuineness.

Cognitive deficiencies versus cognitive distortions

Traditionally, cognitive psychotherapy focuses on cognitive distortions which mar the ability to appraise situations in a realistic and productive fashion. However, individuals with learning difficulties have a generalised developmental delay which means that useful cognitive processes may more often be underdeveloped or inadequate (Fig. 7.1). In addition, there may be specific areas of cognitive deficiency such as the absence of a theory of mind (Baron-Cohen, 1989) and inability to understand and label emotions (Hobson, 1986) in many individuals who have autism. Cognitive deficiencies or distortions may lead to inappropriate and/or detrimental states of mind, behavioural patterns and emotions. However, the cause of such pathological mental states is important because intervention will vary as a result. Cognitive deficiencies can be helped by psycho-educational strategies as well as by tutored exercises in developing the ability to consider different perspectives (e.g. 'Well, maybe somebody else might see things differently. If you were somebody else seeing what you were doing and how you were thinking and feeling, what might *they* think. What would *they* do?'). Cognitive deficiencies can also be remedied partially by focusing on learning from experience and the development of a problem-solving approach (Table 7.2). In contrast cognitive distortions are often better tackled by more traditional techniques of cognitive restructuring.

Table 7.2. The problem-solving approach

- Identify specific problems to be worked on
- Decide in which order to tackle problems
- Negotiate realistic goals
- Clarify steps needed to achieve goal(s)
- Generate as many solutions as possible
- Weigh-up advantages and disadvantages of each solution
- Decide on task required to tackle first step of chosen solution
- Undertake exercise
- Review with evaluation of success and, if necessary, reappraisal of how it could have gone better
- Decide on next step and proceed

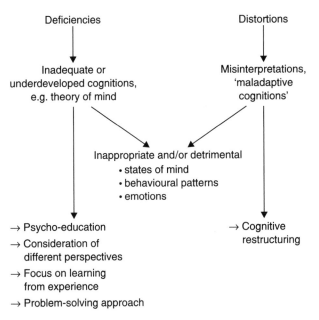

Figure 7.1. Cognitive deficiencies versus cognitive distortions.

The cognitive triad

As with other client groups, maladaptive beliefs in families who have a child with learning difficulties can be grouped into three areas – the so-called cognitive triad (Beck, 1976). This consists of core beliefs relating to oneself, the future and one's surroundings, which underlie most other assumptions and attributions ('core role constructs'). Thus, low self-esteem in the individual with learning difficulties, as well as other family members, is a common occurrence as evidenced by such statements as 'I'm a failure, I'm dim and stupid and ugly. I'm no good at making friends. Every time I try to do something it goes wrong'. A negative view of the future is also frequently witnessed in statements such as 'It's going to go from bad to worse, I know it, you can't pull the wool over our eyes, doctor'. Negative views of people and happenings around the individual are shown in many ways. An example might be 'People are well-meaning but they really don't understand what we're going through and they really can't help'. Although some psychological perspectives may be entirely appropriate, for example awareness of the child's developmental limitations and their implications, others may be unnecessarily maladaptive and detrimental. These often arise from familial depressive tendencies resultant from having a member with a disability, as well as from grief and chronic sorrow issues. There are also often extremely practical considerations such as the family's continuing search for the cause of the child's disability in the absence of any identifiable aetiology. In this respect, the therapist must guard against detrimental instructions to cease this search (which is usually seen as patronising and unhelpful by the family anyway). It is more appropriate in such circumstances to engage the family in discussion of what investigations have been undertaken, what results were obtained and with what meaning, and what value there may be in further similar pursuits. For example, there may be good psychological reasons for undertaking genetic and neuroimaging investigations if this will satisfy the family that all possible avenues of enquiry have been exhausted. There is of course the other issue that such investigations have undergone substantial recent refinement and will sometimes uncover aetiologically important data of use not only in facilitating resolution of the family's grief reaction and orientating them towards the future, but also in terms of possible genetic counselling implications and more appropriate multidisciplinary interventions (see Turk & Sales (1996) for full discussion of the importance of diagnosis).

Given the developmental nature of learning difficulties, and the frequently entrenched family perspectives, the combination of behavioural with cognitive approaches becomes particularly useful. Thus, for a fairly depressed and physically and psychologically inert family, behavioural strategies such as graded task assignments are applicable. For example, a socially isolated and introspective family can be encouraged to undertake outings and other enjoyable activities even if this may be against their nature and inclination and at odds with the prevailing mood ('It doesn't matter if you don't feel up to it. Just do it. Do what you would do if you were happier – or what you used to do when you were happy'). Subsequently, as problems lighten, cognitive approaches can be instituted, thereby shifting the emphasis from activity-based interventions to tackling thoughts and assumptions. It seems that while activity schedules are efficient at producing change, the re-evaluation of long-held thoughts, attributions and assumptions is important in ensuring enduring benefit and avoiding relapse. The critical issue is that behavioural and cognitive approaches are complementary and are usually used simultaneously (the proportion of each varying) whatever the severity of the problem and whatever the child's severity of learning difficulty.

The functional analysis

Much time spent with families who have a child with learning difficulties will be focused on undertaking a functional analysis of the presenting challenging behaviours. Such behaviours are far from being a necessary accompaniment to having learning disabilities. However, they are a common reason for clinical referral. Diary keeping of the nature, frequency and severity of targeted behaviours in vivid detail must be complemented by information on antecedents (where, when, with whom, what was happening?). There must also be data on the consequences of the behaviour (Did she get more attention as a result? Was he allowed to get away with what he was doing? Did she manage to secure solitude and freedom from pressure to interact socially? Did the behaviour seem to serve some self-stimulatory function?). This approach comprises the celebrated ABC chart technique for identifying possible behavioural reinforcers which may be triggering and perpetuating the inappropriate behaviours to the exclusion of more adaptive tendencies (see Oliver (1995) for detailed discussion of the role of functional analyses in evaluating self-injurious tendencies in children with learning difficulties).

The cognitive equivalent of ABC charting is of equal use. In this situation an **activating** event triggers a **belief** based on past experience and attributional tendencies which results in **consequential** behaviour and feelings. The sequence may begin extremely early in the development of the family with a disabled member (e.g. the birth of a child with an obvious learning disability syndrome creating a belief that all family activities will be negative, distressing and unfulfilling, and leading to depressive feelings and withdrawal from social and other enjoyable pursuits) or may be later (e.g. a younger child overtaking the child with learning difficulties academically, creating parental beliefs that there will be little, if any, further intellectual development, and possibly leading to similarly depressive feelings with associated behaviours which may further reinforce family beliefs that all life must revolve around the child with learning difficulties). Documentation of multiple examples of behavioural and cognitive functional analyses, both in the therapy session and as part of homework exercises, helps in gaining understanding of how particular behaviours and beliefs are triggered and reinforced, and how these behaviours and beliefs can in turn encourage either useful or maladaptive mood states and behaviours.

Logical errors

Although human ingenuity would seem to know no bounds in reconstruing events to coincide with developing views of self, surroundings and future, there are a number of recognised logical errors which recur in the assessments made by cognitive psychotherapists. By being alert to these, the therapist can intervene strategically to force discussion of often deeply held belief systems within the family or individual and to seize the moment in an attempt to produce change.

Arbitrary inference describes the tendency to draw a negative conclusion on the basis of subjective impressions even in the absence of concrete evidence to support these views: 'Families are only ever happy with an academically successful child. We will never be happy'.

Selective abstraction is repeatedly judging a situation on the basis of a fragment of information available, focusing only on certain negative aspects and ignoring contradictory factors: 'You say we need to take a long-term view of his development, steering clear of untested fad therapies. Well, he made no progress for two years, but now thanks to the alternative approach we commenced two months ago he is starting to walk and talk after all this time'.

Magnification or catastrophising is exaggerating the intensity, stress or significance of events, and embellishing situations with surplus meaning that is not supported by objective evidence: 'She would not settle to sleep last night. There's no hope for us'.

Personalisation or self-reference is the tendency to relate external events to oneself: 'His autistic features became noticeable when I started back at work part-time. I must be responsible for them'.

Dichotomous or all-or-nothing thinking is thinking in extreme, absolute 'black and white' terms: 'Either you are bright or dim, successful or unsuccessful, a happy fulfilled family or a sad unfulfilled one. There are no in-betweens, there is no middle road'.

Superstitious thinking is the belief in cause–effect relationships between non-contingent events: 'If only we could find a way for her to communicate, then everything would be all right'.

Cognitive techniques

The variety of cognitive techniques available have in common the aim of encouraging more rational appraisal of the evidence for and against the holding of certain beliefs. Recent studies confirm that they can be used successfully with learning-disabled individuals with depression (Lindsay, Howells & Pitcaithly, 1993) and recurrent stereotypic nightmares (Bradshaw, 1991). In addition, the cognitive–behavioural techniques of contingency management, deceleration procedures, verbal instruction, self-management programmes, and visual instruction and imagery have been described as being of particular benefit (Whitman, 1994).

Thought catching describes the active therapist intervention of interrupting the family's or individual's flow of conversation to focus on a particular thought or attribution as a means of evaluating its validity. (For example, 'Hold it right there . . . hang on . . . you just said that the one thing that depresses you most is your son's problems expressing his feelings. Why is that? Did your partner/son/other children know of this? Does this depress him/them? Is this actually true all the time?'.) This can link effectively with *psychoeducational strategies*. Knowledge imparted at strategic points in therapy can be particularly effective in orientating the child and family towards reality. Also, awareness of newly learnt facts may have a direct impact on emotional state and consequently on behaviour. For example, acknowledgement of the behavioural deterioration in adolescents with autism (normal adolescent changes, hormonal fluctuations, changes in routine, increasing awareness of personal limitations and dependency, growing familial anxieties regarding the future) can help alleviate feelings of guilt and reorientate family members towards greater mutual support and more appropriate management and survival strategies.

Hypothesis testing and the generation of alternatives lie at the heart of cognitive problem-solving approaches. They emphasise the shared interactional nature of cognitive–behavioural therapy and the importance of developing valid tests for particular points of view.

Cognitive restructuring is facilitated by a cognitive functional analysis (see above). It can be helped along by the therapist encouraging the rephrasing of sentences to *cut out absolutes* ('never say never') e.g. 'He must attend a mainstream school. We can't cope with the idea of special education'. Parents can be encouraged to reframe such phrases in terms such as 'We would really prefer him to attend mainstream school. The prospect of special education is one we are having particular problems coming to terms with'. Such shifts are, of course, not easy but the appreciation that situations can be viewed in a different light, and with greater flexibility, can be highly beneficial.

Self-monitoring follows on from such approaches. Once the child and family are aware of the importance of cognitive processes and how they can be analysed and adapted, they should be encouraged to develop an automatic tendency to monitor their own thoughts and to become their own cognitive therapists, thereby helping to limit the duration of therapy and to minimise therapist dependency. *Depersonalising* techniques help counteract the tendency to believe that everything revolves around oneself (egocentricity). It is very common for families with a disabled member to hold double standards whereby they judge themselves far more harshly than others ('We should be able to cope; we only have ourselves to blame for not coping'). Directed exhortations to the family to explain the logic underlying such statements can trigger therapeutic discourse. *Reattribution* can be of relevance to professionals as well as to families. A speaker at a scientific meeting, addressing the needs of a family with a learning-disabled member, referred to 'the learning-disabled family'. He did, of course, mean a family with a learning-disabled member. However, there was some curious truth in the speaker's perception of how the family perceived themselves as a result of having a child with learning difficulties, which again opened up areas for cognitive work.

Attributional style

Just as behaviours usually have a situational basis determined by time, location and company, so too do cognitions. It has been appreciated, however, that there is wide individual variability in the extent to which people are influenced by happenings ('It is not things themselves which disturb us but the view we take of them'). There are three dimensions to attributional style which Seligman *et al.* (1984) have identified as contributing to what they term 'the word in your heart'. The *internal-external* dimension is akin to the older notion of locus of control. Some individuals will feel responsible for events happening to them, while others tend to feel themselves the victims of circumstances. Conversely, when things go well some individuals attribute this to their own actions, while others feel them to be the result of lucky coincidence. The more in control of events you believe yourself to be, the more you will feel able to modify things positively. Similarly, the less you habitually feel responsible for negative happenings, the greater your self-esteem. Thus many individuals seem able from early on to appreciate that 'change has to come from within' and that their own appraisal of happenings and their adaptation to them are crucial. Others will feel adrift in a sea of unpredictable currents, wafting them randomly in varying directions. This latter perspective is a common one in adolescents with learning difficulties confronted with the apparently insoluble struggle of continuing dependency versus the apparent impossibility of true autonomy (Kymissis & Leven, 1994). Individual work can be undertaken to challenge the all-or-nothing aspect of this appraisal and to work on areas of life where personal control and influence over events can be usefully developed.

The *global-specific* dimension addresses the situationality of one's mental state, so feeling depressed or helpless may be linked with particular circumstances or situations (which by inference could then be worked on), or may be perceived as a pervasive tendency unrelated to specific events. The view at one extreme could be of one's entire life being blighted and unrewarding, in contrast to a perspective that certain situations or events will produce or rekindle profound feelings of grief and loss while others may promote a sense of reasonable well-being, even if happiness still proves to be elusive. The *stable–unstable* dimension describes the time corollary of the above. Are events always destined to be negative or are they so just at a particular time (for particular reasons)? On the basis of these three dimensions, Seligman has derived an optimism scale. He speculates that those who score highest on this scale tend to be more successful, healthier, to improve under pressure, to endure stress better and even to live longer. Such optimistic claims are extreme, but there is a strong face validity to the notion that the prevailing attributional style on the three dimensions is a useful phenomenon to consider, as well as having some predictive value as to how events will be construed and hence what the prevailing behaviours and emotions are likely to be.

More recent research has confirmed the importance of peoples' habitual patterns of subjective beliefs about the cause of events ('Things going wrong are always the result of her learning difficulties') (Seligman *et al.*, 1990). It does seem that this *explanatory style* can predict not only prevailing mental state but also physical accomplishment, e.g. in athletic pursuits. Seligman *et al.* (1990) have usefully applied the analogy of a habit or addiction to such habitual attribution patterns about causality with families with a learning-disabled child. Most people can appreciate the deeply ingrained nature of ways of thinking and the often painful withdrawal process with intermittent cravings for earlier pathological modes of thinking. It is unclear why this urge to readopt unhelpful cognitive attribution patterns should occur, but it may be linked to the small but compelling literature suggesting a genetic basis to ways of thinking (Schulman, Keith & Seligman, 1993).

Bereavement and chronic sorrow

An essential component of psychotherapy skills when working with families who have a child with learning difficulties is an understanding of the bereavement and grieving process. Families experiencing the arrival of a child with disability will tend to go through a series of psychological stages reflecting their grief at the loss of the antici-pated idealised child and the arrival of the child with disabilities (Bicknell, 1983). Denial of reality is common and varies from a momentary inability to understand or acknow-ledge the news ('shock') to long-term refutation of the child's disabilities and needs. Subsequent protest and anger are often directed towards the breaker of bad news, but may also be inwards to oneself as guilt and depression with irrational self-blame for events seen as having contributed to the problem. Searching behaviour can be directed inwards ('soul-searching') or seen in more concrete terms, for example 'shopping around' for multiple professional opinions or trying out many fad therapies of dubious potential benefit. Usually these phases are replaced by the slow gaining of a new individual and family identity ('adaptation').

As well as bereavement, a phenomenon of 'chronic sorrow' has been recognised. Here, repeated reminders of the disabled family member's problems and differences from others rekindle grief feelings and some of the above processes (Wikler *et al.*, 1981). Such events usually coincide with times that emphasise the child's differences from others, e.g. falling behind a younger sibling developmentally, needing a statement of special educational need, not being able to play sport or socialise like other children, or returning to a dependent life at home after schooling. Wikler and colleagues found that only 25 per cent of parents had experienced time-bound grief, and that most of them were enduring a succession of ups and downs with no general upward course. It also seemed that professionals overestimated how upsetting early experiences were, yet underestimated how upsetting later experiences were. Chronic sorrow rather than time-bound adjustment seemed to characterise the experiences of parents of children with learning disabilities. This sorrow was periodic rather than continuous. The impor-tant cognitive message for therapists and families is that chronic sorrow is not an abnormal response, it is a normal reaction to an abnormal situation. Many of the above-described techniques will be useful in addressing this crucial change of perspective. While chronic sorrow is a normal response, cognitive techniques can facilitate its progress through understanding and the development of useful coping strategies.

Case illustrations

Three case studies are presented to illustrate the applicability of the above processes and interventions to working with families who have a child with learning difficulties.

Case 1

Melanie is a 15-year-old girl who lives with her mother and older brother at home and attends the local secondary school for students with moderate learning difficulties. She was referred to the Child & Adolescent Mental Health Learning Disability Service by her social worker because of self-injury and suicidal statements. Melanie claimed to find school work boring and the class size intimidating. She admitted to finding her peer group rough, loud and aggressive. This had resulted in several bullying incidents. Her mother confirmed Melanie's frustration with having learning difficulties and expressed her concern that this frustration was unnecessarily hindering Melanie's academic progress and behaviour. Indeed, Melanie had demonstrated increasing aggression, roughness, rudeness and social distancing over the preceding year. In one-to-one discussion, Melanie admitted to intense unhappiness, with regular suicidal ideation. She admitted to having taken an overdose in response to alleged instructions from a deceased rock singer she idolised. Melanie also acknowledged frequent tearfulness, sleep disturbance with early morning waking, poor appetite and diurnal mood variation. There were no psychotic features.

Exploration of home life revealed that Melanie's father, a man with an explosive temper who had hit Melanie in anger and as punishment, had lately left the family home following increasing personal awareness of marital incompatibilities. The social worker confirmed her own intensive involvement over a year, providing practical support, help with peer-group relationships, and accessing appropriate clubs. Melanie's mother, although clearly caring, had developed a strong belief that Melanie's behaviour was to attract attention and that therefore she should be ignored. However, she did acknowledge the role of Melanie's problems expressing herself in the development and maintenance of her psychological difficulties. School reports confirmed a marked deterioration in Melanie's articulation skills, which staff attributed to emotional factors.

Discussion of family and early developmental aspects revealed that Melanie's mother still carried substantial guilt relating to Melanie's learning difficulties, despite a comprehensive battery of negative investigations. This related to her failure to focus on her diet while pregnant because of intercurrent stresses.

Meetings with both parents were undertaken, during which the role of their disharmony in aggravating Melanie's distress was explored. Work was also undertaken with the mother to address her continuing guilt regarding Melanie's difficulties and to restructure her belief that Melanie's behaviours were attention seeking and therefore to be ignored. By encouraging dialogue between Melanie and her mother, it became clearer that Melanie had overwhelming anger about her learning difficulties and believed strongly that she should never have been born. Furthermore, she insisted that she should have died soon after birth instead of a much loved and missed cousin who had died in such circumstances some years earlier. This combination of guilt, anger and self-deprecation had created a belief in Melanie that she had been in some way responsible for the cousin's death and that therefore it was only right and proper that she should be punished. Melanie also admitted to believing she was responsible for the recent parental separation and preceding intense marital disharmony. Cognitive restructuring and reattribution work was undertaken, utilising problem-solving strategies to discern what explanations for the above events were in fact the most plausible. Melanie gained awareness of her parents' behaviour being beyond her control, but expressed frustration and distress at her inability to have influenced things for the better ('I *should* have been able to keep Mum and Dad together, I really *should* have done'). However she maintained her deeply-held belief in her responsibility for her cousin's death despite exhortations to explain how this could have possibly been the case. Melanie reflected on her sadness at having not attended the cousin's funeral but rejected the suggestion that she visit the grave.

Because of the persisting intensity of Melanie's depressive symptoms, she was commenced on paroxetine, an antidepressant of the selective serotonin re-uptake inhibitor (SSRI) class. This raised her mood, improved her amount of social interaction and co-operation and seemed to ease her ability to work successfully with cognitive concepts. Melanie started to talk more of future possibilities and the positive arrangement whereby she was spending time with both parents individually. Acceptance of praise still proved difficult, and Melanie's anger and distress worsened again in response to father's admission to having a new partner and hence her awareness of the rapidly diminishing chances of family reconciliation. In response to the therapist's statement 'You're really furious about your learning difficulties and how much this leaves you dependent on other people who don't seem to be able to organise their own lives', Melanie responded sarcastically 'Oh well done'! She then expressed how incensed she had been during a recent visit to the newsagents with her father when he had described her to the shop owner as 'acting like a two year old'. She also expressed her confused emotions when her father visited. She enjoyed his company but became distressed by the unrealistic hopes of family reconstitution this raised in her. Work then focused on Melanie's coming to terms with her father's unpredictable visits and behaviour and the fact that this was part of him and not her fault.

Six months after initial assessment, Melanie had improved to the extent that medication was discontinued. Parental acrimony continued, but Melanie seemed more able to switch off and distance herself from it without feeling in some way responsible. Her self-injurious and suicidal tendencies had stopped and she seemed to be behaving in a more appropriate adolescent fashion – complaining of her mother being over-controlling and expressing her desire for greater autonomy. She expressed her desire to have further help in understanding why certain thoughts preoccupied her and how she could understand why things around her happened in a more rational way.

Case 2

Hubert is a 10-year-old boy who lives with his parents, 10-year-old sister and 4-year-old brother and who attends the local primary school for students with moderate learning difficulties. He was referred for psychiatric assistance because of parental concerns regarding his failure to attain educationally and a bad temper. His parents acknowledged the number of negative investigations which had been undertaken but still expressed their desire for further help in trying to determine the cause of Hubert's difficulties. Hubert was one of triplets. One of the threesome, a girl, had died aged 2 from pneumonia superimposed on her cerebral palsy and severe global developmental delay. The other triplet, Hubert's sister, had displayed unremarkable development. Indeed, it had been noticed from early on that she undertook a very nurturing role with Hubert, doing most things for him. Tantrums were noted when Hubert commenced infant school. These were attributed to difficulties expressing himself. Having always had a quiet and sensitive personality, these tendencies became accentuated with the recurrence of tantrums in response to bullying.

Familial grief over Hubert's learning difficulties and the loss of one of his triplet sisters had been aggravated by his mother having had a number of miscarriages and a stillbirth before her pregnancy with them. This had required fertility treatment, and much of the pregnancy was spent in hospital because of threatened miscarriage. Hubert claimed to like his current school and to want to stay there if the bullying could be stopped. Discussion with his class teacher confirmed that Hubert was usually well-behaved and enthusiastic at school but that he did perceive bullying as a problem.

Tantrums and squabbling with his twin sister persisted. Family exploration of beliefs about this revealed that his sister was intensely jealous of him, believing that he was getting all the attention. Furthermore, his sister admitted to feeling responsible for his learning difficulties and to seeing it as a failure on her part that her intensive efforts to nurture and tutor him had not alleviated his problems. Hubert and his sister's emotional closeness was reflected by their decision to huddle together on the same chair during therapy sessions despite ample seating available. When it was suggested to Hubert's sister that she might benefit from backing off and distancing herself from him a bit, she became tearful, exclaimed 'But I want to help him' and had to leave the room. Following her return, the family members were asked to explore together why she had been so upset and how this might relate to Hubert's frustration. Hubert admitted his awareness and annoyance that his grandmother, at least, did seem to give him undue amounts of attention and to excuse any misdemeanours on the basis that he was 'different'. Homework tasks were agreed whereby the family would discuss their roles together and that the grandmother would be instructed to treat the children similarly. On review three weeks later, his grandmother had indeed responded to requests that she be less sympathetic to Hubert's tantrums and more equal in her affection to Hubert and his sister. Hubert was reported by his parents and sister as much calmer and better behaved, and his sister said she was much happier. She was accepting, with some reluctance, her mother's repeated message that 'You are not your brother's mother, I am'. Hubert's sister was also being encouraged by her parents to spend more time going out with her own friends, while acknowledging that her special relationship with her triplet brother would persist, with its closeness and sense of mutual support. Both Hubert and his sister stated they were looking forward to their new school terms and his sister added (without prompting) that she liked coming for the sessions because they helped family members say important things and to sort out their problems.

Case 3

Quentin is a 12-year-old boy who lives with his parents and attends the local school for students with moderate learning difficulties. He has fragile X syndrome, a common genetic cause of developmental delay, which was felt to have been responsible for his attentional deficits, social interaction problems (notably shyness and social anxiety) and speech and language impairment as well as his intellectual disability. A major aggravation of Quentin's anxiety and self-esteem problems occurred while travelling home on the school bus when a passing policeman on a motor bike noticed one of the pupils on the bus making an obscene gesture to him. Having hailed in the bus and boarded it, the policeman walked down the aisle challenging each pupil as to whether they were responsible. When challenged, Quentin succumbed to the overwhelming urge to avert his gaze as well as trying to turn his head and torso away (a well-recognised behavioural aspect of his condition). This, to the policeman, confirmed Quentin's guilt and he proceeded to mete out a vigorous reprimand. Quentin developed an intense anxiety state with agoraphobia, tearfulness, school refusal, fear of social interaction and a more specific phobia of policemen. He consistently denied having been the perpetrator of the obscene gesture. Following expressions of concern by his parents to the local police force, backed up by supportive letters from his psychiatrist, a desensitisation programme was established whereby a plain-clothed policeman visited the family home with his police dog to befriend Quentin. Over a number of visits, the policeman disclosed his professional identity and engaged Quentin in discussion about police work and let him try on the police helmet and play with bits of police equipment.

Quentin's police phobia, social anxiety and school refusal gradually resolved, but he continued to demonstrate highly anxious tendencies which concerned his parents. These were helped in part by a highly appropriate structured yet caring approach at school, with an emphasis on the emotional welfare of the pupils as well as built-in rewards for positive behaviour and attitudes. However, he continued to display a worrying tendency to try to please everybody and to be extremely apologetic following the slightest misdemeanour. This made his mother, in particular, anxious that she had been too demanding of him and that this may have precipitated his emotional difficulties. Parental discussion with the therapist confirmed that they had indeed been quite rigid and structured with Quentin to bring out the best in him, but they had never smacked him nor placed him under undue pressure to do well at school. A further parental concern uncovered was that Quentin's intermittent extreme unhappiness and anxiety would persist into adolescence where it would consolidate into more enduring personality traits. Bringing Quentin into the discussion revealed that he did experience frustration and unhappiness when unable to do things like his non-learning-disabled peers. He also admitted to finding school work hard and that he did feel some parental insistence to do homework, which lead him to become destructive and tearful.

It transpired that Quentin was struggling academically at school, with problems settling to work. Further family work with collaborative exploration of other possible reasons for his predicament confirmed a number of family difficulties, including the maternal grandfather having experienced a stroke with subsequent personality change, immobility and incontinence. The maternal grandmother had heart disease and was reacting emotionally to the strain of of her own physical condition as well as her husband's state. She would urge Quentin to look after her 'now that Dada is gone'. Quentin's mother's sister had divorced and remarried, leading to radical changes in the extended family routine. In addition, the family had moved house, not a great distance but sufficient for Quentin to have had to change school because the family now resided within the catchment area of a different education authority.

The undeniable impact of these multiple stressors and life events was impressed on the family, along with the fact that Quentin's difficulties were not being caused primarily by parental input. The effects of fragile X syndrome on development and behaviour were reviewed and the relevance of Quentin's impending entry into adolescence discussed. His mother reflected on her own anxious tendencies and agreed with the therapist's suggestion that Quentin was almost certainly becoming increasingly aware of his disabilities and their implications. The parents were congratulated on their unstinting input over the years, and the school staff were praised for their highly appropriate and structured educational input.

> At follow-up three months later, Quentin was progressing well. His school staff expressed pleasure at his progress. Moodiness was less marked and his parents were able to understand much of his behaviour in terms of early adolescence. However, persisting family stressors meant that a high level of continuing anxiety and uncertainty was still being experienced by all family members.

The above case vignettes emphasise the potential for, and importance of, working cognitively with all family members as a whole, in a range of subgroups and individually, as a means of creating enduring changes in familial and individual ways of thinking and appraising events and situations. They also illustrate the importance of combining cognitive with behavioural strategies with a wider network of relatives, friends and professionals to complement the practical collaborative work undertaken between family and therapist.

Specific evaluations and evidence of effectiveness

The potential for individuals with even quite severe learning difficulties to benefit from cognitive approaches has been confirmed (Kuschlik, 1989). Studies have also demonstrated the efficacy of cognitive techniques in helping people with learning difficulties who have depression (Lindsay et al., 1993) and recurrent nightmares (Bradshaw, 1991). Work suggesting benefits from specific cognitive–behavioural techniques has been reviewed above (Whitman, 1994).

From a family perspective, early parental understanding of the nature and implications of their child's disorder is crucial to parental acceptance and the early institution of appropriate remedial and preventative interventions. There is evidence that parental acceptance and reality orientation depend on how and when this delicate information is conveyed. How this information is shared is as important as who does it. Parents want to be told the truth, however painful, and earlier rather than later. Time and multiple meetings are required in order to combat inevitable shock and denial associated with this breaking of bad news (Cunningham, Morgan & McGrucken, 1984). Counselling by a well-informed person is essential. Both overoptimism and underoptimism by the informant can be extremely upsetting (Carr, 1985). Dissatisfaction with disclosure of diagnosis and impairments is not inevitable, but can have profound long-term adverse effects.

Tunali and Power (1993) have emphasised that rather than trying to determine whether families of handicapped children adjust or not, one should identify variables that are associated with family adaptation. In reviewing the literature, they identify several predictors of successful adjustment, including marital satisfaction, harmony and quality of parenting, presence of both parents at home, and acceptance and understanding of the handicapping condition. Active problem-solving approaches are positively associated with adjustment, whereas approaches such as avoidance and wishful thinking are related to higher levels of distress. However, Tunali and Power make the point that it is often difficult to tell whether such 'predictors' are indeed predictors or whether they are consequences of successful coping. They proceed to outline a model of adaptation to inescapable situations where a need is under threat, based on 'redefinition'. The example is given of forced behavioural change in the family (e.g. less time available for leisure pursuits) being associated with additional cognitive changes that parallel the changes in the situation (e.g. devaluation of leisure activities).

Such input can be viewed as tertiary prevention strategies – aimed at reducing the complications and disability associated with established disorders, particularly those which have become chronic (Turk, 1996b). Thus tertiary prevention includes not only active intervention aimed at the presenting condition itself, but also rehabilitation to reduce potential secondary problems, minimise disability and prevent handicaps despite the persistence of impairment.

Future research

There is a need for further structured evaluations of cognitive–behavioural approaches for young people with learning difficulties and their families. The techniques need to be clearly defined, for example problem-solving approaches, psycho-education, hypothesis testing. So too do the presenting difficulties, for example morbid familial grief, chronic sorrow, depression. Long-term follow-up is required to determine how durable gains are. This will require further refinement of rating scales for emotional and behavioural disturbance in young people with learning difficulties. However, there is already good evidence for the benefits of time-limited, problem-focused cognitive approaches with this client group. The applicability of particular approaches to specific problems, and the nature and intensity of therapist training required, still need clarification.

References

Alloy, L.B., Peterson, C., Abramson, L.Y. & Seligman, M.E. (1984). Attributional style and the generality of learned helplessness. *Journal of Personality & Social Psychology*, **46**, 681–7.

Baron-Cohen, S. (1989). The autistic child's theory of mind: a case of specific developmental delay. *Journal of Child Psychology & Psychiatry*, **30**, 285–97.

Beck, A.T. (1976). *Cognitive Therapy and the Emotional Disorders*. International Universities Press, New York.

Bernal, J. & Hollins, S. (1995). Psychiatric illness and learning disability: a dual diagnosis. *Advances in Psychiatric Treatment*, **1**, 138–45.

Bicknell, J. (1983). The psychopathology of handicap. *British Journal of Medical Psychology*, **56**, 167–78.

Bradshaw, S.J. (1991). Successful cognitive manipulation of a stereotypic nightmare in a 40 year old male with Down's syndrome. *Behavioural Psychotherapy*, **19**, 281–3.

Carr, J. (1985). The effect on the family of a severely mentally handicapped child. In *Mental deficiency: the changing outlook*, 4th edn (ed. A.M. Clarke, A.D.B. Clarke & J.M. Berg), pp. 512–48. Methuen, London.

Cunningham, C., Morgan, P. & McGrucken, R.B. (1984). Down's syndrome: is dissatisfaction with disclosure of diagnosis inevitable? *Developmental Medicine & Child Neurology*, **26**, 33–9.

Dupont, A. (1986). Socio-psychiatric aspects of the young severely mentally retarded and the family. *British Journal of Psychiatry*, **148**, 227–34.

Gath, A. (1977). The impact of an abnormal child upon the parents. *British Journal of Psychiatry*, **13**, 405–10.

Gath, A. (1989). Living with a mentally handicapped brother or sister. *Archives of Disease in Childhood*, **64**, 513–16.

Gath, A. & Gumley, D. (1987). Retarded children and their siblings. *Journal of Child Psychology & Psychiatry*, **28**, 715–30.

Hobson, R.P. (1986). The autistic child's appraisal of expressions of emotion. *Journal of Child Psychology & Psychiatry*, **27**, 321–42.

Kendall, P.C. & Lochman, J. (1994). Cognitive–behavioural therapies. In *Child & adolescent psychiatry, modern approaches* (ed. M. Rutter, E. Taylor & L. Hersov), pp. 844–57. Blackwell Scientific, Oxford.

Kuschlik, A. (1989). *Helping caring adults to enjoy working directly with people with learning difficulties who also have severely challenging behaviours.* World Congress of Cognitive Therapy, Abstracts, Oxford.

Kymissis, P. & Leven, L. (1994). Adolescents with mental retardation and psychiatric disorders. In *Mental health & mental retardation – recent advances & practices* (ed. N. Bouras), pp. 102–7. Cambridge University Press, Cambridge.

Lindsay, W.R., Howells, L. & Pitcaithly, D. (1993). Cognitive therapy for depression with individuals with intellectual disabilities. *British Journal of Medical Psychology*, **66**, 135–41.

Oliver, C. (1995). Annotation: self-injurious behaviour in children with learning disabilities: recent advances in assessment and intervention. *Journal of Child Psychology & Psychiatry*, **30**, 909–27.

Romans-Clarkson, S.E., Clarkson, J.E., Dittmer, I.D., Flett, R., Linsell, C., Mullen, P.E. & Mullen, B. (1986). Impact of a handicapped child on mental health of parents. *British Medical Journal*, **293**, 1395–7.

Rutter, M., Graham, P. & Yule, W. (1970). *A neuropsychiatric study in childhood.* Clinics in Developmental Medicine, Nos. 35/36. Heinemann/Spastics International Medical Publications, London.

Schulman, P., Keith, D. & Seligman, M.E. (1993). Is optimism heritable? A study of twins. *Behaviour Research & Therapy*, **31**, 569–74.

Seligman, M.E., Abramson, L.Y., Semmel, A. & von Baeyer, C. (1984). Depressive attributional style. *Southern Psychologist*, **21**, 18–22.

Seligman, M.E., Nolen-Hoeksema, S., Thornton, N. & Thornton, K.M. (1990). Explanatory style as a mechanism of disappointing athletic performance. *Psychological Science*, **1**, 143–6.

Sinason, V. (1992). *Mental handicap and the human condition – new approaches from the Tavistock.* Free Association Books, London.

Tunali, B. & Power, T.G. (1993). Creating satisfaction: a psychological perspective on stress and coping in families of handicapped children. *Journal of Child Psychology & Psychiatry*, **34**, 945–57.

Turk, J. (1996a). Working with parents of children who have severe learning disabilities. *Clinical Child Psychology & Psychiatry*, **1**, 583–98.

Turk, J. (1996b). Tertiary prevention of childhood mental health problems. In *The prevention of mental illness in primary care* (ed. T. Kendrick, A. Tylee & P. Feeling), pp. 265–80. Cambridge University Press, Cambridge.

Turk, J. & Sales, J. (1996). Behavioural phenotypes and their relevance to child mental health professionals. *Child Psychology & Psychiatry Review*, **1**, 4–11.

Whitman, T.L. (1994). Mental retardation. In *Cognitive and behavioral interventions: an empirical approach to mental health problems* (ed. L.W. Craighead, W.E. Craighead, A.E. Kazdin & M.J. Mahoney), pp. 313–33. Allyn & Bacon, Boston.

Wikler, L., Wasow, M. & Hatfield, E. (1981). Chronic sorrow revisited: parent vs. professional depiction of the adjustment of parents of mentally retarded children. *American Journal of Orthopsychiatry*, **51**, 63–70.

8
Post-traumatic stress disorders

P. Smith, S. Perrin and W. Yule

Research over the last two decades has shown that children and adolescents who have been exposed to extreme stressors manifest a range of short-term and long-term reactions, including anxiety, fears and depression, as well as post-traumatic stress disorder. The diagnosis remains controversial, particularly as applied to children, but has proven to be a useful framework for describing and understanding children's reactions to a variety of life-threatening experiences. This in turn has led to the refinement of interventions for children: broadly based cognitive–behavioural therapies within a multi-modal, family-based approach are the treatments of choice.

Post-traumatic stress reactions in children and adolescents

Post-traumatic stress disorder was first recognised by the American Psychiatric Association (1980) in the third edition of the *Diagnostic and Statistical Manual*, and in the 1987 revision it was acknowledged that PTSD can also occur in children. The most recent edition, DSM-IV (American Psychiatric Association, 1994), describes in more detail the way in which a number of symptoms may manifest in children. PTSD is defined as: (a) exposure to an event in which the person experienced, witnessed, or was confronted with actual or threatened death or serious injury, or a threat to the physical integrity of self or others, and in which the person's response involved intense fear, helplessness or horror; (b) persistent re-experiencing of the event; (c) persistent avoidance of related stimuli or numbing of responsiveness; and (d) persistent symptoms of increased arousal.

Work with children who have survived a variety of life-threatening experiences has demonstrated that they do indeed show this tripartite grouping of symptoms –

re-experiencing, avoidance and increased arousal. Cardinal symptoms manifest differently at different ages, and a range of other reactions is also common (e.g. Terr, 1979; Kinzie *et al.*, 1986; McFarlane, 1987; Yule & Williams, 1990; Pynoos *et al.*, 1993).

Most children are troubled by repetitive, intrusive thoughts about the trauma. Such thoughts can occur at any time, but particularly when trying to fall asleep. At other times, intrusive thoughts and images are triggered by reminders in the environment. Bad dreams and nightmares are common. Younger children may show repetitive play and drawing involving themes related to the traumatic event. Many children develop fears associated with specific aspects of the traumatic event, with phobic levels of avoidance of trauma-related stimuli and reminders. Children may avoid thinking about the event because it is overwhelmingly distressing. Survivors often experience a pressure to talk about their experiences, but find it very difficult to talk with parents and peers. Child survivors can become very alert to danger in their environment, being adversely affected by reports of other related traumatic events. Sleep disturbances are very common, particularly within the first few weeks of the event, and children often wake through the sleep cycle. Separation difficulties are frequent, even among teenagers. Many children become much more irritable and angry both with parents and peers, and younger children are likely to show regressive and anti-social behaviours. Children commonly experience difficulties in concentration, especially in school work.

Children also report a number of cognitive changes. Post-trauma, many feel that the world is a much more dangerous place. Survivors learn that life is fragile, and may not envision themselves living to adulthood. Life priorities frequently change in response to trauma. Some children feel that they should live each day to the full and not make any plans for the future. Others realise that they have been over-concerned with materialistic or petty matters and resolve to rethink their values, frequently taking on the image of themselves as helpers to others. Many experience 'survivor guilt', attributing blame to themselves about others dying or being seriously injured, and thinking that they should have done more to help others to survive. In addition, a range of other reactions is also common, including depression, anxiety, oppositional behaviour, and prolonged grief reactions.

Despite refinements and revisions in the major diagnostic systems, PTSD remains a controversial diagnosis. Indeed, the notion that PTSD is a 'normal reaction to an abnormal situation' has led some to question whether it is a psychiatric disorder at all (see O'Donohue & Elliot, 1992). PTSD is included under the anxiety disorders in DSM because of the predominant symptoms of fear, avoidance and hyperarousal. But the presence of a specified external aetiological agent has led to its inclusion under adjustment reactions in the WHO classificatory system (ICD 10; World Health Organisation, 1992). Whichever subcategory of disorder PTSD best falls under, it is widely recognised that current criteria poorly reflect the wide variety of major stress responses reported in the literature. This has led to the proposal for a spectrum of disorders to be delineated more closely, including Disorders of Extreme Stress Not Otherwise Specified (DESNOS; Herman, 1992). In children, Terr (1991) has proposed a similar distinction between Type I and Type II PTSD, the former characterised by intrusive recollections, the latter by denial, numbing and dissociation. The diagnosis of PTSD is nowhere more controversial than in its application to children living through armed conflict and political violence. Richman (1993) cautions against an uncritical approach to using a PTSD framework in such situations, pointing out that the diagnosis fails to capture adequately the effects of repeated and chronic stressors on whole communities, and ignores the centrality of children's interpretations of the meaning of violence (Dawes, 1994).

Behavioural and cognitive accounts of post-traumatic stress disorder

It is apparent from the above description that children can and do develop PTSD, but it is becoming clearer that: (a) children's reactions range more broadly than the narrow confines prescribed in DSM (American Psychiatric Association, 1994); and (b) not all exposed children go on to develop PTSD (Schwarz & Kowalski, 1991). Exposure to a traumatic event is thus a necessary but insufficient cause of development of disorder: the aetiology and course of PTSD in childhood are likely to be complex functions of developmental stage, prior experiences and temperament, family functioning, subsequent coping, and reactions to secondary adversity (Pynoos, 1994). With this broad context in mind, several classes of model have been proposed to account for the development and maintenance of PTSD symptomatology. Most relevant to cognitive–behaviour therapies are those derived from learning theory (e.g. Keane, Zimmering & Caddell, 1985), and those based on information-processing theory (e.g. Foa, Steketee & Olasov-Rothbaum, 1989).

Initially helpful in explaining PTSD in combat veterans (Keane *et al.*, 1985), Mowrer's (1960) two-factor learning theory has proved useful in conceptualising the development of PTSD in children (see Saigh, 1992). Mowrer's is a conditioning model, incorporating elements of both Pavlovian and operant conditioning. As applied to PTSD, the traumatic event is an unconditioned stimulus that elicits certain involuntary responses: (1) orientation to the threat cue; (2) autonomic arousal; (3) fear; and (4) the behavioural 'flight or fight' response. Because of their proximity to the threatening event (the unconditioned stimulus – UCS), previously neutral stimuli become conditioned stimuli (CS), capable of eliciting the same involuntary responses (conditioned response – CR) as the trauma itself. Under normal conditions, repeated exposure to the CS alone should lead to extinction of the conditioned anxiety response (CR). However, in PTSD, extinction fails to occur because the traumatised individual is negatively reinforced for avoiding the CS. Other previously neutral stimuli associated with the CS may also elicit the conditioned anxiety response through the process of stimulus generalisation; and the conditioned stimuli themselves may go on to condition other non-trauma-related stimuli (higher order conditioning). Thus, the traumatised person is confronted with a wide array of anxiety-eliciting cues in the environment that cause persistent hyperarousal, intrusive recall of the traumatic event, and behavioural avoidance of the conditioned cues. The prediction from such an account is that prolonged therapeutic exposure to traumatic memories or reminders (CS) in the absence of the original UCS will lead to extinction of the anxiety response and a reduction in intrusive recall of the event.

Learning theory has been fundamental in formulating interventions for PTSD (see below), but cannot help in explaining individual differences in reactions (Foa et al., 1989). Information-processing models seek to do this: recognising that stressors cannot be completely defined in objective terms (Rachman, 1980), they take into account individual differences in threat appraisal, attributions, and the meaning ascribed to trauma. Common to most cognitive conceptualisations is the notion that individuals bring to the traumatic event a set of beliefs and models of the world, themselves and others (Janoff-Bulman, 1985, 1992). Exposure to trauma provides information which is incompatible with these models, and yet highly salient. Post-traumatic reactions result when there is a failure to integrate this new information into pre-existing meaning structures (see Dalgliesh, in press). Foa and Kozak (1986) give an example of one such model.

Based on Lang's (1977) theory of network memory, Foa and Kozak (1986) propose that traumatic events lead to the development of fear structures in long-term memory which encompass stimulus information about the traumatic event, information about the cognitive, behavioural and physiological reactions to the event, and information which links these stimulus and response elements together. Such fear networks are large, intense and readily accessible. Activation of the fear structure leads to increases in arousal and re-experiencing, and attempts to suppress such activation lead to avoidant behaviours. Successful resolution of the trauma can only occur by activating the fear network and providing corrective information (both cognitive and affective) which is incompatible with that in the fear network, thereby integrating the fear network into existing memory structures. Foa and Kozak's model emphasises that the uncontrollability and unpredictability of the traumatic event violate fundamental assumptions about safety and self-efficacy.

Although developed from work with traumatised adults, there is emerging evidence that the role of threat appraisal, attributional processes, and attitudinal changes central to cognitive accounts of PTSD in adults are also important factors which mediate the re-integration of traumatic memories in children. In line with adult work (e.g. Foa et al., 1991; Thrasher, Dalgliesh & Yule, 1994), Moradi (1996) has reported a specific attentional bias to trauma-related material in children with PTSD, using a modified Stroop task. Attributional processes can also mediate symptoms: in young survivors of a shipping accident, Joseph et al. (1993) found that more internal and controllable attributions were associated with intrusive thoughts and depressive feelings one year after the accident. Consistent with the adult literature regarding the 'shattering' of pre-trauma assumptions (Janoff-Bulman, 1992), Johnson et al. (1996) reported evidence of attitudinal changes in children who survived an earthquake, which were related specifically to PTSD symptomatology.

Behavioural and cognitive accounts of PTSD are broadly compatible. Both imply that exposure to trauma-related cues and memories in tolerable doses is necessary to reduce PTSD symptoms, and this forms the basis for cognitive–behavioural interventions.

Assessing post-traumatic stress disorder in children and adolescents

Because PTSD overlaps several domains of functioning, assessment is necessarily broad, and incorporates direct interview with the child, information gathering from family and teachers, and the use of self-report inventories and diaries.

When interviewing children, it is important to remember that, often, this will be the first time they have discussed the event in detail. In some senses, then, the first interview comprises imaginal exposure (see below) and must be handled with care. Pynoos and Eth (1986) describe in detail a broadly applicable technique for interviewing young children shortly after they have witnessed a traumatic event. The therapist must be skilled in balancing the needs of obtaining accurate information while at the same time ensuring that the first interview is a therapeutic one.

A number of standardised self-report measures and semi-structured interviews is now available (see McNally (1991) and Nader (1995) for comprehensive reviews). Probably the most widely used measure of PTSD symptomatology is the Impact of Events Scale (IES; Horowitz, Wilner & Alvarez, 1979) which assesses symptoms of intrusion and avoidance, and has been used with children as young as 8 years old (Yule & Williams, 1990; Yule & Udwin, 1991). It is usual to screen for co-morbidity, and commonly used measures of childhood depression, anxiety and fears include the Birleson Depression Inventory (Birleson, 1981), the Children's Manifest Anxiety Scale (Reynolds & Richmond, 1978), and the Fear Survey Schedule for Children (Ollendick, 1983). Semi-structured interviews based on DSM criteria can aid the interviewer in diagnosing PTSD. The Clinician Administered PTSD Scale for Children (CAPS-C; Nader *et al.*, 1994), the Diagnostic Interview Schedule for Children (DISC; Shaffer *et al.*, 1996), and the Diagnostic Interview for Children and Adolescents Revised (DICA; Reich, Shakya & Taibelson, 1991) all require the interviewer to be trained in the administration of the scale, and have been shown to possess adequate validity and reliability. Unfortunately there has been a dearth of standardised approaches to the assessment of stress reactions in children under 8 years of age. While children between 3 and 8 years can often give adequate verbal responses to questions from standardised measures used with older children, there is a need to develop measures particularly suited to young children.

Comprehensive interview with the child's carers is necessary if treatment formulation and planning are to be successful. Most semi-structured diagnostic interviews include both child and parent versions, which allows the interviewer to cover all symptoms systematically with carers. This is particularly important where the symptom may be of a particularly embarrassing nature or where the child may be unaware of his or her behaviour. Beyond coverage of current symptom state, a full pre-trauma history from carers will help in understanding the child's usual reactions to stress and ways of coping; whether current symptomatology is in part a function of prior temperament; what changes in behaviour the traumatic event precipitated; and in setting appropriate treatment goals. Taking the child's developmental level into account will allow one to assess which, if any, of the presenting complaints are normal, age-appropriate behaviours (for example separation anxiety), as well as guiding the choice of treatment strategies. Given the important mediating role of parental reactions and fears (e.g. McFarlane, 1987), assessment of all family members is usually necessary to determine whether adults or siblings also require intervention, and to advise carers on management of their children.

Finally, effective intervention will depend also on a thorough assessment of the child's or family's living situation. In cases where the traumatic event is relatively discrete and the family remains intact (such as, for example, in some road traffic accidents), crucial family resources will still be available to the child. In cases where other family members have beeen involved in the traumatic event, work with them will probably be necessary to assist them to help their children more effectively. In yet other cases, for example where the child has suffered a parental bereavement, very practical issues of social welfare will arise. In situations of ongoing community violence or armed conflict, taking account of the context in which the child is living will allow judgement as to whether, when, and what kind of intervention is most appropriate.

Treatment

Derived from behavioural and cognitive models of PTSD, at the core of CBT is the use of imaginal and in-vivo exposure techniques within a safe therapeutic environment (Keane *et al.*, 1985) to allow adequate emotional processing of traumatic memories (Rachman, 1980). The problem for the clinician is how to help the survivor remember and re-experience the event and the emotions that it engenders in such a way that the distress can be mastered rather than magnified. This will depend foremost on the establishment of a safe and trusting environment in which the traumatic event can be remembered and discussed. Therapists must be prepared to ask children about the most difficult aspects of the traumatic experience, but at the same time ensure that exposure to traumatic memories is paced in such a way that the child does not experience overwhelming anxiety. For many children, talking directly about the traumatic event may be too difficult, and other means of accessing traumatic memories must be found.

Asking children to draw their experiences often assists in the recall of both the event and the accompanying emotions (Pynoos & Eth, 1986), and with younger children, play may be used similarly (Misch *et al.*, 1993).

During imaginal exposure, children are asked to imagine and recount their traumatic experience, whereas in-vivo exposure refers to real-life confrontation of traumatic cues or reminders. Exposure work may be preceded by coping-skills enhancement or training: children may be taught deep muscle and breath relaxation, and positive imagery training, among other skills. Children are instructed in the use of SUDS (Subjective Units of Distress scales) to rate their anxiety, and a 'script' of the event is developed with their therapist. The child is then asked to recount the experience while the therapist prompts for SUDS. Particular attention is paid to points in the account which are poor in detail or which elicit high SUDS. Here, the child will be asked to provide greater detail and to hold the image in mind until SUDS scores decrease. It is crucial that the child feels in control of exposure sessions, and that they are paced appropriately. At the end of every session, children will practise their relaxation skills so that they can leave the session without feeling unduly aroused. Concurrently, and usually with parents' involvement, between-session homework assignments utilising gradual in-vivo exposure to traumatic reminders will be designed to address behavioural avoidance.

Yule (1992) has described the combined use of imaginal and in-vivo exposure in the treatment of a 16-year-old boy who had survived a shipping accident two years earlier. Following relaxation training, the boy was asked to describe accurately, in first person present tense, what he had observed, heard, felt, smelled and thought during the accident. The session was audio taped and the boy listened to the tape at home between sessions. Following treatment, significant gains were observed on standardised measures of anxiety and depression, and on the Impact of Events Scale. After treatment, the boy could travel on a boat again for the first time in two years.

Using a behavioural approach, Saigh (1987a) was the first to show that, as Rachman (1980) had predicted, longer exposure sessions than normal are needed if desensitisation and symptom reduction are to occur. He used flooding to treat a 14-year-old Lebanese boy who met criteria for PTSD after having been abducted and tortured. The imaginal flooding process consisted of 10 minutes of deep muscle relaxation, followed by 60 minutes of therapeutic stimulation during which the boy was instructed to imagine the particular details of four anxiety-evoking scenes. SUDS ratings were elicited at 2-minute intervals during the aversive scene presentations. After seven flooding sessions, SUDS levels decreased appreciably. Post-treatment and at four-month follow-up, there were clinically significant treatment gains in self-reported anxiety, depression and misconduct, and virtually no arousal to the anxiety-provoking scenes. Saigh (1992) has subsequently summarised a five-stage intervention process involving education, imagery training, relaxation training, the presentation of anxiety-provoking scenes, and debriefing.

Case illustrations

The following case illustrates in some detail the use of exposure-based techniques.

Case 1

Alex (13 years old) was involved in a serious gang attack and was referred to therapy by his mother, who accompanied him to the first interview. Seven months prior to assessment, Alex and two friends had been hospitalised following an attack by a gang of youths. He had been stabbed and severely beaten, and required surgery for perforations to his intestines and spleen.

Alex presented as a markedly anxious and withdrawn boy. He was having nightmares almost every night, and intrusive thoughts and images daily. Fearful that he would meet his attackers again, he refused to leave the house alone and had been absent from school since the attack. His mother described him as having undergone a personality change. He showed great fluctuations in mood, cried frequently, and was short tempered with his parents and siblings. He had been interviewed by the police soon after the attack, but had not been able to talk to anyone about it since then. Alex felt out of control and feared that he was 'going mad'. His scores on standardised assessment, as follows, confirmed high levels of post-traumatic stress symptomatology, depression and anxiety.

Impact of Events	45
Birleson	24
Revised Manifest Anxiety Scale	28

Alex was praised for his incredible bravery at the time of the attack and for his decision to seek treatment. His symptoms were explained as a normal but very distressing reaction to an abnormal situation. He was provided with an explanation of how trauma can effect thoughts, feelings and behaviours, based on Mowrer's two-factor model (see above). Examples were given of how his attempts to forget were largely unsuccessful and perhaps unhelpful. Alex was presented with a treatment rationale focusing on several sessions of coping-skills training followed by gradual exposure to trauma-related stimuli through imaginal and in-vivo techniques. It was emphasised that he would learn more effective coping skills and would be in control of his level of exposure at all times. A treatment contract for five sessions of coping-skills training was developed, and it was agreed that Alex could terminate treatment if he did not wish to do exposure work.

Alex was instructed in the use of a daily self-monitoring form that focused on the frequency of intrusive recall and nightmares, his level of arousal during recall (SUDS), and any negative thoughts or emotions. The SUDS was explained and Alex developed detailed anchor points for anxiety at 0, 50 and 100. To facilitate his understanding of the relationship between traumatic cues, avoidance and symptoms, the form was structured so that it identified antecedents (A), behaviours/emotions/thoughts (B), and consequences (C). Alex practised using the form during the session. Finally, he was asked to complete a weekly diary, 'How I cope with stress' to record any positive coping skills learned during the previous week. His mother was asked to review the weekly diary with Alex, and to provide plenty of encouragement.

Over the next five sessions, Alex was instructed in the use of various anxiety-management techniques, including muscle group and breath control relaxation, positive imagery training, and thought stopping. Particular attention was paid to his use of the SUDS to evaluate the effectiveness of anxiety management techniques. During positive imagery training, Alex was encouraged to provide great detail about the scene, focusing on all aspects of sensory awareness as well as thoughts and emotions. This was done to increase the salience of the positive image and to shape behaviour around reporting all details of a scene from memory. The therapist met with Alex's mother at the end of every session to discuss Alex's improvement and to develop ways in which she could reinforce his coping behaviour.

Standardised questionaries were re-administered at the beginning of the fifth session. His scores were as follows:

Impact of Events	34
Birleson	10
Revised Manifest Anxiety Scale	12

These scores indicated that Alex was still experiencing high levels of traumatic recall and avoidance, but his depressive and anxiety symptoms had significantly decreased. It was explained that Alex's scores suggested that he could benefit from exposure work. He was provided with a very detailed account of how sessions would be structured and his ability to control the level of exposure. Homework assignments would continue and be reviewed in every session. Alex agreed to try exposure and a new contract was signed for an additional six sessions.

In the sixth session, Alex was asked for his SUDS score and to relax himself as much as possible (i.e. SUDS < 50). It was explained that he would develop a script of the trauma that would increase in detail during every session, and that by filling in the detail, Alex's distress when remembering the trauma would decrease. Alex's first run through of the trauma was uninterrupted by the therapist. At the end of recall, Alex's SUDS score was taken and he was asked to use relaxation skills to reduce any anxiety. The therapist then guided Alex through the trauma again, using the script, and prompted for SUDS scores at points that seemed particularly difficult for him to describe. These scores were recorded on the script. Again, Alex was asked to use his relaxation skills. The script was reviewed, highlighting those parts that were poor in detail or where Alex had reported high SUDS scores. It was explained that in future sessions there would be a pause at such points and he would be asked to provide much greater detail and then to hold the image until his SUDS had decreased. The last part of the session was left to discuss Alex's experiences of talking about the trauma in the session. He was nervous but felt that it had been helpful to talk about it. He was asked to use his relaxation skills again at the end of the session.

Sessions seven through ten continued in a similar fashion. The trauma was usually reviewed at least twice in each session. The session was never terminated without Alex engaging in his relaxation skills and a self-reported SUDS score below 50. By the end of session ten, Alex could recall the entire traumatic event in great detail with his SUDS rating never reaching above 50. Alex agreed that this was a very tolerable level of anxiety which he could quickly reduce with his relaxation skills. The therapist provided Alex with considerable praise for his efforts. Alex's mother was also impressed with his progress. She reported that he was making more attempts to leave the house on his own and seemed much less nervous when left alone.

At session 11, Alex completed the questionnaires again:

Impact of Events	12
Birleson	6
Revised Manifest Anxiety Scale	8

These scores were all comparable to those found in normal children and indicated a significant reduction in his symptomatology. This was made clear to Alex and his mother. Alex was also asked to describe how his life had improved more generally and his plans for the future. He reported increased satisfaction with himself, felt he was getting out more with friends, and was satisfied that he would be able to concentrate better on his school work. It was agreed that maximum benefit from therapy had been gained for the present. Alex was presented with a diploma indicating his successful completion of a coping-skills programme.

This case illustrates a very structured approach to the reduction of PTSD symptoms through coping-skills training and exposure work. Alex's initial reluctance to talk about the trauma was circumvented by increasing his sense of mastery over his own anxiety symptoms. With successful completion of this aspect of therapy, he was more willing to try the more difficult exposure work.

Therapeutic exposure under supportive circumstances seems to deal well with intrusion symptoms and behavioural avoidance. Nevertheless, given the breadth of reactions to trauma, a flexible approach to treatment is called for, and in clinical practice a range of techniques is included in a CBT package. Addressing the central trauma through therapeutic exposure, as above, is essential to effective treatment. In addition, intervention will usually include components to treat other common reactions such as sleep disturbance, separation anxiety, anger and conduct problems, prolonged grief reactions, and generalised anxiety. In older children and adolescents, guilt, self-blame, helplessness and vulnerability are common themes, and cognitive restructuring may be used to counter misattributions of predictability, causality and responsibility. When working with younger children, it is important that any misunderstandings about the causes of the event are clarified.

A multi-modal approach to treatment, where symptom management and family issues are addressed in conjunction with therapeutic exposure, is illustrated by the following case.

Case 2

Ben was a 7-year-old boy, referred by his GP following a road traffic accident two years earlier. His mother had been driving Ben and his older brother to school when they were involved in a three car pile-up. Nobody was killed in the accident, but his mother sustained fractured ribs and his brother bruising and cuts to the mouth. Ben was unhurt.

Immediately after the accident, Ben became very frightened of cars and refused to travel in them. He had difficulty separating from his mother. He became withdrawn and bad tempered, getting into fights with siblings and other children. His attention and concentration worsened and he had difficulty settling at school. Immediately after the accident, Ben became enuretic. At referral, Ben's avoidance of cars had diminished, although he still became nervous when being driven by mother. His concentration and behavioural problems persisted. He was enuretic at night, some four or five times a week, and woke up crying most nights having had nightmares. Some two years after the accident, Ben continued to suffer from distressing intrusive (nightmares) and arousal (disrupted sleep, poor concentration, irritability) symptoms of PTSD which were having a marked impact on his functioning, and that of his family.

In the first session, Ben was withdrawn, and rather than talking about the accident, he demonstrated it hesitantly using toy cars, becoming anxious as he did so. He remembered the accident clearly, but thought that he was responsible for his brother's injuries having bumped into him when the car was hit. The misunderstanding was cleared up by mother, and she reported that Ben had talked to her about the accident for the first time soon after the first session. Ben became more distressed when telling about and drawing his dreams. They were not about cars, but anxiety related in that he was chased by a monster. Ben was asked to think about his favourite superhero who would help him face up to the monster in the dream, and he drew Sonic the Hedgehog shouting at the monster to go away. He was taken with the idea that he could 'fight back' against his bad dreams.

Over five fortnightly treatment sessions, Ben's mother kept accurate diaries of his sleep patterns and enuresis. A star chart system was implemented to tackle bedwetting, and advice was given to his mother as to what to do when Ben woke up distressed. Ben was instructed in some brief relaxation techniques to use before he went to bed. Further rehearsal of dreams with positive outcomes was carried out during sessions. Ben played out the accident in sessions, supplying more detail and showing less anxiety on each subsequent occasion. Ben's school was unaware of the accident, and were informed, with permission; his teachers were able to reduce demands on Ben temporarily and supply additional one-to-one assistance which improved his concentration and performance at school.

Treatment thus comprised therapeutic exposure, star charts, dream restructuring, relaxation techniques, and supportive counselling and advice on behavioural management for Ben's mother, as well as liaison with school. Enuresis resolved quickly after implementation of star charts, and this had a positive effect on the whole family's sleep. Initially, Ben continued to have nightmares, but was less upset by them; and their frequency gradually diminished. As Ben's sleep improved, so did his behaviour and concentration, and he was less irritable with his siblings. By the end of treatment, Ben was able to talk about and play out the accident without evident distress. At four-month follow-up, he was no longer bedwetting, nightmares had ceased, and school performance had improved.

This case illustrates some of the issues raised when working with younger children, and highlights the necessity for multi-faceted intervention to target particularly distressing symptoms. However, despite using multi-modal treatment approaches, intervention may be unsuccessful for a number of reasons. Our third case illustrates how post-traumatic stress reactions may affect whole families, and describes some of the difficulties in engaging clients some years after the event when symptoms are chronic and diffuse.

Case 3

Claire (aged 17) worked as a shop assistant and lived with her parents and younger sister. She went to see her GP because of frequent headaches, which had started soon after a serious road traffic accident five years earlier. Investigations revealed no organic cause, and her GP referred Claire for assessment of PTSD.

Claire came to assessment with her mother. She was able to describe the accident without upset. The family had been going on summer holiday when their car was struck by a lorry. Father sustained spinal injuries which left him paralysed from the waist down. Mother was badly bruised and knocked unconscious. Claire, aged 12 at the time, was thrown against the side windows and knocked out. She remembered coming round to see her father being cut from the car by firemen.

Soon after the accident, Claire had frequent intrusive thoughts and occasional nightmares, but they subsided within a year. She was fearful of cars, and still preferred to take public transport. She denied any symptoms of depression or anxiety, but reported chronic headaches that caused her to be laid up in bed for days at a time. Headaches had caused considerable problems at school and she decided not to attend college. It transpired that there had been considerable tension and frequent arguments at home since the accident, and Claire's biggest concern was finding enough money to move to a flat of her own so that she could be away from her father, whom she said was depressed and belligerent to all family members. However, she felt guilty about leaving home. This was reinforced by her mother, who asked Claire to show more respect towards her father and to help to care for him. Claire felt resentful towards her mother, and they had been fighting repeatedly over the last year.

Claire accepted that her headaches might be stress related, and was willing to learn some anxiety-management techniques, but thought that moving out of the family home was the only real solution. The possibility of family therapy to discuss how the accident had affected the family as a whole was discussed, but Claire was doubtful that this would help: she thought that her father would not come to therapy, as repeated attempts to engage him in the past had been unsuccessful.

It was agreed with Claire and her mother that therapy would focus on improving the quality of their relationship. Attempts were made to identify their common experiences of the trauma and its aftermath. They were given specific homework assignments designed to increase their awareness of the cascade effects of the father's post-traumatic anger on their emotional states and communication with each other. It appeared at times that improvements were made, as they reduced the frequency of negative comments to each other.

However, over the next few sessions, it became increasingly clear that Claire's mother had become locked into the role of protecting her husband at all costs. She could not acknowledge the significant impact that the accident had had on herself, and whenever this issue was broached, she became tearful and quickly shifted the topic back to Claire's problems. This in turn prompted Claire to accuse her mother of being insensitive to everyone's feelings except those of her husband. Her mother could not break free of her role as caretaker for her injured husband in order to acknowledge her own pain and suffering. This in turn prevented her from recognising the pain and suffering that her daughter experienced. Despite repeated attempts, Claire's father could not be engaged in either family or individual therapy.

After seven sessions, it was agreed that treatment was not going to be effective in reducing family conflict without the presence of Claire's father. Furthermore, Claire thought that the stress-reduction techniques she had learned were only short-term measures: she had found a flatshare with friends and was determined to move out. The therapist encouraged them to stay in therapy until they worked through this difficult transition, but Claire was adamant about terminating treatment. Her mother remained in a high state of avoidance, and saw no point in continuing treatment without either her husband or Claire. The case was closed with little change in Claire's headaches.

In this case, the accident had had individual effects on all family members, and had caused major disruptions to family communication and roles. Although anxiety-management techniques had some small impact, the cascade effect of the trauma on the whole family was acknowledged by Claire as the major maintaining factor in her presenting symptoms. However, it proved impossible to engage the whole family in therapy.

In summary, therapeutic exposure in the context of a safe and trusting relationship is at the heart of cognitive–behavioural techniques for treating PTSD in children. Care must be taken that exposure sessions are sufficiently long for desensitisation to occur and for emotional processing to be promoted: repetitive retelling alone is not enough. In addition, depending on the age of the child, the time since the traumatic event, and the pattern of symptom presentation, a variety of other techniques is commonly used, both to target particularly distressing symptoms and to bolster coping strategies for the future. We have concentrated in this chapter on individual work within a family context, but it should be noted that a variety of other cognitive–behaviourally derived interventions, such as critical incident stress debriefing, a preventative intervention (Dyregrov, 1991), and group therapy (e.g. Galante & Foa, 1986; Yule & Udwin, 1991) are advocated, with the choice of treatment strategy depending mainly on the nature of the traumatic event and the time since its occurrence.

Efficacy of treatment

As yet, there have been no randomised, controlled treatment trials of CBT for PTSD in children, and no long-term treatment follow-up studies. However, Saigh's series (1987a, 1987b, 1989) of single case multiple baseline across traumatic scene studies is promising for behaviourally based exposure treatments. In an uncontrolled trial of a 12-session CBT programme with 19 sexually abused and traumatised children (comprising coping-skills training, gradual exposure, and educative/preventative work), Deblinger, McLeer and Henry (1990) found that all symptoms showed some improvement: each major category of PTSD symptoms improved, and although some children were still symptomatic, none met criteria post-treatment. Regarding group treatment and debriefing, recent evidence from the adult literature is mixed (e.g. see Kenardy et al., 1996). Few outcome studies have been conducted with children. Yule (1992) observed that children who attended debriefing meetings after a shipping accident fared better on a range of outcome measures than children who were not offered such help. Inferences from this uncontrolled study must be limited, however, since the debriefing group also received additional treatment. Better evidence comes from Stallard and Law's (1993) uncontrolled trial of debriefing showing significant improvements on standardised self-report measures in a small group of young children involved in a road traffic accident. At present, it is not known whether all survivors benefit, nor when best to offer such debriefing.

Future research

Further research is needed in a number of areas. Refinement of the phenomenology and long-term course of post-traumatic stress reactions by age and type of trauma is needed, but hampered at present by the lack of age-appropriate standardised measures for younger children. Analysis of the way that children explain and ascribe meaning to traumatic events, descriptions of their post-traumatic attitudes towards the world and themselves, and investigation of changes in (preconscious) information processing will contribute to a fuller understanding of traumatic stress reactions. Most important, there is a need for treatment-outcome studies of PTSD in children and adolescents. Studies of both referred and non-referred children with PTSD, and carefully selected control groups, are necessary before firm conclusions can be reached about the chronicity of symptoms and the effectiveness of current treatments.

References

American Psychiatric Association (1980). *Diagnostic and statistical manual of mental disorders*, 3rd edn. American Psychiatric Association, Washington, DC.

American Psychiatric Association (1994). *Diagnostic and statistical manual of mental disorders*, 4th edn. American Psychiatric Association, Washington, DC.

Birleson, P. (1981). The validity of depressive disorder in childhood and the development of a self-rating scale: A research report. *Journal of Child Psychology and Psychiatry*, 22, 73–88.

Dalgleish, T. (in press). Cognitive theories of post-traumatic stress disorder. In *The post-traumatic stress disorders* (ed. W. Yule). Wiley, Chichester.

Dawes, A. (1994). The emotional impact of political violence. In *Childhood and adversity – psychosocial perspectives from South African research* (ed. A. Dawes & D. Donald), pp. 177–99. David Phillips, Cape Town.

Deblinger, E., McLeer, S.V. & Henry, D. (1990). Cognitive behavioral treatment for sexually abused children suffering posttraumatic stress: Preliminary findings. *Journal of the American Academy of Child and Adolescent Psychiatry*, 19, 747–52.

Dyregrov, A. (1991). *Grief in children: a handbook for adults*. Jessica Kingsley Publishers, London.

Foa, E.B., Feske, U. & Murdock, T.B. (1991) Processing of threat related information in rape victims. *Journal of Abnormal Psychology*, 100, 156–62.

Foa, E.B. & Kozak, M.J. (1986). Emotional processing of fear: Exposure to corrective information. *Psychological Bulletin*, 99, 220–35.

Foa, E.B., Steketee, G. & Olasov-Rothbaum, B. (1989). Behavioral/cognitive conceptualizations of post-traumatic stress disorder. *Behavior Therapy*, 20, 155–76.

Galante, R. & Foa, D. (1986). An epidemiological study of psychic trauma and treatment effectiveness after a natural disaster. *Journal of the American Academy of Child Psychiatry*, 25, 357–63.

Herman, J.L. (1992). Complex PTSD: A syndrome in survivors of prolonged and repeated trauma. *Journal of Traumatic Stress*, 5, 377–91.

Horowitz, M.J., Wilner, N. & Alvarez, W. (1979). Impact of event scale: A measure of subjective stress. *Psychosomatic Medicine*, 41, 209–18.

Janoff-Bulman, R. (1985). The aftermath of victimization: Rebuilding shattered assumptions. In *Trauma and its wake* (ed. C.R. Figley), pp. 70–90. Brunner/Mazel, New York.

Janoff-Bulman, R (1992). *Shattered assumptions: towards a new psychology of trauma*. The Free Press, New York.

Johnson, K.M., Foa, E.B., Jaycox, L. H. & Rescorla, L. (1996). Post trauma attitudes in traumatised children. Poster presented at the XIIth ISTSS Annual Meeting, San Fransisco.

Joseph, S., Brewin, C., Yule, W. & Williams, R. (1993) Causal attributions and psychiatric symptoms in adolescent survivors of disaster. *Journal of Child Psychology and Psychiatry*, 34, 247–53.

Keane, T.M., Zimmering, R.T. & Caddell, J.M. (1985). A behavioral formulation of PTSD in Vietnam veterans. *Behavior Therapist*, **8**, 9–12.

Kenardy, J.A., Webster, R.A., Lewin, T.J., Carr, V.J., Hazell, P.L. & Carter, G.L. (1996). Stress debriefing and patterns of recovery following a natural disaster. *Journal of Traumatic Stress*, **9**, 37–49.

Kinzie, J.D., Sack, W.H., Angell, R.H., Manson, S. & Rath, B. (1986). The psychiatric effects of massive trauma on Cambodian children: I. The children. *Journal of the American Academy of Child and Adolescent Psychiatry*, **25**, 370–6.

Lang, P. J. (1977). Fear imagery: an information processing analysis. *Behaviour Therapy*, **8**, 862–86.

McFarlane, A.C. (1987). Family functioning and overprotection following a natural disaster: The longitudinal effects of post-traumatic morbidity. *Australia and New Zealand Journal of Psychiatry*, **21**, 210–18.

McNally, R.J. (1991). Assessment of posttraumatic stress disorder in children. *Psychological Assessment*, **3**, 531–7.

Misch, P., Phillips, M., Evans, P. & Berkowitz, M. (1993). Trauma in preschool children: A clinical account. *Association of Child Psychology and Psychiatry: Occasional Papers*, **8**, 11–18.

Moradi, A.R. (1996). Cognitive characteristics of children and adolescents with PTSD. Unpublished PhD thesis, University of London.

Mowrer, O.H. (1960). *Learning theory and behavior*. Wiley, New York.

Nader, K.O. (1995). Assessing traumatic experiences in children. In *Assessing psychological trauma and PTSD: A handbook for practitioners* (ed. J.P. Wilson & T.M. Keane), pp. 291–348. Guilford Press, New York.

Nader, K.O., Kreigler, J., Keane, T., Blake, D. & Pynoos, R. (1994). *Clinician administered PTSD scale: child and adolescent version (CAPS-C)*. National Centre for PTSD, White River Junction, VT.

O'Donohue, W. & Elliot, A. (1992). The current status of posttraumatic stress disorder as a diagnostic category: Problems and proposals. *Journal of Traumatic Stress*, **5**, 421–39.

Ollendick, T.H. (1983). Reliability and validity of the Revised Fear Survey Schedule for Children (FSSC-R). *Behavior Therapy*, **21**, 685–92.

Pynoos, R.S. (1994). Traumatic stress and developmental psychopathology in children and adolescents. In *Posttraumatic Stress Disorder: A Clinical Review* (ed. R.S. Pynoos), pp. 65–98. Sidran Press, Lutherville, MD.

Pynoos, R.S. & Eth, S. (1986). Witness to violence: The child interview. *Journal of the American Academy of Child and Adolescent Psychiatry*, **25**, 306–19.

Pynoos, R.S., Goenjian, A., Karakashian, M., Tashjian, M., Manjikian, R., Manoukian, G.,

Steinberg, A.M. & Fairbanks, L.A. (1993). Posttraumatic stress reactions in children after the 1988 Armenian earthquake. *British Journal of Psychiatry*, **163**, 239–47.

Rachman, S. (1980). Emotional processing. *Behaviour Research and Therapy*, **18**, 51–60.

Reich, W., Shakya, J.J. & Taibelson, C. (1991). *Diagnostic Interview for Children and Adolescents (DICA)*. Washington University, St Louis, Mo.

Reynolds, C.R. & Richmond, B.O. (1978). What I think and feel: A revised measure of children's manifest anxiety. *Journal of Abnormal Child Psychology*, **6**, 271–280.

Richman, N. (1993). Annotation: children in situations of political violence. *Journal of Child Psychology and Psychiatry*, **6**, 1286–302.

Saigh, P.A. (1987a). In-vitro flooding of an adolescent's posttraumatic stress disorder. *Journal of Clinical Child Psychology*, **16**, 147–50.

Saigh, P.A. (1987b). In-vitro flooding of a childhood posttraumatic stress disorder. *School Psychology Review*, **16**, 203-211.

Saigh, P.A. (1989). The use of in-vitro flooding in the treatment of a traumatized adolescent. *Journal of Behavioural and Developmental Paediatrics*, **10**, 17–21.

Saigh, P.A. (1992). The behavioral treatment of child and adolescent posttraumatic stress disorder. *Advances in Behaviour Research and Therapy*, **14**, 247–75.

Schwarz, E.D. & Kowalski, J.M. (1991). Posttraumatic stress disorder after a school shooting: Effects of symptom threshold selection and diagnosis by DSM-III, DSM-III-R, or proposed DSM-IV. *American Journal of Psychiatry*, **148**, 592–7.

Shaffer, D., Fisher, P., Dulcan, M., Davies, M., Piacentini, J., Schwab-Stone, M., Lahey, B., Bourdon, K., Jensen, P., Bird, H., Cacino, G. & Regier, D. (1996). The NIMH diagnostic interview schedule for children (DISC-2.3): Description, acceptibility, prevalences, and performance in the MECA study. *Journal of the America Academy of Child and Adolescent Psychiatry*, **35**(7), 865–77.

Stallard, P. & Law, F. (1993). Screening and psychological debriefing of adolescent survivors of life threatening events. *British Journal of Psychiatry*, **163**, 660–5.

Terr, L.C. (1979). The children of Chowchilla. *Psychoanalytic Study of the Child*, **34**, 547–623.

Terr, L.C. (1991). Childhood traumas: An outline and overview. *American Journal of Psychiatry*, **148**, 10–20.

Thrasher, S. M., Dalgleish, T. & Yule, W. (1994). Information processing in posttraumatic stress disorder. *Behaviour Research and Therapy*, **32**, 247–54.

World Health Organisation (1992). *International classification of diseases*, 10th edn. WHO, Geneva.

Yule, W. (1992). Post traumatic stress disorder in child survivors of shipping disasters: The sinking of the 'Jupiter'. *Psychotherapy and Psychosomatics*, **57**, 200–5.

Yule, W. & Udwin, O. (1991). Screening child survivors for post-traumatic stress disorders: Experiences from the 'Jupiter' sinking. *British Journal of Clinical Psychology*, **30**, 131–8.

Yule, W. & Williams, R. (1990). Post traumatic stress reactions in children. *Journal of Traumatic Stress*, **3**, 279–95.

9
Pain in childhood

Patrick J. McGrath and Julie E. Goodman

Introduction

Cognitive–behavioural approaches have contributed to major advances in the areas of health psychology and behavioural medicine. These contributions have enhanced our understanding and improved our management of many different disorders including epilepsy (Dahl, Brorson & Melin, 1992), reflex vomiting (Sokel *et al.*, 1990), eczema (Sokel *et al.*, 1993), juvenile rheumatoid arthritis and sickle cell disease (Varni, Walco & Katz, 1989), asthma (Colland, 1993), and chronic illness (Wallander & Marullo, 1993), but this approach has not yet been universally applied to all areas of health. Because of the broad and scattered application of cognitive–behavioural approaches to medical conditions, this chapter will limit its focus to pain in children and adolescents. We feel that the application of cognitive–behavioural methods to pain provides an excellent template for similar treatment of other medical conditions.

The International Association for the Study of Pain has established a standard definition of pain as: 'An unpleasant sensory and emotional experience associated with actual or potential tissue damage or described in terms of such damage' (Merskey & Bogduk, 1994, p.210). Cognitive–behaviour therapy has been used both to influence the presumed cause of pain (usually when the cause is related to 'stress') and to ameliorate the sensory and emotional aspects of pain. We will examine cognitive–behaviour therapy in relation to both of these elements in specific pain problems.

There is a wide diversity of pain problems in children and adolescents that can be assisted by cognitive–behaviour therapy. However, we will focus our discussion on those problems that are common, and for which there is most clinical experience and research. These include: pain from procedures, headache, recurrent abdominal pain, and fibromyalgia. Similar strategies used to treat these problems can also be applied to neuropathic pain, pain from sickle cell disease, irritable bowel syndrome, and pain from cancer.

Pain from procedures

Pain from procedures includes the pain from relatively common and minor procedures such as injection and venepuncture, as well as pain from more uncommon and major procedures such as bone marrow aspiration and lumbar puncture. The most predominant strategies used for reducing pain from procedures are distraction and hypnosis. In addition to giving control to the child, relaxation training, breathing exercises, and positive reinforcement have been used to augment the positive effects of these strategies. Distraction has been commonly used for minor procedures such as finger pricks, immunisation and venepuncture. Hypnosis has been used for major procedures such as bone marrow aspiration.

Distraction

The rationale underlying the use of distraction is that it divides or limits the child's attention to painful stimuli. Thus, there is limited attentional capacity available to feel pain: if attention is focused elsewhere, pain will be noticed less. It is important, however, to ensure that the distraction technique being used is captivating enough to be effective.

Case illustration

James is a 3-year-old child with diabetes who requires repeated finger pricks, up to four times daily, for blood tests to assess his blood sugar levels and gauge his insulin requirements. He has become quite resistant to and apprehensive of these tests. Whenever his mother approaches him with the test kit he cries and tries to run away. As a strategy to prevent him from running from her, his mother had tried using the 'sneak attack' approach, trying to surprise him, and assumed that this approach would give him less time and opportunity to become upset. He subsequently became very suspicious of his mother, and avoided her whenever he suspected a surprise finger prick. As a result, each finger prick turns into a one-hour battle. Unfortunately, his blood sugar levels are somewhat erratic and frequent testing is necessary to enhance good control. His mother consulted the psychologist from the diabetes clinic, who developed the following, individualised programme for her.

1. Do not try to fool James about what is to happen.
2. Set up a bowl of his favourite 'diabetic' ice cream for him to eat immediately following the finger prick.
3. Allow him to watch his favourite video during the finger prick (reserve his favourites for this).
4. Let James choose the finger that will be pricked.
5. Hold his hand firmly; wait until he is involved in the video and then proceed with the prick.

6. Ignore any crying.
7. Give lots of praise and the ice cream immediately when finished.

This programme was effective in reducing the turmoil surrounding the finger pricks, but it still took 20 minutes to complete a finger prick. Gradually, over the following two weeks, finger pricks became more routine, and much more predictable for James. He no longer feared 'sneak attacks' and the process became less onerous. James' mother sometimes omitted the ice cream reward, or the video distraction. However, two months later, the problem recurred and the full programme was reinstated for two weeks.

As described in the above vignette, distraction is usually embedded in the context of other behavioural methods. For example, being forthcoming with James about exactly what was going to happen and when it would happen probably reduced excessive anticipatory anxiety. Further, the videotape distraction was combined with an immediate positive tangible reward (ice cream) as well as positive, verbal feedback, regardless of James' crying behaviour. Crying behaviour was ignored, so that he was not scolded for crying, nor was he given excessive sympathy for crying. For longer and more invasive procedures such as venepuncture or lumbar puncture, distraction can be combined with EMLA, a topical analgesic containing lidocaine and prilocaine (Halperin *et al.*, 1989).

Research examining the use of distraction has generally shown that there is a measurable, but small, treatment effect size. For example, Fowler-Kerry and Lander (1987) found a small effect ($d = 0.39$) when using music distraction to reduce self-reported pain in 200 4.5–6.5-year-old children undergoing intramuscular immunisation. Two other studies have evaluated the use of distraction during venepuncture. Vessey, Carlson and McGill (1994) found a medium effect ($d = 0.65$) of kaleidoscope distraction in reducing pain in 100 3–11-year-old children undergoing venepuncture. Arts *et al.* (1994) found no significant effect of music distraction in reducing pain in 180 4–16 year olds undergoing routine venepuncture.

Tips to ensure good distraction
1. Allow enough time for the child's attention to be as fully engaged as possible by the method of distraction being used. Clinical judgement and the age and developmental level of the child should be used to gauge how long the pre-procedure distraction time should be.
2. Choose a method of distraction that is interesting and appropriate to the age and developmental level of the child. Potential distractors include: blowing bubbles or other blowing games, listening to music, singing, watching videos or mobiles, reading aloud to the child, or playing with toys. For example, watching videotapes of cartoons during a finger prick may be appropriate for pre-school or younger, school-aged children, whereas listening to a favourite CD might be more appropriate for adolescents.

3. Allow the child to have some choice in selecting the method of distraction to give the child a sense of control over the procedure.
4. Do not try to deceive the child with distraction.

Hypnosis

There is considerable controversy in the literature on hypnosis. Some believe it is an altered state of consciousness (e.g. Hilgard & LeBaron, 1984), whereas others (e.g. Spanos, 1986a, 1986b) regard the hypnotic state simply as a state of heightened suggestibility. Both sides to the argument agree that hypnosis involves a focusing of attention with suggestions. As such, attention is diverted away from pain and pain-inducing stimuli. The focusing of attention has included the use of 'favourite stories' in young children (Kuttner, 1988), and the more conventional techniques of visual or cognitive focusing that are widely used with adults. Although many believe it is clinically useful to assess hypnotic suggestibility prior to using hypnosis as a form of intervention, no clear relation has been identified between hypnotic suggestibility and effectiveness of hypnosis in children. Some families may have religious objections to the use of hypnosis, and therefore, the family's view of hypnosis should be known before recommending its use.

Case illustration

Marie, age 5, has acute lymphoblastic leukaemia and is required to have numerous and frequent finger pricks and other invasive procedures. Pain from bone marrow aspirations and lumbar punctures is prevented by using conscious sedation, an anaesthetic procedure whereby the child is given a very brief anesthesia in the treatment room. Generally, Marie does not show excessive anticipatory anxiety to these procedures. However, she often becomes distressed for up to an hour prior to each finger prick. In collaboration with the unit psychologist, Marie's mother developed a form of hypnosis that incorporated guided imagery to help Marie dissociate from the pain of the finger prick. The story described a medieval knight, whose suit of armour protected her from a dragon's fiery breath. In a variation on this story, Marie's mother suggested that Marie was the knight, whose suit of armour would protect her from the pain from the finger prick. Although this strategy did not eliminate the pain from the needle pricks, Marie reported that they felt less painful when she was 'wearing' her suit of armour.

Hypnosis can be combined with other medical and psychological therapies. Hypnosis is often conceptualised in other terms such as distraction, relaxation or guided imagery. Moreover, there is no reason not to use pharmacotherapeutic procedures, in addition, if they are warranted.

There is good evidence that hypnosis can reduce pain from medical procedures. For example, in a randomised trial, Kuttner (1988) found that hypnosis in the form of favourite stories was superior both to a distraction treatment and to standard care in reducing behavioural distress in response to bone marrow aspirations.

Headaches

The two most common types of headaches that children and adolescents experience are tension-type headache and migraine. Tension-type headaches are typically associated with dull or pressing pain, often bilateral, not aggravated by physical activity, not accompanied by vomiting or severe nausea, and generally less severe than migraine (Olesen *et al.*, 1988). Migraine headaches are of several types, but the most frequent are migraine with aura, previously known as classic migraine, and migraine without aura, previously known as common migraine. Migraine headaches are often well-defined attacks of severe throbbing pain that is often unilateral. Significant nausea and vomiting are common and the pain is made worse by physical activity. The aura of migraine is usually visual and occurs about half an hour prior to the headache itself.

The reported prevalence of headaches occurring once a month or more has varied from 23 per cent to 51 per cent (Egermark-Eriksson, 1982; Sillanpaa, 1983; Kristjansdottir & Wahlberg, 1993). More frequent unspecified headaches occurring once a week or more have been reported among 7 per cent to 22 per cent of schoolchildren (Egermark-Eriksson, 1982; Sillanpaa, 1983; Larsson, 1988; Kristjansdottir & Wahlberg 1993). A smaller proportion of schoolchildren experience almost daily headaches (2.5–6 per cent) and about 0.3–1.2 per cent of the children report daily headaches (Egermark-Eriksson, 1982; Sillanpaa, 1983). A very marked increase in the prevalence of headache with age has been noted. In children below 10 years of age, headache is approximately equally distributed in both sexes. However, during adolescence, the prevalence of headache increases in both males and females, but generally increases more in females until there is a marked preponderance of female headache sufferers. This trend is maintained in adulthood. Clinical impressions suggest that there is a secular trend of increasing prevalence of headache. This has been confirmed by Sillanpaa, who did a 20-year follow-up survey in which he examined children in the same schools using the same instrument (Sillanpaa & Anttila, 1996). The authors found a striking increase of the prevalence of migraine as well as unspecified headaches over a 20-year time period. The greatest increase in prevalence was observed in areas with high social instability. The authors suggested that changes in the psychosocial environment might explain the increase in headache prevalence in the children.

The rationale for using CBT for children who have recurrent headaches is to reduce psychosocial stress that often triggers migraine, to reduce perceived pain intensity and severity, and to reduce or prevent disability from headache. Three major techniques have been used: hypnosis, progressive muscle relaxation, and cognitive restructuring. However, although headaches from pathological causes are rare, a careful history and physical examination by a physician should be completed prior to beginning CBT.

Hypnosis

There are many different forms of hypnosis. All of them involve the focusing of attention and usually also suggest relaxation and reduction of pain. Hypnosis is sometimes indistiguishable from forms of relaxation training.

Progressive muscle relaxation

Relaxation typically consists of a combination of relaxation with tension, relaxation without tension, and abbreviated relaxation using breathing exercises. Although relaxation training has been shown effectively to reduce the frequency of migraine and overall headache activity in children (e.g. Richter *et al.*, 1986), relaxation training alone, in the absence of additional, concurrent cognitive behavioural strategies such as cognitive restructuring or coping-skills training, may not be sufficient as a consistently effective therapy (McGrath *et al.*, 1988). Audiotaped instructions of relaxation exercises may also be used between sessions to facilitate training (e.g. McGrath *et al.*, 1990).

Cognitive–behavioural approaches to headaches often include a psycho-educational component to teach children about the relation between their headaches and psychosocial stress. Most programmes incorporate a series of steps and should include the following elements:

1. Rationale of the relationship between headache and psychosocial stress.
2. Prospective recording of pain and coping strategies prior to treatment, during treatment, and following treatment.
3. Learning to identify negative thoughts and to replace them with more positive thoughts.
4. Examining unrealistic beliefs.
5. Distraction strategies.
6. Imagery, behaviour rehearsal, mental activities.
7. Problem solving.

The major form of assessment needed prior to the implementation of cognitive–behaviour therapy for headaches is the determination of whether the patient has the cognitive ability and the motivation to complete the programme. For example, it is unlikely that children under 9 or 10 years of age have the metacognitive ability to use cognitive restructuring. Hypnosis and relaxation may be used with children over the age of 7 or 8 years, but a younger child would probably require considerable parental involvement and assistance with the exercises. Further, children with only occasional headaches are unlikely to be motivated enough to undertake such a demanding programme.

Relaxation and cognitive restructuring are often combined. Both of these methods have been delivered in a reduced-therapist-contact model in which the adolescent moves through the treatment programme by means of telephone contact and a manual. The programme is introduced to the adolescent in one or two introductory sessions, and compliance is encouraged and maintained through regular follow-up telephone calls. The reduced-therapist-contact approach is about three times more cost efficient and equally effective to the therapist-directed approach (McGrath *et al.*, 1992).

Case illustration

Kerry is 15 years old and has had recurrent headaches that occur about twice a week for two years. They began just after she started to menstruate. She has two types of headaches: 'regular' headaches and 'killer' headaches. Her 'regular' headaches, which occur about 80 per cent of the time, are tension-type headaches, while her 'killer' headaches are migraine headaches without an aura. Kerry usually does not miss school from her tension-type headaches but often must go home when she has a migraine. The tension-type headaches usually make it difficult for her to concentrate. She tries to keep up in school but feels she could work better if she had fewer headaches. Her mother also has had chronic tension-type and migraine headaches since about the same age. Kerry uses paracetamol sparingly because she is afraid of becoming addicted. When her doctor suggested a referral to the psychologist at the local hospital for treatment of her headaches, both she and her family were reluctant because they did not feel it was a psychological problem. However, Kerry decided to try it for a few sessions.

   The treatment was a combination of psycho-education, relaxation training, hypnosis, and cognitive restructuring. Kerry found that the best part of the treatment was meeting the other five girls who had the same problem. They learned all about headaches and were very supportive in encouraging each other to do the exercises and manage their headaches. Kerry learned to recognise the stressors that were most likely to trigger her headaches. These were skipping meals (i.e. not eating) and being worried about her school work. She really enjoyed the relaxation exercises and found the hypnosis and imagery exercises, as directed by the audiotape, to be very helpful. She also learned to use a full dose of paracetamol or ibuprofen as soon as her headache began, rather than waiting until the pain became unbearable. Over the 12 weeks of the programme, Kerry's migraines declined by about half in severity and about half in frequency. She almost eliminated the occurrence of her tension-type headaches. She attended booster sessions every three months for one year. On her own, she kept in contact with three of the other headache group members. She described the treatment group as a positive and helpful experience.

Cognitive–behaviour therapy should be combined with education about headache and, when indicated, appropriate use of over-the-counter analgesics (usually paraceta-mol/acetaminophen). Many parents are wary of the use of paracetamol for pain in children, with about 15 per cent fearing drug abuse or addiction and about 30 per cent fearing the development of tolerance (Forward, McGrath & Brown, 1996). As a result, parents frequently delay the administration of medication for over an hour after the headache begins (Forward *et al.*, 1996). Early aggressive use of over-the-counter analgesics may reduce the pain of significant headache.

Several randomised, controlled trials have been conducted to evaluate the effect of cognitive–behavioural treatment of migraine and tension-type headache. For example, Larsson and colleagues (e.g. Larsson & Melin, 1986, 1988, 1989; Larsson *et al.*, 1987a, 1987b; Larsson, Melin & Doberl, 1990) have demonstrated that relaxation delivered in a school-based programme to children with tension-type headache was significantly more effective than a control condition. Similarly, Richter *et al.* (1986) showed that relaxation and cognitive interventions, alone or combined, were more effective than a placebo control for migraine headaches. McGrath *et al.* (1992) demonstrated that a therapist-reduced treatment, in which the adolescents used a manual and tape in combination with two appointments and telephone calls from the therapist, was at least as effective as the same treatment delivered by a therapist.

Recurrent abdominal pain

Recurrent abdominal pain refers to pain in the abdomen that occurs on at least three occasions over a period of greater than three months and that interferes with normal activities and for which no organic cause can be found (Apley, 1975). The rationale for the use of cognitive–behavioural techniques in treating recurrent abdominal pain is that stress may be important in triggering attacks in susceptible children. Moreover, children may have secondary gain, most notably school avoidance, and increased parental attention from having recurrent abdominal pain. The techniques used have included stress management and operant approaches. Sanders and his colleagues (Sanders *et al.*, 1994) have demonstrated the effectiveness of these strategies in well-designed trials.

The assessment should include a thorough history and physical examination conducted by a physician to rule out significant pathology causing recurrent abdominal pain. Approximately 10 per cent of children who present with recurrent abdominal pain have an underlying organic pathology which explains the pain (e.g. lactose intolerance, appendicitis, parasites, etc.; Rappaport & Leichtner, 1993). In addition, the relation between stressful life events and pain, and between secondary gain and pain should be determined. The developmental capacity of the child to learn and use cognitive–behavioural methods must be ascertained. Finally, the ability of the parents to function as effective agents of change must be assessed.

Case illustration

Mona, a 12-year-old child, has experienced bouts of abdominal pain since she was 7 years old. The pain has waxed and waned over the years, and there has been no apparent relation to obvious stressors. Her parents are concerned because she has started to miss a significant amount of school. Until this year, she had reported pain once every week or so, and has been absent from school about one day per month. This year she has been absent from school about 25 per cent of the time. Her teacher reported that she is a quiet student who works hard. However, she is falling behind this year. Assessment revealed that she was very afraid of being embarrassed in school by vomiting (although she rarely vomited with her pain) and there was some concern expressed by her parents that she was 'enjoying' the time she spent at home watching television.

She was cooperative and compliant with cognitive–behaviour therapy, able to learn to relax well. Her fear of vomiting was directly attacked and her parents were encouraged to make sick time at home boring, with no access to television, and to reward every two weeks of perfect school attendance with a movie for her and her friend. She was coached to increase her activity as she had a very sedentary lifestyle and was also helped to increase her consumption of dietary fibre (she especially liked popcorn). Her bouts of pain gradually decreased and her attendance at school increased dramatically.

The only other validated treatment for recurrent abdominal pain is supplementary dietary fibre (Feldman *et al.*, 1985). Cognitive–behaviour therapy can be combined with an increase of dietary fibre (about 10 g per day), but no empirical studies have been done to determine whether this combined approach improves long-term outcome.

The evidence for the effectiveness of cognitive–behaviour therapy for recurrent abdominal pain is a series of randomised trials by Sanders and colleagues (1989, 1994) that have shown excellent outcome.

Fibromyalgia

Fibromyalgia is a non-inflammatory, soft tissue, rheumatic disorder of unknown aetiology which is characterised by widespread aches, pains, and stiffness. The presence of an excessive number of tender points, identified by pressure dolorimeter or thumb palpation, is typically noted. Fibromyalgia occurs both on its own and in conjunction with other rheumatic disorders. It is also often exacerbated by fatigue, stress, inactivity, and cold, damp weather. Those affected have also reported experiencing sleep disturbances, headaches, irritable bowel syndrome, feelings of numbness, and subjective feelings of swelling. Standard diagnostic criteria for fibromyalgia have been developed by the American College of Rheumatology (Report of the Multicenter Criteria Committee, 1990), and by the International Association for the Study of Pain (Merskey & Bogduk, 1994). Fibromyalgia is a chronic pain disorder and most adults seen in rheumatology clinics with fibromyalgia are significantly disabled.

Very little research on the prevalence, natural course and treatment of fibromyalgia in children and adolescents has been conducted. Malleson, Al-Matar and Petty (1992) reported a retrospective chart review of children with idiopathic, musculoskeletal pain presenting at a tertiary care children's rheumatology clinic. Most of the children (35/40) with diffuse pain fulfilled Yunus and Masi's (1985) diagnostic criteria for fibromyalgia. They found that these children had frequent recurrences and many had significant psychological morbidity. A recent epidemiologic study (Buskila *et al.*, 1993) studied 338 healthy Israeli schoolchildren, aged 9 to 15 years, from a single school and found 6.2 per cent to have fibromyalgia using the American College of Rheumatology's criteria (Report of the Multicenter Criteria Committee, 1990). There were no age or gender differences noted. Children with fibromyalgia had lower thresholds for tenderness than children without fibromyalgia at both tender point and control sites. There were seven children who had low pressure-pain thresholds at tender points who did not report widespread pain, and thus were not diagnosed as having fibromyalgia. A

30-month follow-up (Buskila *et al.*, 1995) found that 73 per cent of the children origin-ally diagnosed with fibromyalgia no longer fulfilled its diagnostic criteria. None of the children with low pain thresholds had developed fibromyalgia. The authors concluded the prevalence of fibromyalgia in a community sample of adolescents to be 1.7 per cent.

The underlying cause of fibromyalgia is unknown. A very wide variety of causes has been suggested, but none has been firmly established. Depression and sleep problems are common, but it is unclear if they are the cause or result of the disorder. Case control studies of clinical samples have found mixed results regarding the psychological con-comitants of fibromyalgia in adolescents. Yunus and Masi (1985) compared 33 fibro-myalgia patients and controls and found that the children with fibromyalgia had higher rates of sleep problems, fatigue, depression, anxiety, chronic headaches, numbness, and irritable bowel symptoms compared to the controls. However, they used psychometri-cally weak measurements of anxiety, depression and sleep problems. Reid, Lang and McGrath, (1996) found no differences between adolescents and their families with fibromyalgia, juvenile rheumatoid arthritis and pain-free controls on a variety of well-validated instruments measuring clinical psychopathology.

The one treatment trial of cognitive–behaviour therapy for fibromyalgia in adoles-cents was a clinical series with seven patients (Walco & Ilowite, 1992). The authors found that four of the five patients who completed more than four sessions of treatment were pain-free, and the remaining patient who completed treatment had sharply reduced pain. Their treatment programme was comprised of four to nine sessions of instruction, focusing on progressive muscle relaxation and guided imagery, or self-regulatory techniques directed at reducing pain, and improving sleep and mood. They concluded that a cognitive–behavioural approach may be useful in treating the pain and other symptoms, such as sleep and/or mood disturbances, associated with fibromyalgia in children.

Cognitive–behaviour therapy might be effective in fibromyalgia by increasing restorative sleep, by decreasing pain sensitivity, and by increasing physical fitness. The CBT strategies used with fibromyalgia have included cognitive restructuring, improving sleep hygiene, and increasing activity.

Case illustration

Jill is a 14-year-old girl who has had widespread pain, fatigue and difficulty sleeping for two years. She has gradually become less physically active, quitting the swimming team, and more socially withdrawn, sharply limiting her contact with her peer group. Her family doctor had thought that her symptoms would remit or significantly improve because she could find no physical basis for Jill's complaints. In addition, although Jill was a bit unhappy, she was not depressed. After a year without improvement, Jill's parents asked that she be referred to a specialist. Her doctor gave her parents the choice of seeing either a psychiatrist or a rheumatologist. Jill's parents chose to see a rheumatologist. A thorough physical examination showed that Jill's pressure-pain tolerance was lower than normal, and that she had 12 of 18 tender points. A series of blood tests revealed nothing abnormal. Jill was diagnosed with fibromyalgia and referred to a psychologist for treatment.

The treatment package consisted of a 10-week, time-limited treatment that included:

1. An explanation of fibromyalgia as a non-articular rheumatic disorder that is negatively influenced by poor sleep, lack of exercise, and increased psychosocial stress.
2. Daily recording of pain, mood and fatigue using a detailed diary.
3. Relaxation training using diaphragmatic breathing.
4. Identification of negative thoughts.
5. Assistance in changing negative, self-defeating thoughts to more realistic and positive thoughts.
6. Instruction in appropriate sleep hygiene.
7. Assistance in gradually increasing activity level and developing a programme of mild exercise and activity to enhance physical fitness, endurance and tolerance.
8. Training in guided imagery, and distraction from pain.

Jill had individual sessions with a psychologist, who also had three sessions with her parents. Jill made good progress with her sessions and was able to decrease her pain and fatigue. She began a programme of mild exercise and increased her number and frequency of social contacts. She still had a sufficient number of tender points necessary for a diagnosis of fibromyalgia but had much less widespread pain and fatigue. She was followed for one year by telephone calls and remained relatively well.

When she was 16 years old she was in a car accident and sustained a whiplash injury. Her doctor said the pain would just go away with time. When it did not, Jill became more withdrawn and depressed. Her sleep deteriorated and her pain returned. She declined further treatment, saying that it would not help her. Her family moved and she was lost to follow-up.

Cognitive–behaviour therapy for fibromyalgia is often combined with low-dose amitriptyline and physiotherapy. There are no data to determine the effectiveness of these combinations in children and adolescents.

Conclusions

Cognitive–behaviour therapy has been applied to many areas of children's health. Pain management provides an excellent model of the application of cognitive–behavior therapy with medical problems. A major challenge for the future is to integrate cognitive–behaviour therapy into medical practice. Although cognitive–behavioural approaches are widely accepted by mental health practitioners, there are still significant barriers to their implementation in medical settings. These barriers include: (1) physicians and nurses are often unaware of cognitive–behavioural approaches and are therefore unlikely to refer for them; (2) because it is commonly believed by professionals and the lay public that psychological interventions such as CBT are appropriate only for disorders that are psychologically based, most medical disorders are thought not to benefit from these approaches; (3) many psychologists are not familiar enough with medical conditions to develop treatment strategies for them; (4) in some countries, funding for the use of CBT for medical conditions or symptoms is either difficult to obtain or unavailable.

The reduced-therapist-contact methods that have proven extremely effective in headache may have applications to other disorders and have the advantage of being cost effective. Further, reduced-therapist-contact methods can be delivered to children who, because of distance from major centres, do not have ready access to specialist care. There is also a need for a great deal more systematic clinical work applying cognitive–behavioural treatments to children's medical conditions. As wider experience is gained, single-subject studies, clinical series, and well-designed clinical trials need to be developed to ensure an evidence-based approach to treatment.

References

Apley, J. (1975). *The child with abdominal pains*, 2nd edn. Blackwell, London.

Arts, S. E., Abu Saad, H. H., Champion, G. D., Crawford, M. R., Fisher, R. J., Juniper, K. H. & Ziegler, J. B. (1994). Age-related response to lidocaine–prilocaine (EMLA) emulsion and effect of music distraction on the pain of intravenous cannulation. *Pediatrics*, **93**, 797–801.

Buskila, D., Neumann, L., Hershman, E., Gedalia, A., Press, J. & Sukenik, S. (1995). Fibromyalgia syndrome in children: An outcome study. *The Journal of Rheumatology*, **22**(3), 525–8.

Buskila, D., Press, J., Gedalia, A., Klein, M., Neumann, L., Boehm, R. & Sukenik, S. (1993). Assessment of nonarticular tenderness and prevalence of fibromyalgia in children. *Journal of Rheumatology*, **20**, 368–70.

Colland, V.T. (1993). Learning to cope with asthma: A behavioural self-management program for children. *Patient Education and Counselling*, **22**(3), 141–52.

Dahl, J., Brorson, L. O. & Melin, L. (1992). Effects of a broad-spectrum behavioral medicine treatment program on children with refractory epileptic seizures: An 8-year follow-up. *Epilepsia*, **33**(1), 98–102.

Egermark-Eriksson, I. (1982). Prevalence of headache in Swedish schoolchildren: A questionnaire survery. *Acta Paediatrica Scandinavica*, **71**, 135–40.

Feldman, W., McGrath, P. J., Hodgson, C., Ritter, H. & Shipman, R. T. (1985). The use of dietary fiber in the management of simple, childhood, idiopathic, recurrent, abdominal pain. Results in a prospective, double-blind, randomized, controlled trial. *American Journal of Diseases of Children*, **139**, 1216–18.

Forward, S.P., McGrath, P.J. & Brown, T.L. (1996). Mothers' attitudes and behaviour towards medicating children's pain. *Pain*, **67**, 469–75.

Fowler-Kerry, S. & Lander, J.R. (1987). Management of injection pain in children. *Pain*, **30**, 169–75.

Halperin, D.L., Koren, G., Attias, D., Pellegrini, E., Greenberg, M. L. & Wyss, M. (1989). Topical skin anesthesia for venous, subcutaneous drug reservoir and lumbar punctures in children. *Pediatrics*, **84**(2), 281–4.

Hilgard, J.R. & LeBaron, S. (1984). *Hypnotherapy of pain in children with cancer*, Kaufmann, Los Altos, Calif.

Kristjansdottir, G. & Wahlberg, V. (1993). Sociodemographic differences in the prevalence of self-reported headache in Icelandic school-children, *Headache*, **33**(7), 376–80.

Kuttner, L. (1988). Favorite stories: A hypnotic pain-reduction technique for children in acute pain. *American Journal of Clinical Hypnosis*, **30**, 289–95.

Larsson, B. S. (1988). The role of psychological, health behaviour and medical factors in adolescent headache. *Developmental Medicine and Child Neurology*, **30**, 616–25.

Larsson, B. S., Daleflod, B., Hakansson, L. & Melin, L. (1987a). Therapist-assisted versus self-help relaxation treatment of chronic headaches in adolescents: a school-based intervention. *Journal of Child Psychology and Psychiatry*, **28**, 127–36.

Larsson, B. S., & Melin, L. (1986). Chronic headaches in adolescents: treatment in a school setting with relaxation training as compared with information–contact and self-registration. *Pain*, **25**, 325–36.

Larsson, B. S. & Melin, L. (1988). The psychological treatment of recurrent headache in adolescents – short-term outcome and its prediction. *Headache*, **28**, 187–95.

Larsson, B. S. & Melin, L. (1989). Follow-up on behavioral treatment of recurrent headache in adolescents. *Headache*, **29**, 249–53.

Larsson, B. S., Melin, L. & Doberl, A. (1990). Recurrent tension headache in adolescents treated with self-help relaxation training and a muscle relaxant drug. *Headache*, **30**, 665–71.

Larsson, B. S., Melin, L., Lamminen, M. & Ullstedt, F. (1987b). A school-based treatment of chronic headaches in adolescents. *Journal of Pediatric Psychology*, **12**, 553–66.

Malleson, P. N., Al-Matar, M. & Petty, R. E. (1992). Idiopathic musculoskeletal pain syndromes in children. *Journal of Rheumatology*, **19**, 1786–9.

McGrath, P. J., Cunningham, S. J., Lascelles, M. A. & Humphreys, P. (1990). *Help yourself – A treatment for migraine headaches: Professional handbook*. University of Ottawa Press, Ottawa

McGrath, P. J., Humphreys, P., Goodman, J. T., Keene, D., Firestone, P., Jacob, P. & Cunningham, S. J. (1988). Relaxation prophylaxis for childhood migraine: A randomized placebo-controlled trial. *Developmental Medicine and Child Neurology*, **30**, 626–31.

McGrath, P. J., Humphreys, P., Keene, D., Goodman, J. T., Lascelles, M. A., Cunningham, S. J. & Firestone, P. (1992). The efficacy and efficiency of a self-administered treatment for adolescent migraine. *Pain*, **49**, 321–4.

Merskey, H. & Bogduk, N., Eds. (1994). *Classification of chronic pain: descriptions of chronic pain syndromes and definitions of pain terms*, 2nd edn. IASP Press, Seattle.

Olesen, J., Bes, A., Kunkel, R., Lance, J.W., Nappi, G., Prarrentath, V., Rose, F.C., Shoenberg, B.S., Soyka, D., Tfelt-Hansen, P., Welch, K.M.A. & Wilkinson, M. (1988). Classification and diagnostic criteria for headache disorders, cranial neuralgias and facial pain. *Cephalagia*, **8**, supplement 7, 1–96.

Rappaport, L. & Leichtner, A. M. (1993). Recurrent abdominal pain. In *Pain in infants, children, and adolescents* (ed. N.L. Schecter, C.B. Berde & M. Yaster), pp. 561–70. Williams & Wilkins, Baltimore.

Reid, G. J., Lang, B. A. & McGrath, P. J. (1996). Primary juvenile fibromyalgia: psychological adjustment, family functioning, coping and functional disability. *Arthritis and Rheumatism*, **40**(4), 752–60.

Report of the Multicenter Criteria Committee (1990). The American College of Rheumatology 1990 criteria for the classification of fibromyalgia. *Arthritis and Rheumatism*, **33**, 160–72.

Richter, I. L., McGrath, P. J., Humphreys, P. J., Goodman, J. T., Firestone, P. & Keene, D. (1986). Cognitive and relaxation treatment of paediatric migraine. *Pain*, **25**, 195–203.

Sanders, M. R., Rebgetz, M., Morrison, M. & Bor, W. (1989). Cognitive–behavioral treatment of recurrent nonspecific abdominal pain in children: An analysis of generalization, maintenance, and side effects. *Journal of Consulting and Clinical Psychology*, **57**, 294–300.

Sanders, M. R., Shepherd, R. W., Cleghorn, G. & Woolford, H. (1994). The treatment of recurrent abdominal pain in children: A controlled comparison of cognitive-behavioral family intervention and standard pediatric care. *Journal of Consulting and Clinical Psychology*, **62**, 306–14.

Sillanpaa, M. (1983). Prevalence of headache in prepuberty. *Headache*, **23**, 10–14.

Sillanpaa, M. & Anttila, P. (1996). Increasing prevalence of headache in 7-year-old schoolchildren. *Headache*, **36**, 466–70.

Sokel, B., Christie, D., Kent, A., Glover, R., Lansdown, R., Knibbs, J. & Atherton, D. (1993). A comparison of hypnotherapy and biofeedback in the treatment of childhood atopic eczema. *Contemporary Hypnosis*, **10**, 145–54.

Sokel, B. S., Devane, S. P., Bentovim, A. & Milla, P. J. (1990). Self hypnotherapeutic treatment of habitual reflex vomiting. *Archives of Disease in Childhood*, **65**, 1–2.

Spanos, N. P. (1986a). Hypnotic behavior: a social-psychological interpretation of amnesia, analgesia and 'trance logic'. *Behavioral and Brain Sciences*, **9**(3), 449–67.

Spanos, N. P. (1986b). More on the social psychology of hypnotic responding. *Behavioral and Brain Sciences*, **9**(3), 489–502.

Varni, J. W., Walco, G. A. & Katz, E. R. (1989). Assessment and management of chronic and recurrent pain in children with chronic diseases. *Pediatrician*, **16**(1–2), 56–63.

Vessey, J.A., Carlson, K.L. & McGill, J., (1994) Use of distraction with children during an acute pain experience. *Nursing Research*, **43**(6), 369–72.

Walco, G. A. & Ilowite, N. T. (1992). Cognitive-behavioral intervention for juvenile primary fibromyalgia syndrome. *Journal of Rheumatology*, **19**, 1617–19.

Wallander, J. L. & Marullo, D.S. (1993). Chronic medical illness. In *Handbook of prescriptive treatments for children and adolescents* (ed. R.M. Ammerman, C.G. Last & M. Hersen), pp. 402–16. Allyn and Bacon, Boston.

Yunus, M. B. & Masi, A. T. (1985). Juvenile primary fibromyalgia syndrome. A clinical study of thirty-three patients and matched normal controls. *Arthritis and Rheumatism*, **28**, 138–45.

10
Clinically depressed adolescents

Richard Harrington, Alison Wood and Chrissie Verduyn

Over the past decade, evidence from a variety of different research approaches has supported the validity of the concept of major depressive disorder (MDD) in adolescents. Longitudinal studies have shown that the concept has predictive validity, to the extent that young people with depressive conditions have a greater risk of subsequent depression (Kovacs et al., 1984; Harrington et al., 1990) and suicidality (Rao et al., 1993; Harrington et al., 1994) than non-depressed psychiatric cases. Family studies suggest that juvenile affective disorders show, at least in part, a specific association with a family history of affective disorders (Strober et al., 1988; Puig-Antich et al., 1989; Harrington et al., 1993). Epidemiological data support the idea of a specific aetiology, in that depressive disorders in young people show a pattern of age trends and sex differences during early adolescence (rates increase with age in girls, and remain stable in boys) that distinguishes them from most other mental disorders (Fleming, Offord & Boyle, 1989; Fleming & Offord, 1990; Rutter, 1991; Cohen et al., 1993b).

Progress in establishing the predictive and discriminant validity of the concept of depressive disorder in young people is now being matched by the identification of effective forms of treatment. Thus, although early controlled trials failed to find any specific benefit of tricyclic antidepressant medication over placebo (Harrington, 1992), recent reports indicate that the 'new' antidepressants may be effective (Emslie et al., 1995). Psychological treatments, too, have produced encouraging findings both for group treatments such as therapeutic group support (Fine et al., 1991) and for family interventions (Beardslee et al., 1996).

This chapter is concerned with one of the most promising of the psychological treatments for depression in young people, cognitive–behaviour therapy. The term cognitive–behaviour therapy includes many therapeutic techniques that are based on a variety of different theoretical models of depression. Some formulations emphasise the cognitive aspects of both the treatment and its theoretical basis. For instance, Beck states that cognitive therapy 'is based on an underlying theoretical rationale that an individual's affect and behavior are largely determined by the way in which he structures the world' (Beck, 1967). Behavioural techniques are a component of treatment, but are 'a means to an end – cognitive change' (Beck *et al.*, 1979). Other formulations take a broader approach that includes not only cognitive techniques but also a range of behavioural methods, including graded exposure to feared situations and problem-solving techniques (Andrews, 1996). For reasons that will become clear later on, in the present chapter we shall be concerned with this broader model of CBT.

The chapter is divided into two parts. In part one, the *principles* underpinning cognitive–behaviour therapies are outlined. Part one begins with a brief critical review of cognitive–behavioural theories and treatments of depression in adults. The relevance of these theories to depression in adolescence is then described, together with the modifications that are necessary when using cognitive–behaviour therapies with young people. Part one concludes with a meta-analysis of the efficacy of CBT in clinically depressed children and adolescents.

In part two, the *practice* of CBT with depressed adolescents is described. Assessment procedures and the basic elements of CBT are outlined. The approach described is pragmatic, relying more on evidence of what is possible and what works than on cognitive or behavioural theories *per se*. Cognitive–behaviour therapy is conceptualised as just one part of a treatment strategy for depression. The chapter concludes with a section on how CBT can be combined with other interventions.

Principles

Behavioural and cognitive theories of depression

Although it is beyond the scope of this chapter to review psychological models of depression in detail, a sense of these models is relevant to understanding the basis of CBT. Early psychological models of depression attributed the symptoms to a reduced frequency of social reinforcement (Lazarus, 1968). Probably the best known of the behavioural formulations of depression is Lewinsohn's theory that depression is the result of a low rate of response-contingent positive reinforcement (Lewinsohn, Weinstein & Alper, *et al.*, 1970). Depressed people are seen as lacking in social skills. In the early stages of depression, symptoms may be maintained by reinforcement from others, but later on close family and friends may try to avoid the depressed person altogether, thus further reducing the frequency of rewards in the environment.

Later psychological models of depression focused much more on the role of cognitions – thoughts, images and attitudes – on mood. When psychologists talk about cognitive models of depression, they are usually referring to one of two theories (Williams, 1992), Beck's cognitive theory and Seligman's learned helplessness formulation.

Beck's cognitive theory

Beck's cognitive theory of depression (Beck, 1967; Beck *et al.*, 1979) arose out of clinical observations on depressed patients. According to Beck, the individual's view of himself and the world is an important determinant of behaviour. At the heart of Beck's cognitive models of depression are three ideas: the cognitive triad, cognitive errors, and cognitive schemata.

The *cognitive triad* includes the person's views of him or herself, of the future and of the world. Depressed people often believe that they are defective or incompetent in some way. They think that they are worthless and frequently criticise themselves for what they perceive as deficits. Depressed people also have a negative view about the future. They expect that things will never get better and that nothing that they can do will change the future. Cognitive theory also suggests that depressed people misinterpret the world around them. They feel acted upon by the world and take a negative view of most situations.

Cognitive theory proposes that these negative styles of thinking lead to many of the symptoms of depression. For example, if people see themselves as failures and as rejected by peers, then negative emotional reactions such as depression and irritability are likely to follow. Similarly, suicidal feelings can be understood as arising from feelings of hopelessness about the future and from the erroneous view that the person is a burden to others and therefore better off dead. Loss of energy is thought to arise from the person's view that his or her efforts will inevitably fail.

The second component of Beck's theory is the so-called *cognitive errors*, also known as cognitive distortions. Cognitive distortions are habitual errors in the logic of thinking that alter reality and lead to an unnecessarily negative view of one's self, the future and the world. A variety of slightly different classifications of these distortions exist (Beck *et al.*, 1979; Burns, 1980), but the most common are arbitrary inference, selective abstraction, personalisation and over-generalisation. Arbitrary inference occurs when a depressed person jumps to conclusions that are not supported by the evidence. In selective abstraction, a detail is focused on and taken out of context. Personalisation refers to a process in which a person relates external events to him or herself without a good reason for doing so. Over-generalisation occurs when someone makes a general deduction on the basis of a single incident. Cognitive errors therefore lead individuals to distort their experience systematically in line with their negative view of themselves.

These cognitive errors are thought to arise out of *cognitive schemas*. Cognitive schemas are relatively stable patterns of thinking that govern the ways in which external situations are interpreted. In cognitive theory, when someone faces a situation, a schema related to that situation is activated. Schemas provide rules for evaluating situations and are thought to be activated by particular environmental events. Cognitive theory hypothesises that a person's liability to depression arises out of early experiences, which form the basis for that person developing a negative view of self and the world. The schemas are generally latent, but can be activated by experiences that are similar to those that led to the negative schema in the first place.

Seligman's learned helplessness theory

A variety of other cognitive formulations of depression exists, of which probably the best known is Seligman's theory of *learned helplessness*. This theory was originally based on experiments with dogs in which it was observed that animals exposed to uncontrollable electric shocks failed subsequently either to learn a response to stop the shocks or to initiate as many escape attempts. In human terms, there was an expectation of helplessness that was generalised to the new situation (Seligman & Peterson, 1986). Learned helplessness theory, and its various reformulations (Abramson, Seligman & Teasdale, 1978; Abramson, Metalsky & Alloy, 1989), posit that the expectation of uncontrollable adverse events leads to depression, but only if the person attributes them to internal, stable and global causes. In this respect, they have much in common with other cognitive theories.

Problems with cognitive theories

Cognitive theories of depression have been of enormous value in generating effective treatments for depression. They have also been useful to the extent that their descriptions of depressive thinking seem accurate. For instance, depressive cognitions discriminate depressed patients from those with anxiety disorder (Beck *et al.*, 1987). However, cognitive models have also encountered a number of difficulties.

The first is that there is evidence that negative styles of thinking may be as much a consequence of depression as a cause. Thus, most measures of depressive thinking recover towards normal after remission from the depressive episode (Simons *et al.*, 1986) as do measures of dysfunctional attitudes (Teasdale, 1988). In addition, psychological treatments that aim to change behaviours rather than cognition are just as effective at altering negative thinking and attributional styles as cognitive therapy (Rehm, Kaslow & Rabin, 1987; Jacobson *et al.*, 1996). Indeed, one study has found that during cognitive therapy the therapist's focus on the impact of distorted cognitions on depressive symptoms correlated negatively with the outcome (Castonguay *et al.*, 1996). These findings are not consistent with the view that negative thoughts are only causing depressed mood, but suggest that they are also either a consequence of depression or a part of the disorder, or both. The second difficulty is that early cognitive models were often interpreted to mean that environmental events are only important to the extent that they trigger negative styles of thinking. This neglects the large body of evidence that social and environmental factors are important in the aetiology of depression.

These problems have led to a number of reformulations of cognitive theories. For instance, cognitive theories now acknowledge the importance of environmental stressors, while retaining the idea that there may be specific cognitive vulnerabilities (Beck, 1983). There has also been much interest in the role that negative cognitions could have in maintaining depression. Thus, Teasdale and Barnard (1993) have presented an analysis of depression in which negative schemata are both a cause and a consequence of depression. Their formulation of depression has a much greater emphasis on understanding how depression is maintained. Individuals who are vulnerable to depression are hypothesised to have a tendency to establish a 'depressive interlock' in which an initial mild depressive reaction becomes intensified.

Cognitive–behaviour therapy in depressed adults

Cognitive therapy includes a variety of cognitive and behavioural techniques designed to identify and resolve the problems of depressed patients. These methods have been described elsewhere (Beck *et al.*, 1979; Burns, 1980), but the following points are relevant to this chapter.

Cognitive–behaviour therapy is a relatively short-term form of treatment, which in the United Kingdom seldom takes more than 15 to 20 sessions and may be as brief as eight sessions (Shapiro *et al.*, 1995). The therapy is active in the sense that the therapist directs the sessions towards the discussion of certain selected problems. There is an emphasis on questioning of the patient by the therapist, both to elicit negative styles of thinking and to reveal inconsistencies in this thinking. However, CBT is a *collaborative* process in which the patient and the therapist are jointly engaged in identifying and solving specific problems. Much use is made of homework assignments in which the patient is asked to carry out certain tasks outside of the sessions, such as generating several alternative interpretations of a situation. Therapy sessions typically begin with a review of homework tasks, and then with explicit tasks for that session. Each session concludes with the setting of further homework.

There are many independently developed cognitive–behavioural programmes. Some have a focus on increasing the depressed person's level of activity using behavioural methods. Others focus on changing negative cognitions. However, there is a great deal of overlap between these programmes and, as they have evolved, they have tended to become more similar to one another (Rehm, 1995). The following account of cognitive–behavioural therapy with depressed adults is taken from a standard text on the topic (Fennell, 1989).

In the early sessions there is often an emphasis on improving mood and other symptoms of depression. Therapy tends to focus on behavioural changes such as increasing activity levels. This is because many of the symptoms of depression, such as poor concentration, make it difficult for the patient to focus on abstract concepts such as attitudes. As the therapy progresses, the process focuses more on cognitions. Patients are encouraged to investigate systematically their own thoughts and circumstances using techniques such as thought diaries. Once negative thoughts are identified, the patient and therapist work out ways of dealing with them. For example, the therapist will often teach the patient ways of identifying and correcting negative automatic thoughts. The patient may also be helped to identify the negative schema and attitudes that usually underlie these negative thoughts, such as that 'I shall never be happy until I am loved by everyone'. The therapist then helps the patient to challenge these negative assumptions, – 'cognitive restructuring'.

The cognitive–behavioural therapies have been evaluated in numerous studies of depressed adults. Rehm (1995) identified 44 studies in which cognitive or behavioural treatment programmes were compared either with no treatment or with other forms of therapy. There were no substantial differences between the four categories of CBT identified by Rehm – behavioural, social skills, cognitive and self-management therapies. In 27 studies it was found that CBT was superior to no treatment, with just five studies finding it equal.

There are, however, some important unresolved issues regarding the efficacy of CBT. The first is that little of the research conducted up to now has been based on clinically representative samples (Hollon, Shelton & Davis, 1993). The second issue is whether CBT is any better than the current standard of treatment for clinically depressed adults, antidepressant medication. Although CBT has usually done quite well when compared with pharmacotherapy (Jacobson & Hollon, 1996), there are concerns about the methods used in these comparative trials. For instance, few of these studies have included a pill-placebo group, so it is unclear as to whether the sample was drug responsive (Klein, 1996). In the NIMH comparative study, CBT appears to have been less effective than drugs in severely depressed cases (Klein & Ross, 1993). There are now doubts as to whether CBT has a prophylactic effect. The findings from early studies that CBT was better than drugs at preventing relapse (e.g. Evans et al. (1992) were based on small samples that may have been particularly responsive to CBT. In the NIMH study, none of the treatments produced full recovery and lasting remission for most cases of depression (Shea et al., 1992).

We can conclude that although CBT appears to be an effective short-term treatment for moderately depressed adults, it probably does not work in the way that cognitive theory suggests. Moreover, the claim that CBT is the only treatment, psychological or otherwise, to prevent relapse has not yet been proven.

Cognitive theories of depression in young people

Support for cognitive–behavioural theories of depression in children and adolescents comes from: (a) evidence of cognitive and behavioural abnormalities in these young people, and (b) data on cognitive development in the general population.

Cognitive and behavioural abnormalities in depressed young people

Several cross-sectional studies have documented an association between depression in young people and negative cognitions similar to those described in depressed adults (reviewed by Harrington, 1993). For instance, McCauley and colleagues (1988) found that depressed children showed significantly lower self-esteem and more hopelessness, externalised locus of control and negative attributional style than children with other psychiatric disorders. Depressed young people also have less social self-confidence than youngsters with other psychiatric problems (Marton et al., 1993) and more negative cognitions than adolescents with anxiety disorder (Laurent & Stark, 1993). This association between depression and negative cognitions is present from early adolescence, with little in the way of age trends (Garber, Weiss & Stanley, 1993).

Although these associations are reasonably robust, their meaning is still unclear. Some longitudinal studies have shown that negative styles of thinking such as attributional style can precede depressive *symptoms* (Seligman & Peterson, 1986; Nolen-Hoeksema, Girgus & Seligman, 1992; Robinson, Garber & Hilsman, 1995) but studies of children with depressive *disorders* have generally shown that depressive cognitions are often transient phenomena, closely linked to depression itself. For instance, in a study of the children of women with affective disorders, Hammen and co-workers (Hammen, Adrian & Hiroto, 1988) found that depressive disorder at follow-up was best predicted by initial symptoms and life events, but not by negative attributions. Asarnow and Bates (1988) reported that inpatient children whose depressive disorder had remitted did not show negative attributional patterns. Similarly, in a large cross-sectional study of adolescents in the community, Gotlib and colleagues (1993) reported that both negative cognitions and negative attributional style were more common in depressed adolescents than in adolescents whose depressive disorder had remitted. In addition, preliminary findings indicate that the response of depressed adolescents to CBT is not linked to changes in negative cognitions (Lewinsohn *et al.*, 1990; Jaycox *et al.*, 1994).

The empirical status of cognitive theories of depression among the young is therefore similar to that of adults. There is substantial support for cognitive theory's descriptive account of the thinking of depressed young people to the extent that, as predicted, depressed youngsters have more negative cognitions than non-depressed people. However, at present there is little support for a role of these cognitions in causing depressive disorder.

It should be borne in mind, however, that some cognitive theories hypothesise that dysfunctional beliefs are latent, unless primed by a stressor (Beck, 1983). It may be that the studies conducted so far on depressed children and adolescents have not been an appropriate test of cognitive theory's predictions. A more pertinent test could be to use some kind of mood induction procedure that would uncover the hypothesised latent cognitions. Moreover, there are several reasons for thinking that straightforward downward extensions of psychological models developed with adults may not be appropriate for young people. First, the reliability of many measures of negative cognitions that were first developed for use in adults is low in children (Robins & Hinkley, 1989). Second, in many cognitive theories (e.g. Beck) negative styles of thinking are the result of childhood adversity. As Cole and Turner (1993) point out, this implies that in childhood negative cognitive style does not exist before adversity, but arises out of it. Cognitive style may not be a stable trait-like characteristic in young people. Third, there are developmental changes in children's abilities both to experience and to report many depression-related cognitions (Rutter, 1986).

Developmental changes in depressive cognitions

There is evidence that children are capable of recognising their own emotional states from as young as two years (Kagan, 1982), and during the pre-school years children start to differentiate the basic emotions and to understand their meaning (Kovacs, 1986). However, even if they experience repeated failure, pre-school children are not easily discouraged and they only rarely show evidence of learned helplessness (Rholes *et al.*, 1980; Harter, 1983). According to Piaget, children in this stage of pre-operational thought (age 18 months to 7 years) have an egocentric view of life. Their thinking is often slow and they have difficulties seeing the wood for the trees.

With the onset of concrete operational thinking (age range 7 to 11 years) the child begins to discover what is consistent in the course of any change or transformation (Piaget, 1970). Thus, when faced with a contradiction between thought and perception (a central idea in cognitive theories of depression – see above), the child can start to make logical decisions. Egocentrism declines at around the age of 7 to 8 years. The child starts to develop self-consciousness (Harter, 1983) and begins to evaluate his or her own competence by comparison with others (Dweck & Elliot, 1983). Self is perceived more and more in psychological terms than in physical terms (Cicchetti & Schneider-Rosen, 1986) and concepts such as guilt and shame become more prominent. Enduring and relatively stable negative attributions about the self therefore become possible. At the same time the child's emotional vocabulary expands, and children start to make fine-grain distinctions between emotions such as sadness and anger. In other words, by around the age of 8 to 11 years, children can experience many of the cognitions that are found in adult depression (Kovacs, 1986).

Modifications of cognitive–behaviour therapy when used with children and adolescents

Developmental level

It does not necessarily follow, however, that 8–11-year-old children are mature enough to undergo cognitive therapy in the same way as adults. For a patient to have cognitive therapy in the way described above it is necessary to have not only the ability to experience negative cognitions, but also the capabilities to reflect on these cognitions and to engage in complex reasoning in which different hypotheses are evaluated and alternative solutions to problems are generated. It seems that children have limitations in some of these respects.

Thus, a key feature of many cognitive therapies with adult patients is the ability to reflect on one's psychological interior and to consider private attributes of the self such as thoughts and feelings. Some of these are real and concrete but others are hypothetical. For instance, dysfunctional assumptions such as 'my value as a person depends on what others think of me' (Beck *et al.*, 1979) are abstract higher-order generalisations about the self that require the integration of the construct of personal value in relation to the opinions of others. In many accounts of cognitive therapy, the identification and challenging of such assumptions or schemes are important components of treatment (Beck *et al.*, 1979), particularly of preventative interventions (Fennell, 1989). Indeed, it has been suggested that the cognitive therapies should have an increasing focus on the schematic level (Teasdale & Barnard, 1993). Yet in Piagetian theory this kind of abstract generalisation is only made possible by the advances in logicomathematical operations that Piaget called *formal operational thought*, which occur during middle adolescence.

Now, it is important to note that recent evidence has raised questions about the validity of the original formal operations theory. For instance, it is unclear whether changes in logical abilities are the source of these age-related changes or whether they stem from other changes such as memory capacity. In educational circles there has been a move away from the view that these developments place intrinsic limits on the ability of adolescents to think logically and an increasing recognition that early attention to the development of critical thinking can increase the likelihood of its emergence (Keating, 1990). Moreover, many components of cognitive–behaviour therapy do not require abstract thinking, but rather the ability to reason effectively in relation to concrete, practical matters.

There are, however, also developmental changes in young people's ability to reason that extend into adolescence and that are likely to influence the ability to undertake CBT. Thus, a key task in many of the cognitive therapies is to evaluate the evidence for and against a particular belief, such as the automatic thought 'my friends don't want to know me' (Beck *et al.*, 1979; Burns, 1980). In a series of studies that explored the growth of scientific reasoning, Kuhn and colleagues (Kuhn, Amsel & O'Loughlin, 1988) found that the ability to hold mental representations of the 'theory' versus the 'evidence' emerged only gradually during adolescence. Children tended to ignore the evidence against their beliefs. Early adolescents still had difficulty keeping theory and evidence separate, and it was only by middle adolescence that most individuals had developed some skill at separating theory from evidence.

It will be appreciated that many adults have problems in evaluating evidence for and against theories. Cognitive therapists, for example, have not always been able to assimilate the evidence that contradicts their belief that CBT is the most effective treatment for depression! However, the data suggest that adolescence is a transitional period in cognitive development and that therefore CBT cannot be applied unmodified to children and adolescents, but must be flexible and shaped for the young person's developmental level. The therapeutic programme cannot be prescribed in a set order, cookbook fashion. This does not mean that complicated cognitive hypotheses cannot be discussed with adolescents. Many adolescent patients are very interested in talking about thinking. But it does mean that no assumptions should be made about the kinds of techniques that may or may not be useful.

Therapist stance

It follows that the therapist's stance must be as an *educator*. In describing the posture of the cognitive therapist with children and adolescents, Kendall (1991) puts this nicely: '. . . educator here is intended to communicate that we are talking about interventions for learning behaviour control, cognitive skills, and emotional development, and we are talking about optimal ways to communicate to help someone to learn. A good educator stimulates the students to think – to think for themselves'. It is particularly important that the therapist works *collaboratively* with the patient. No hypotheses about the causes of depression should be imposed by the therapist. For instance, there can be no assumptions about the presence of hypothetical, fixed underlying cognitive schemata that cause the disorder. There is little empirical evidence for such schemata in children.

The context of cognitive–behaviour therapy

It is also very important to recognise that CBT with adolescents does not take place in a vacuum, but in a social context. There are several implications. First, it may be necessary to involve the family in the therapy. In our programme (see below) the family has relatively little direct involvement in individual therapy, though it is very common for some other kind of work to take place with the family or with the wider social milieu. Other CBT programmes include the parents in parallel sessions in which they are given information about depression and the possible contributing factors and instructed on how to be supportive during the therapy (Hops & Lewinsohn, 1995).

The second point is that CBT with adolescents should not neglect the importance of environmental factors in precipitating and maintaining depression. Therapists need to remember that sometimes the thinking of depressed adolescents is realistic. It may be true that their parents hate them! In such cases it is usually better to use treatments that aim to alleviate depressive symptoms and which help patients to solve their relationship problems rather than dwelling on their thinking patterns.

Efficacy of cognitive–behaviour therapy in depressed young people

No psychological treatment for depressed children and adolescents has been as thoroughly evaluated as CBT. Three kinds of studies provide information on the efficacy of CBT in depressed young people – case studies, randomised comparative studies in non-diagnosed school-based samples, and randomised studies in clinically diagnosed samples.

Case studies

There have been a number of case reports about CBT in depressed children and adolescents (Petti *et al.*, 1980; Frame *et al.*, 1982; Asarnow & Carlson, 1988; Wilkes & Rush, 1988; Vostanis & Harrington, 1994) and several books contain detailed descriptions of CBT with depressed young people (Stark, 1990; Wilkes *et al.*, 1994). These illustrate how CBT can be used with a variety of different kinds of depression, including psychotic depression (Asarnow & Carlson, 1988) and depression in children with mild intellectual retardation (Petti *et al.*, 1980).

Studies in non-diagnosed school-based samples

At least five randomised comparative studies have investigated the value of cognitive–behavioural therapies in samples selected from school settings on the basis of cut-off scores on depression questionnaires, but without diagnostic assessments (Reynolds & Coats, 1986; Stark, Reynolds & Kaslow, 1987; Kahn *et al.*, 1990; Liddle & Spence, 1990; Stark, Rouse & Livingston, 1991). The results are summarised in Table 10.1. In four of the five studies, cognitive–behavioural interventions have been significantly more effective in reducing depressive symptoms than no-treatment, with an effect size (the difference between the mean score for the CBT group and the mean score for the no treatment group, divided by the standard deviation) in most studies exceeding 1.0 (Vostanis & Harrington, 1994). This is considered relatively large in psychological therapy outcome research (Kazdin & Bass, 1989). In two non-randomised comparative studies, CBT was found to be significantly superior to a waiting-list control condition (Butler *et al.*, 1980; Jaycox *et al.*, 1994).

Studies in clinically diagnosed samples: preliminary results from a meta-analysis

It will be appreciated that the results from non-diagnosed samples, which clearly show that CBT is better than no treatment, may not apply to clinically diagnosed cases. Indeed, the results from diagnosed samples have been less clear-cut, with some studies showing that CBT is significantly better than the comparison condition and others not.

Many of these studies have been based on relatively small sample sizes and therefore it is difficult to tell if negative results were really negative or whether they were due to insufficient statistical power. This is a common problem in treatment outcome research across the whole of medicine and psychology, where it has become common practice to obtain a more definitive conclusion by combining the results from different studies using a set of techniques called meta-analysis. Meta-analysis comprises two stages, a systematic search of the literature and other sources to identify all eligible studies, and the statistical combination of the data from these studies. The statistical part of a meta-analysis can be conducted either on continuous data (e.g. a depression score) or on categorical data (e.g. depressive disorder or not). In the present chapter, we have confined our analysis to the question of whether or not cases still had depressive disorder because (a) the key issue in studies of clinically diagnosed cases is not whether they are a little less depressed but whether they still have the disorder, and (b) two studies (Hops & Lewinsohn, 1995; Brent *et al.*, submitted) have not yet published their full quantitative results but have published data on clinical improvement. To avoid publication bias, it is important such studies are included.

The meta-analysis was carried out with methods similar to those used by Hazell and colleagues (1995), who conducted a meta-analysis of the efficacy of tricyclic drugs in child and adolescent depression. The literature was searched using Medline (1966–94),

Table 10.1. Randomised comparative studies of cognitive or behavioural interventions in non-diagnosed depressed children in school samples

Reference	Age (years)	n	Selection criteria	Outcome criteria	Results*
Reynolds & Coats (1986)	Mean 15.6	30	BDI BID RADS	BDI BID RADS	CBT = RT > NT
Stark et al. (1987)	9–12	29	CDI	CDI	SC = BPS > NT
Kahn et al. (1990)	10–14	68	BDI BID RADS	BDI BID RADS	CBT = RT = SM > NT
Liddle & Spence (1990)	7–11	31	CDI CDRS	CDI CDRS	CBT = AP = NT
Stark (1990)	Approximately 9–12	24	Self-report Interview	Interview	CBT > AP

* =, not significantly different; >, significantly better than.
Therapy conditions: CBT = cognitive–behaviour therapy; RT = relaxation training; NT = no treatment (e.g. waiting list); AP = attention placebo (e.g. non-specific counselling); SC = self-control; SM = self-modelling; BPS = behavioural problem solving.
Depression assessment instruments: BDI = Beck Depression Inventory; BID = Bellevue Index of Depression; CDI = Children's Depression Inventory; RADS = Reynold's Adolescent Depression Scale; RCDS Reynold's Child Depression Scale. CDRS = Children's Depression Rating Scale.

Psych-lit and Excerpta Medica. Abstracts of English papers were reviewed. Reference lists from recent reviews and book chapters were searched. Authors of abstracts identified in conference proceedings were contacted for details of their studies. Studies were included in the meta-analysis if they described subjects between 6 and 18 years who were diagnosed as suffering from a depressive disorder and if they randomised to a cognitive–behavioural intervention or to a comparison condition. In line with recent reviews of CBT in both adults and children (Kendall, 1991; Andrews, 1996), a broad definition of CBT was used that included behavioural (e.g. social skills training) as well as cognitive interventions. Most studies used multiple outcome measures and for the purposes of pooling results, a single best estimate of the proportion who had 'improved' in each study was obtained. In all instances this meant that the subjects no longer had a depressive disorder.

Seven studies were identified (Lewinsohn *et al.*, 1990; Fine *et al.*, 1991; Clarke *et al.*, 1995; Hops & Lewinsohn, 1995; Vostanis *et al.*, 1996; Wood *et al.*, 1996b; Brent *et al.*, submitted) for inclusion in the meta-analysis and Table 10.2 summarises the descriptive information for each study. Six of these studies were based on cases with a current diagnosis of depressive disorder. One was based on cases with high levels of depressive symptoms, of whom nearly a half had a previous diagnosis of depressive or other emotional disorder (Clarke *et al.*, 1995). Six of the studies used the term 'cognitive–behaviour therapy' to describe the treatment, but the study of Fine and co-workers on social-skills training was included because such training is a well-recognised component of some of the cognitive–behaviour therapies (Rehm, 1995), such as the Coping with Depression Course of Lewinsohn and his colleagues (1985).

Usable data on the proportion of cases who improved with each intervention could be extracted from all the studies, and are summarised in Table 10.3. For each study we estimated the ratio of the odds of improvement in the group having CBT compared with the group having another intervention. An odds ratio greater than one indicates that a larger proportion improved in the CBT group than in the comparison group. In six out of seven studies, the odds ratio was greater than one, and in three studies the 95 per cent confidence interval did not include one, indicating a significant difference in favour of CBT.

Following the methods of Hazell *et al.* (1995), we pooled the data from these studies to calculate the overall proportion improved with the cognitive–behaviour therapies (171/257 or 66.5 per cent) and the overall proportion improved with the comparison conditions (123/253 or 48.6 per cent). We then calculated the pooled odds ratio, which was 2.10 (95 per cent confidence interval 1.47 to 3.00), meaning that across the pooled studies CBT was significantly superior to the comparison interventions.

In interpreting the results of these studies, it is important to bear in mind that because of the high rate of improvement in the combined comparison groups (average 49 per cent), a trial would require around 145 cases per group to detect an odds ratio for improvement of 2.0 with a power of 80 per cent. This meta-analysis therefore had more than enough power to detect a significant difference between CBT and the comparison

Table 10.2. Overview of outcome studies of cognitive or behavioural interventions in clinically diagnosed samples of depressed children or adolescents

Reference	Age (years)	Gender (F:M)	Comparison condition/s	Outcome measure	Sample
Lewinsohn et al. (1990)	Mean 16.3	36:23	Waiting list	K-SADS	Various community samples
Fine et al. (1991)	13–17	83% female	Therapeutic support	K-SADS	Outpatients
Clarke et al. (1995)	Mean 15.3	105:20	Usual care	K-SADS	Community
Hops & Lewinsohn (1995)	Adolescent	Not known	Waiting list	K-SADS	Various community samples
Vostanis et al. (1996)	8–17	32:25	Non-focused intervention	K-SADS	Outpatients
Wood et al. (1996b)	9–17	33:15	Relaxation training	K-SADS	Outpatients
Brent et al. (submitted)	Mean 15.7	81:26	Family therapy or supportive therapy	K-SADS	Outpatients

K-SADS = Schedule for Affective Disorders and Schizophrenia for School aged Children.
In the study of Fine et al. (1991), allocation to treatment was not strictly random, but rather was based on the near-random method of allocating consecutive cases to the next available group.

Table 10.3. Results, expressed as numbers improved in each group, in studies of cognitive or behavioural interventions in clinically diagnosed samples of depressed children or adolescents

	Criteria for improvement	Number improved with CBT	Number improved with intervention	Odds ratio (95% confidence interval)
Lewinsohn et al. (1990)	No depressive disorder	18/40	1/19	14.73 (1.79–121.21)
Fine et al. (1991)	K-SADS rating < 4 on dysphoric or anhedonic ratings	4/10	8/16	0.66 (0.13–3.30)
Clarke et al. (1995)	No depressive disorder	47/55	52/70	2.03 (0.81–5.11)
Hops & Lewinsohn (1995)	No depressive disorder	43/64	15/32	2.32 (0.97–5.53)
Vostanis et al. (1996)	No depressive disorder	25/29	21/28	2.08 (0.53–8.10)
Wood et al. (1996b)	K-SADS rating < 3 on depression and anhedonia	13/24	5/24	4.49 (1.26–16.00)
Brent et al. (submitted)	No depressive disorder and BDI < 9 on at least three occasions	21/35	21/64	3.07 (1.31–7.22)
Pooled results		171/257	123/253	2.10 (1.47–3.00)

Hops & Lewinsohn (1995): the numbers were estimated from percentages in the text.
Clarke. et al. (1995): significant differences between the two groups were found in respect of time to the next episode of depression.
BDI, Beck Depression Inventory.

conditions, but none of the trials published thus far has even approached this figure. The high rate of improvement in some of the comparison groups also underlines the point that many depressed cases will improve either with other interventions or with no treatment at all. This suggests that in many instances it would be better that CBT is preceded by other, simpler forms of treatment and that CBT is reserved for those cases who fail to respond.

Conversely, the finding that a third of cases fail to improve after CBT underlines the importance of either using longer-terms forms of CBT or of combining CBT with other forms of treatment. It is also worth noting that two studies in clinical samples have found that although, as a group, adolescents who have had CBT retain the gains that they have made during treatment, a significant proportion of individuals (around one third) relapse during the six months after treatment has finished (Wood *et al.*, 1996b). There are grounds, then, for giving some individuals CBT for at least six months after apparent remission, and an uncontrolled pilot study has shown that this is both feasible and effective (Kroll *et al.*, 1996).

At first sight, the findings from the present meta-analysis might seem to suggest that CBT is superior to medication. In their meta-analysis of the efficacy of tricyclic medication in child and adolescent depressive disorder, Hazell and colleagues (1995) found that tricyclic medication was not significantly better than placebo (pooled odds ratio of 1.08 across five studies) and that the overall improvement rate with active drug was just 38 per cent, considerably less than the overall improvement rate found in the CBT studies (60 per cent). However, it must be borne in mind that there have so far been no published randomised comparisons of drug and placebo, and that cases admitted to CBT trials have often been less severely affected than those admitted to trials of medication. Indeed, in an analysis of predictors of response to CBT we found that adolescents with severe depressive disorders seldom improved with CBT (Jayson *et al.*, in preparation).

In summary, the data reviewed here suggest that the cognitive–behavioural therapies are an effective treatment for many clinically depressed adolescents. However, the data also suggest that CBT should be used as part of a treatment strategy that includes both an initial brief supportive intervention and other interventions for the cases in which CBT is ineffective. Moreover, it cannot be assumed that CBT will be useful in severely depressed adolescents.

Who responds to the cognitive–behaviour therapies?
Information is lacking about which depressed adolescents respond to CBT. Three main kinds of predictors have been examined thus far: factors within the child, factors in the child's environment, and characteristics of the therapy or therapist.

Child factors
Probably the most consistent finding has been that severely depressed adolescents are less likely to respond to CBT than moderately depressed cases. Thus, using data from the first Oregon study (Lewinsohn *et al.*, 1990), Clarke and colleagues (1992) found that

better outcome was associated with lower initial levels of self-reported depression. Similarly, in an analysis of the combined data from the two Manchester studies (Kroll *et al.*, 1996; Wood *et al.*, 1996b), Jayson *et al.* (in preparation) found that adolescents with high levels of social impairment were less likely to respond to CBT than those with low levels of impairment. Adolescents with a Global Assessment Scale (Shaffer *et al.*, 1983) score of 30 or less (unable to function in most areas) were unlikely to respond to CBT. Both the Oregon studies and the Manchester studies have shown that younger age is associated with an increased likelihood of remission, but this may be a non-specific effect of the high placebo response rates that occur in the younger age groups. In the first Oregon study, better outcome was associated with a lower level of initial anxiety.

Environmental factors
There is some evidence that greater involvement of parents in therapy is associated with a better response to CBT (Lewinsohn *et al.*, 1996) and that children who come from backgrounds with higher levels of psychosocial stress are less likely to respond (Jayson *et al.*, 1997).

Therapist and therapy factors
Little is known about how the quality of therapy relates to outcome. Jayson *et al.* found seniority of therapist did not predict outcome. Feehan and Vostanis (1996) reported that greater compliance with therapy was associated with a better outcome, but they did not control for severity of initial disorder.

Practice: the adolescent Depression Treatment Programme

Characteristics of the Depression Treatment Programme
Over the past seven years, groups in Manchester and Birmingham in the UK have been developing a cognitive–behavioural programme for the treatment of depressive disorders in clinical samples of depressed adolescents (Vostanis & Harrington, 1994; Feehan & Vostanis, 1996; Kroll *et al.*, 1996; Vostanis *et al.*, 1996; Wood *et al.*, 1996b). The Depression Treatment Programme (DTP) has several characteristics.

First, it is based on a theoretical model of depressive disorder that acknowledges the role of a variety of different factors (Fig. 10.1). It is assumed that the depressive syndrome is the result of both environmental and genetic influences. These can act directly to produce the syndrome or indirectly through their effects on certain dimensions of personality. Environmental factors are seen as important precipitants of the disorder, but it is acknowledged that depressed people can act in ways that increase stress. The treatment programme is therefore concerned not only with the alleviation of depressive symptoms but also with how depressed people deal with adversity. It is also presumed that once the depressive syndrome has become established, the symptoms can

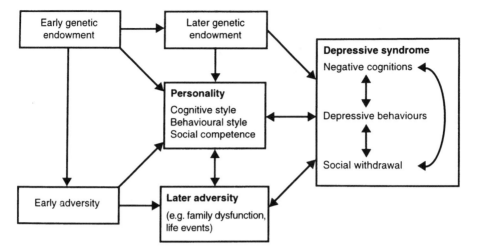

Figure 10.1. Theoretical model of depressive disorder in adolescence. Arrows show the direction of a causal relationship.

have substantial self-perpetuating properties. For instance, negative self-evaluations lead to increasing social withdrawal, which in turn leads to lower self-esteem, and so on.

Second, it is assumed that depressive disorder has heterogeneous causes and that children and adolescents will vary in their abilities to understand and use cognitive–behavioural techniques. Therefore, the programme contains a set of treatment modules that can be tailored to the needs of the individual patient. Thus, the young person who has difficulties forming relationships is taught social skills and social problem solving; the young person whose negative cognitions are prominent will be taught self-monitoring, and so on. Treatment that is relevant to the needs of the individual will enhance compliance. There is no assumption that every child will complete all of the modules.

Third, the programme has been specifically designed to tackle the problems that are found in clinically diagnosed depressed young people. Descriptive studies have consistently shown that such people have three main sets of symptoms: (a) negative styles of thinking, which include low self-esteem, negative attributions and negative cognitions (Hammen et al., 1988; McCauley et al., 1988; Gotlib et al., 1993; Lewinsohn, Rohde & Seeley, 1993); (b) difficulties with social relationships (Puig-Antich et al., 1985a, 1985b, 1993; Goodyer et al., 1991); and (c) behavioural symptoms of depression, such as poor sleep and inactivity (Ryan et al., 1987; Mitchell et al., 1988; Kolvin et al., 1991). The programme has a particular emphasis on dealing with these problems, as well as on problems that are closely linked to depression in clinical samples, such as suicidal attempts.

Fourth, because in the UK there are few training opportunities for child care professionals to learn cognitive–behavioural approaches, the programme is designed for use by child mental health professionals who need have only some knowledge of cognitive–

behavioural theory and therapies. In the studies we have conducted so far, therapists go on a brief two-day introductory course and then have supervised training on at least three cases. The DTP has an emphasis on relatively simple and easy-to-learn behavioural and cognitive tasks, and a version for non-mental health professionals is currently being evaluated.

Development of the Depression Treatment Programme

The programme is similar to the group-based forms of psychological treatment that have been used in non-clinical samples (Butler *et al.*, 1980; Reynolds & Coats, 1986; Stark, 1990; Stark *et al.*, 1987; Kahn *et al.*, 1990; Lewinsohn *et al.*, 1990; Jaycox *et al.*, 1994) but is an individual rather than a group therapy. There were two main reasons for developing an individual therapy. First, depressed patients often present in crisis, such as occurs after an overdose, and require immediate help. Even in large centres it can take weeks to accumulate enough cases to set up a group. Second, in individual therapy it is possible to tailor the programme to the therapeutic and developmental needs of the child.

Like many of the CBT programmes developed for use with adult patients, the DTP has been revised on several occasions to reflect the lessons learned from clinical trials. The first version (Vostanis & Harrington, 1994), which was based on treatment programmes used for the group treatment of depression in non-clinical samples (Reynolds & Coats, 1986; Stark, 1990), had ten treatment modules and there was an expectation that the patient would usually complete all of the modules. This was found to be an effective treatment for children with mostly minor depression (Feehan & Vostanis, 1996; Vostanis *et al.*, 1996), though not significantly better than the comparison intervention (any other finding would have been difficult given that 75 per cent of the comparison group remitted). In the next revision of the programme, there was a greater emphasis on assessment and on tailoring the programme to the needs of the child. It was not assumed that all patients would complete all of the modules. The revised programme was tested in another clinical trial, this time with adolescents diagnosed as having major depression, and was found to be significantly superior to a psychological control treatment, relaxation training (Wood *et al.*, 1996b). However, in the study of Wood and colleagues, which was based on a five-to-eight session programme over eight weeks, there was a high rate of relapse within the two months following apparent remission. Therefore a longer-term version of the programme was piloted in an uncontrolled trial and was found to be associated with a significantly lower relapse rate than in the study of Wood and co-workers (Kroll *et al.*, 1996). The current version of the DTP therefore lasts for some 10 to 14 sessions spread over 10 to 12 weeks and includes four booster sessions over the next eight weeks.

Components of the Depression Treatment Programme

The DTP is mainly intended for use with adolescent patients aged between 11 and 18 years who have a diagnosis of major depression. The assessment procedures and the treatment components have been specified in a manual, and a training videotape is also available.

General assessment

Assessment of adolescents who present with symptoms of depression begins with diagnosis. Standardised diagnostic systems such as the *Diagnostic and statistical manual* (American Psychiatric Association, 1994) and structured psychiatric interviews can help in deciding whether the patient has serious symptomatology that requires treatment. Unfortunately, these diagnostic systems tend to be overinclusive in this age group, and many dysphoric adolescents who meet criteria for so-called major depression remit within a month (Kerfoot *et al.*, 1996). It is important, then, that careful enquiry is made about the impact that the adolescent's symptoms have had on everyday functioning and about the presence of symptoms of unequivocal psychopathological significance, such as suicidal planning or marked weight loss. Probably the best single indicator of whether or not an adolescent has a serious depressive disorder is the duration of the problem. Polysymptomatic depressive states that persist for more than four weeks usually require treatment. In our clinic, severity of depression is also assessed by a depression scale, the Mood and Feelings Questionnaire (MFQ; Angold *et al.*, 1987), which has been validated in clinical trials with depressed adolescents (Wood *et al.*, 1995). The MFQ is also a useful way to monitor treatment response.

Assessment of the depressed adolescent should also include careful enquiry about comorbid disorders, particularly anxiety and conduct disorders. In research settings it is common to diagnose depressive disorder in adolescents *regardless* of comorbid disorders. However, in clinical practice it is much better to reserve the diagnosis for cases in which depression is a prominent part of the clinical picture. Such cases are more likely to persist (Harrington *et al.*, 1990).

Although the accurate diagnosis of depressive disorder is an important part of clinical management, assessment only starts with the diagnosis, not stops with it. Aetiology should be assessed next, with respect to precipitating, predisposing and maintaining factors. No attempt to allocate the syndrome to an exclusively endogenous or reactive category should be made. Instead the importance of both external and internal causes should be assessed in every case. Depressed adolescents usually have multiple problems such as educational failure and impaired psychosocial functioning. They find it harder to make and maintain friendships than their peers and they tend to come from families with high rates of mental illness. There is often a precipitant for the episode of depression and some depressed adolescents have been maltreated or abused. All these problems need to be identified and the causes of each assessed.

The final part of the general assessment involves the evaluation of the adolescent's personal and social resources. There is evidence that being successful at school or in other areas of life can protect young people from the effects of adverse life experiences (Quinton, Rutter & Liddle, 1984). The best guide to the adolescent's ability to solve future problems is his or her record in dealing with difficulties in the past. The ability of the family to support the adolescent should also be evaluated.

Cognitive–behavioural assessment

The cognitive–behavioural assessment is sometimes conducted at the same time as the general assessment, but more often requires a separate session. This session begins by setting meeting days and times. The therapist helps the adolescent to identify specific concerns and perceptions of why he or she is in therapy. The adolescent's reasons for attendance and objectives for the therapy are then defined. It is important for the therapist to help the adolescent identify the main problems. The focus of therapeutic intervention (goals of therapy) should be at the target symptom level. These target symptoms may be broken down into the following categories (Beck *et al.*, 1979): affective symptoms, motivational (e.g. wish to harm self), cognitive (e.g. concentration impairment, memory problems), behavioural (e.g. social withdrawal) and vegetative (e.g. sleep, appetite disturbance).

The therapist determines with the patient which symptom is most distressing and will be most amenable to therapeutic intervention. When goals of therapy have been negotiated, the child is encouraged to record these, and the emphasis of future therapy sessions can be determined. Using information from the general assessment, information is obtained on symptoms, life problems, interpersonal and social problems, associated negative thoughts, context of depression and hopelessness or suicidal thoughts. It is not necessary at this stage to know everything about the patient. The goal is to get an overall picture of the present situation as the adolescent sees it. This involves pinpointing major problems, and gathering enough information about associated thoughts to make a preliminary formulation of the case.

A problem list is then drawn up. Drawing up an agreed problem list gives the patient immediate experience of CBT as a collaborative enterprise. It helps the therapist to understand the patient's perspective, and allows the patient to feel that a genuine effort is being made to grasp his or her personal difficulties. It is crucial when working with depressed children to identify hopelessness and suicidal thoughts.

Goals in relation to each problem area are then defined. It is very important to explain to children that the aim of therapy is to try to help with just some of their difficulties. Some adolescents feel completely better after the treatment, but most are helped in a few, but not all, areas (depressed people have multiple difficulties). This is a most important message because unless adolescents have a realistic view of the likely efficacy of treatment, they may become disappointed that they are not completely better at the end of treatment and blame themselves for not improving more.

There are ten treatment sessions. Each includes a *review* of homework instructions, an *introduction* to the themes of the session, *tasks*, *practice* and *homework* assignments.

Emotional recognition and self-monitoring

Depressed young people may have difficulties in identifying their own or other people's emotions. They also have difficulty in distinguishing between different types of emotions. They tend to perceive thoughts, emotions and activities as part of the same factor, which is well beyond their control. The opportunity to define and identify the way they feel, as well as linking feelings, thoughts and activities, often helps them to feel less helpless and more in control of their mood.

In the first session/s the therapist helps the child or adolescent to distinguish between different emotional states and to start linking behaviour and thoughts. This is achieved by encouraging children to describe recent examples of their own experience. In addition, they are asked to recall events and the thoughts that occurred at the time. As the sessions progress, patients are encouraged to monitor their thoughts in more detail and to practise detecting automatic thoughts. This is achieved using various techniques, such as the idea of the 'thought detective'.

Self-reinforcement

All patients should learn about emotional recognition and self-monitoring. The content of the remaining sessions will, however, depend both on the adolescent's capacities and on the nature of the presenting problems. As a general rule, the next two to three sessions are spent on behavioural tasks such as self-reinforcement. The aim is for patients to be able to reinforce desired behaviours and thus gain a sense of control over their symptoms. Adolescents are asked to reward themselves when they complete an agreed task. Parents are often asked to participate in this part of the programme.

Self-reinforcement is often combined with *activity scheduling*, in which patients are urged to increase the number of pleasant activities that they engage in. They are taught to set realistic goals, with small steps towards achieving them, and to reward themselves at each successful step along the way. At this stage, it is quite common to introduce other behavioural techniques to treat behavioural or vegetative symptoms of depression, such as sleep-hygiene measures.

Social problem solving

The idea of setting realistic goals and developing a plan to achieve them is central to social problem solving, which is very commonly the next technique in the programme. The main aim is to give the patient the message that there are several possible solutions to a problem, such as making or repairing a friendship. The adolescent is helped to generate several possible solutions, to choose between them, to put one into effect and to monitor the results. The youngster may also be encouraged to recall examples of previously successful solutions to problems.

Reducing depressive thinking

The DTP also includes several sessions on techniques for reducing depressive thinking, which follow the techniques described by Beck and colleagues (1979). Thus, the adolescent is helped to identify cognitive distortions and to challenge them using techniques such as pro–con evaluation. Techniques to reduce negative automatic thoughts, such as 'focus on object', are also employed.

Final session/s

In the final session or sessions, the adolescent is prepared to deal with future problems. Potentially difficult situations that might arise in the near future are discussed and possible solutions outlined.

Parental involvement and combination with other treatments

Parents are kept fully informed about their child's progress and will often have some involvement in behavioural tasks such as self-reinforcement and activity scheduling. However, unlike some programmes for the treatment of depression in adolescents (Hops & Lewinsohn, 1995), we do not run a full parallel version of the course for parents. The empirical evidence suggests that parallel parental versions of cognitive–behavioural courses for adolescents do not lead to a significantly better outcome than when the course is just given to the adolescent (Lewinsohn *et al.*, 1990). Rather, in the DTP it is assumed that cognitive–behavioural therapy with the adolescent will occur as part of a wider programme that includes a variety of other interventions, including family interventions.

Treatment of comorbid problems

Depression in adolescents frequently occurs in conjunction with other problems, such as educational failure, anxiety symptoms, and problems with peer relationships (Ryan *et al.*, 1987; Kolvin *et al.*, 1991). It is not possible in this chapter to discuss the management of all of these comorbid problems, but two require special consideration: suicidal behaviour and anti-social problems.

Suicidal behaviour

Suicidal behaviour is very common in adolescent major depression. In our treatment studies, around one third of depressed adolescents have presented after an episode of deliberate self-harm (Wood *et al.*, 1996a).

The first step in managing depressed and suicidal adolescents is accurate assessment of the risk of suicidal behaviour. To do this it is necessary to prepare a detailed formulation of the reasons for suicidality. This will mean obtaining a good history from the adolescent and parents, and examining the mental state for features such as suicidal planning and hopelessness. It is important that the risk assessment is repeated regularly and the results recorded in the case notes.

The risk assessment may show that suicidality is part and parcel of a depressive disorder. In such cases, treatment of depressive symptoms with the techniques described above will usually reduce suicidal thinking. In many young people, however, the motives for deliberate self-harm are more complex and imbedded in chronic family or interpersonal difficulties. In such instances it is usually better to direct attention to the alleviation of these problems. It can, however, be difficult to remedy the kinds of problems that are associated with deliberate self-harm, such as chronic family discord, and direct reduction of suicidal thinking with individual therapy is therefore a legitimate form of treatment.

Several cognitive and behavioural techniques are particularly useful in reducing suicidal thinking. Many adolescents have realistic problems that contribute to their feelings of hopelessness and depression and will be helped by problem-solving strategies (Hawton & Catalan, 1982). For others, cognitive techniques can be used to deal with cognitions such as hopelessness. For example, some adolescents regard attempting suicide as the only way out of an intolerable situation. Helping them to become aware of logical inconsistencies in their beliefs using cognitive techniques such as 'what's the evidence' (Beck *et al.*, 1979) will improve their sense of self-competence.

Anti-social behaviour

Around one fifth of depressed children and adolescents also have a conduct disorder, and more than a third have some anti-social symptoms (Puig-Antich, 1982; Marriage *et al.*, 1986; Dadds *et al.*, 1992; Caron *et al.*, 1993). This overlap between depression and conduct disorder raises two important issues concerning the administration of CBT for the depression.

First, does treatment of depression influence the course of the conduct disorder? Follow-up studies suggest that the outcomes of young people with depression and conduct disorder are identical to those of children with conduct disorder – they have high rates of anti-social behaviour and low rates of depression (Harrington *et al.*, 1991). The implication is that the depressive symptoms are in some sense secondary to the conduct disorder. It would not, therefore, be expected that treatment of depression would have much impact on the course of the conduct disorder, and indeed this is exactly what we find in treatment trials of CBT. For instance, in the study of Wood and co-workers (1996b) conduct problems were not significantly reduced either by CBT or by relaxation training. Comorbid conduct disorder therefore requires a separate intervention.

Second, do conduct symptoms alter the response of depressed adolescents to CBT? Our research suggests that they do not, to the extent that conduct disorder does not predict response to CBT (Jayson *et al.*, 1997). However, in our studies we have excluded cases in which anti-social behaviour was so severe that it dominated the clinical picture. The most common examples of such behaviour are serious aggression (e.g. repeated assaults, fire setting) and persistent running away. These kinds of problems make it very difficult to set up and sustain a CBT programme for depression. Moreover, since depression is sometimes the result of environmental factors that have been precipitated by conduct problems, such as hostility from members of the family (Dadds *et al.*, 1992), interventions for conduct problems may eventually reduce depressive symptoms. Therefore, although the presence of conduct disorder is not an absolute contraindication to giving CBT for comorbid depression, when anti-social symptoms dominate the clinical picture it is usually best to deal with these symptoms first. CBT is best reserved for those cases in which either anti-social symptoms are mild or in which interventions for conduct disorder have not led to a reduction of depressive symptoms.

Algorithm for the treatment of moderately severe major depression

The DTP is designed to be combined with other treatments. It is also conceived as part of a *strategy* for managing major depression in adolescents that includes several other stages.

Figure 10.2 shows an algorithm for the management of moderately severe depressive disorder in adolescents. Adolescents with severe depression, which we define as a Global Assessment Scale (Shaffer *et al.*, 1983) score of 30 or less (which means that the adolescent is unable to function in most activities of daily life), seldom respond to the DTP (Jayson *et al.*, 1997).

Line 1. In clinical samples, mild and moderately severe depressive disorders in adolescents remit rapidly in some one third of cases (Harrington & Vostanis, 1995; Kerfoot *et al.*, 1996).

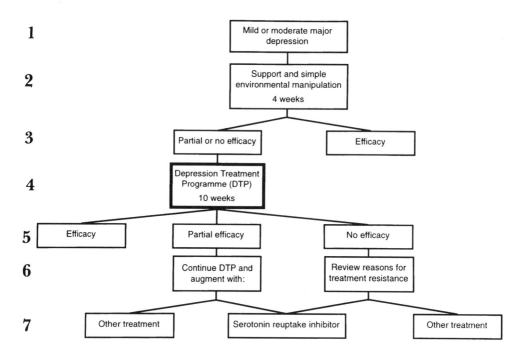

Figure 10.2. Algorithm for the treatment of mild or moderately severe depressive disorder in adolescence.

Line 2. This suggests that a sensible initial approach should consist of a thorough assessment, sympathetic discussions with the adolescent and the family, and encouraging support. These simple interventions, especially if combined with measures to alleviate stress, are often followed by improvement in mood.

Line 3. However, about two thirds of depressed adolescents will not remit within a month, and these cases should be offered further treatment.

Line 4. The best treatment for major depression in adolescence is not yet clearly established, but the meta-analysis presented earlier suggests that CBT is an effective intervention for clinically depressed adolescents. No other psychological intervention for major depression in adolescents has been studied so thoroughly, and therefore although treatments such as interpersonal psychotherapy (Mufson *et al.*, 1993), therapeutic support groups (Fine *et al.*, 1991) and family psycho-educational packages (Beardslee *et al.*, 1993, 1996) are promising, CBT is probably the first-choice psychological treatment. Moreover, controlled studies of the tricyclic antidepressants suggest that they are not significantly better than placebo (Hazell *et al.*, 1995) and tricyclics can be very toxic in overdose (Henry, 1992). Therefore, the cognitive–behavioural therapies are currently the treatment of first choice for moderately severe depression.

Line 5. The meta-analysis suggests that around one third of clinically depressed adolescents will not have improved by the end of the CBT course. However, some of these will have shown a partial response and in such cases we recommend that CBT is continued for a month. Partial response can be defined as improvement in depressive symptoms but still meeting criteria for major depression.

Line 6. By this stage, there are likely to be two groups who still need help, those who have failed to respond or are getting worse and those who have partially improved but are still symptomatic. If an adolescent is resistant to the effects of CBT, then the reasons for this should be reviewed. It may be that other problems besides depression are present. Common causes of treatment resistance include undiagnosed psychosocial stressors such as abuse, chronic family difficulties, and emerging personality problems. Less common but important causes are undiagnosed physical disorders such as endocrine disturbances and drug abuse. Review may also indicate some specific reasons for the failure of CBT. For example, CBT is less effective when given by an inexperienced therapist who tells the adolescent what to do rather than giving the patient the opportunity to work it out on his or her own.

Line 7. If the review does not show a simple way of improving the adolescent's mental state, then a different line in treatment should be pursued. In some instances, this means starting an antidepressant, such as a serotonin specific re-uptake inhibitor. These drugs seems to be less toxic than the tricyclics and there have been encouraging preliminary reports about their efficacy in adolescents (Emslie *et al.*,

1995). In other cases, it may be necessary to provide treatments such as family therapy.

Conclusions

This chapter has summarised the main features and empirical status of cognitive–behaviour therapy in depressed adolescents as well as the theory on which it is based. There is strong support for cognitive theory's descriptive account of symptoms during the acute episode, but this theory has not yet been clearly supported in longitudinal research. Similarly, although cognitive–behaviour therapy has considerable effects on adolescent depressive symptoms, it seems that response to treatment is not dependent on changes in negative cognitions (Lewinsohn *et al.*, 1990; Jaycox *et al.*, 1994). This failure to find a relationship between outcome and changes in putative causal factors is a common issue in all kinds of outcome research, and suggests that more work is required on the mechanisms of therapeutic change. In the meantime, it will be necessary to integrate cognitive–behavioural theories and therapies with other models of the causes and treatment of depression. Cognitive–behaviour therapy is an effective treatment for many depressed young people but it is not a cure-all and needs to be conceptualised as just one part of the treatment strategy.

Case illustrations

Case 1: transition to secondary school and parental separation

This case illustrates the management of a patient who became depressed and anxious in the context of the transition to secondary school and parental separation. The case illustrates the use of simple behavioural and mood-elevating techniques in younger adolescents. It also demonstrates the value of brief, psycho-educational work with the parents.

Background

Neil, aged 11 years, lives with his mother. Neil's mother used to work as a GP's receptionist but has not worked since Neil started school. She describes a depressive illness during her adolescence, for which she received treatment, and has recently been depressed following arguments with her husband and their separation six months ago. She is very religious and has had counselling through her local church. She is reluctant to seek medical treatment. Neil, now the only child, was born after his eldest brother died of a cot death at the age of four months. Both parents acknowledge that they have not grieved for Paul's death and that when Neil was young, they were over-concerned about his health. Neil's father is an engineer and works very long hours. He is a quiet man of few words and Neil's mother has always taken a leading role in parenting Neil. Neil's parents describe a long history of problems in their relationship. They plan to divorce. Neil's birth and early development were normal but he has always been shy and has found it difficult to make friends.

Recent events and problems

For the last year at primary school, Neil was bullied and he was 'devastated' when his best friend left at the end of primary school and moved to another town. He has sided with his mother following the separation. He has found it difficult to settle into grammar school, and has become increasingly depressed for the two months prior to being seen in the child psychiatry department.

Neil was referred to child psychiatry by a consultant paediatrician as he had been extensively investigated for 'funny turns'. Both parents attended the initial appointment. In addition to the fainting episodes, which Neil and his parents accepted were caused by anxiety and panic, Neil described feeling very depressed and being preoccupied with the loss of his friend for the past few months. He had a severe sleep disturbance, poor appetite and concentration and at home isolated himself in his bedroom. At interview Neil presented as a small, immature boy, wearing glasses and a school uniform.

Assessment

The initial assessment consisted of interviewing Neil individually and together with his parents. Individual interview provided an in-depth assessment of Neil's symptoms, including suicidality, an assessment of his family and social relationships and interests. During this interview, Neil became very distressed and tearful when talking about the loss of his friend, the separation of his parents and his experiences of bullying at secondary school. He described occasional suicidal thoughts and hopelessness for the future. Neil denied any acts of deliberate self-harm. The assessment interview with Neil's parents completed Neil's family, social and developmental history. Neil's parents were aware of Neil's symptoms of depression and anxiety. They were not aware of his suicidal thoughts. The parental interview revealed that Neil's mother was low in mood and very concerned about the stigma of psychiatric treatment for Neil. Neil's parents had disagreed about attending the assessment and there was a high level of conflict between them, focused on all aspects of Neil's management.

Cognitive–behavioural formulation

Neil presents with the following difficulties: **affective**: sadness, anxiety; **behavioural**: inactivity, avoidance of social situations, increasing difficulties attending school, panic attacks in school; **physical**: sleep difficulties, tiredness, loss of appetite, dizziness; **cognitive**: self-blame, guilt, hopelessness, suicidal thoughts, sense of failure, loss of confidence. Neil had functioned normally in primary school with the support of a long-standing close friend. Neil's mother has always been overanxious and overprotective of him and they were very close, to the exclusion of Neil's father whilst Neil was a child. Neil had been aware of the sad loss of his brother and his mother's inability to adjust to this. He took away from this the belief that he was a substitute and not quite 'good enough' for his mother. He was also aware of his parents' arguments despite these occurring late at night, and further blamed himself for these. Neil had become increasingly introspective and unable to talk to either parent and had spent more and more time with his friend. When Neil's friend told him that he was moving house, Neil was devastated and felt rejected by the only person whom he felt understood. Neil's lack of control over this loss, which was followed closely by his parents' separation, further exacerbated his feelings of not being good enough, his self-blame and isolation.

Neil had experienced his first 'funny turn' waiting to go into the science laboratory on his own. He was taken to the sick bay and his mother was called in to school to pick him up. The way his mother treated him reminded him of when he was a young child. Neil had always been aware of his mother's worries about his health, and he further blamed himself for making her even more worried on top of everything else which was happening. Neil had been reluctant to see a psychiatrist or a psychologist as he had felt that this implied that everyone else agreed with his father and the school that he was 'putting all of it on'. These thoughts further added to his self-blame and sense of inferiority. Neil therefore displayed over-generalisation, catastrophising, personalisation and arbitrary inference in his thinking.

Problem list
1. Feelings of depression.
2. Poor sleep.
3. Impending divorce.
4. Problems with peer relationships.

Treatment of the child
Eight to ten sessions of CBT were offered to Neil, with involvement of the parents as necessary. The programme was problem oriented and targeted at Neil's cognitive level.

The initial phase of treatment took place over two sessions. The aims were to engage Neil in individual cognitive therapy, to identify a list of goals, and to teach self-monitoring. This section ended with work on emotional recognition, which is helpful in providing a starting point for cognitive techniques.

Neil was reluctant to accept the need for psychological help initially, but over the course of the assessment had begun to engage with the therapist in a collaborative approach to his problems. With the help of the therapist, Neil identified the above list of four problems and recorded the severity of each using a simple ten-point Likert scale. To encourage ownership of his problems, Neil wrote them down at the beginning of the diary which he had been given to accompany the treatment sessions. The theme of the second session was 'emotional recognition'. Neil found this exercise difficult, but was able to describe his experience of feeling depressed in terms of the bodily sensations and the negative automatic thoughts accompanying these. He was able to differentiate between emotional states, for example depression and anger, and between emotional states and the thoughts accompanying them. At the end of the session, the therapist set the first homework task. Neil was asked to record in his daily diary, depressed moods, negative automatic thoughts and recordings of concurrent situations. The therapist rehearsed a recent example with Neil.

Neil brought his diary along to the third session. The therapist set an agenda, spending the first half of the session concentrating on Neil's diary, and moving on to spend time on problems identified by Neil in his diary. Neil had made daily entries in his diary of his moods and happenings. He had not recorded his thoughts. The diary highlighted Neil's severe sleep disturbance and that he had spent long periods of time alone and unoccupied. As Neil had identified his sleep as a goal of therapy, it was agreed that the session would be focused around helping Neil overcome this. Simple sleep-hygiene measures were outlined and Neil was asked to complete a sleep diary for the following session. Neil's mum was invited to join in the final 15 minutes of this session. Neil fed back to his mother the main points of the session and the therapist sought her support with Neil's sleep difficulties. He was given a relaxation tape.

The fourth session was conducted jointly with Neil and his mother. In the previous session, the therapist had been concerned about Neil's levels of hopelessness and the lack of structure and support at home. First, the therapist reviewed Neil's sleep diary and then went on to enquire about his levels of activity at home. The activity schedule was described and Neil and his mother were asked to spend prescribed times together. Neil's mother provided helpful suggestions for how Neil could fill his time, and agreed to support him by taking him to a swimming club. She acknowledged that she had worried that Neil was not 'well enough' to undertake any of his previous pastimes.

Neil was seen for the next two sessions alone. Each time, to begin with Neil and the therapist reviewed his diary/homework task. The focus of these sessions was Neil's moods. The therapist helped him to identify negative automatic thoughts and taught him simple distraction techniques. Neil began to challenge his thoughts and re-evaluate them. Self-re-enforcement was introduced to give Neil a sense of internal control. At the end of each session, Neil's mother was invited to join Neil and the therapist to provide feedback of Neil's progress and help re-enforce the content of the session.

By session six, Neil's mood had improved and he had resumed some of his previous activities. Together, Neil and the therapist re-rated the problems which he outlined at the beginning of therapy. This highlighted Neil's continuing difficulties with peer relationships and the loss of his best friend. Using a problem-solving approach and role-play techniques, Neil and the therapist rehearsed common social relationship difficulties. Neil was able to describe his experiences of bullying and social isolation.

By the end of the eighth session, Neil was significantly improved and attending school fulltime. His mother was pleased with his progress and agreed that the final few sessions should be spaced over two to four weeks. Over the final sessions, the therapist reviewed treatment themes with Neil and encouraged him to predict future problems and identify strategies for dealing with them.

Sessions with the parents

Neil was living with his mother during his treatment. He was having contact with his father, but acknowledged angry feelings towards him. Neil did not want his father to be actively involved in his treatment sessions but, in parallel with treatment, the therapist met with his parents separately on two occasions. These meetings provided an opportunity for the therapist to advise the parents on the importance of them both maintaining relationships with Neil and of their explaining to him that he is not to blame for their separation. Neil needs to understand that they have decided to separate and that it is not possible for therapy to change that. Both parents should re-enforce to Neil their continuing love for him and commitment to him. His parents were also advised regarding minimising conflict and providing a consistent approach to Neil's management. During these meetings, the therapist advised Neil's mother to seek individual help in dealing with her own childhood and the loss of Neil's brother. She arranged counselling via her church.

Case 2: overdose and chronic family problems

Depression and suicidal behaviour in adolescents commonly occur in the context of family difficulties. However, this case shows how individual therapy can be valuable even when it is not possible to work with the family as a unit. It also illustrates the use of cognitive techniques with adolescents who have been abused.

Background

Laura, aged 15 years, lives with her mother. Her parents separated when she was small. From around the age of 11 years through to 13 years she was sexually abused by a boyfriend of her mothers. Laura tried to tell her mother on several occasions what had been going on, but on each occasion her mother had seemed not to listen. She had never forgiven her mother for what she saw as her mother's failure to protect her. She had become increasingly alienated from her mother and they rowed a great deal, especially about boyfriends. They communicated little, and Laura felt she could not talk to her mother about anything. Laura stated that she felt she was unlovable and that the world was rejecting her for her role in being abused. She was harder and harder to control and had been staying out late with a series of boyfriends.

Recent events and problems

On the day of the overdose, Laura had arranged to see her current boyfriend without telling her mother. When she returned home at 10 in the evening, she and her mother had a row. Laura ran upstairs, wrote a note saying that she loved her boyfriend, and took an overdose of 30 paracetamol tablets.

Assessment and initial treatment

When she was seen the next day in hospital, Laura said that she had wanted to die and that she had been depressed for around two months. She was hopeless and said that she could not see any future without her current boyfriend. She believed that she was ugly, unlovable and that no one would ever love her. When interviewed together, there was much tension between Laura and her mother. Her mother was very critical of Laura and implied that Laura had brought most of these problems on herself. Laura was hostile and angry with her mother.

The therapist decided that the main problem was poor communication between Laura and her mother and offered them both an appointment for the following week. They failed to attend, but did come to another appointment ten days after that, when Laura was still depressed and suicidal and had taken another small overdose. Another family session was held, but this finished abruptly when Laura walked out. She agreed to see the therapist individually but did not want to have any more joint meetings with her mother.

Cognitive–behavioural formulation

Laura's depression was precipitated by actual rejection by her mother. Her mother was probably too caught up in her own self-blame to listen to Laura when the abuse was first disclosed, and subsequently interpreted Laura's reckless behaviour with boys as evidence that Laura had brought the abuse on herself. This reinforced Laura's own view that she herself had caused the abuse. In fact, Laura's behaviour with boys stemmed from an exaggerated perception of powerlessness and incompetence that was the result of the abuse. She believed that she was worthless and 'used goods' once she had been abused. This perception, together with a strong sense of being unloved, led to an over-intense desire to form intimate relationships. Her mother's increasingly hostile reactions to what she regarded as Laura's promiscuous behaviour confirmed Laura's belief that she was unwanted. Laura's sense of' isolation was perpetuated by her anger, an understandable reaction to being rejected and abused. Laura therefore had several depressogenic assumptions, which included that she caused the abuse, that she was worthless, and that in order to be happy she must be loved.

Problem list
1. Depression.
2. Negative assumptions.
3. Poor relationship with mother.

Treatment of the child

At the first individual session with the therapist, Laura began to identify two interrelated areas of goals. She wanted to work at her negative feelings about herself and acute problems in her relationship with her mother. With careful exploration, it became clear that Laura related some feelings about herself and her appearance with her previous abusive experiences. She had been aware recently of thinking more and more about sexual abuse, and felt that she had never been able to talk it through. She also expressed some ambivalence about doing so. Laura demonstrated an ability to talk about her feelings and to discriminate between thoughts and feelings.

At the conclusion of the first session, it was agreed that Laura would attend for a series of weekly individual sessions, which would aim to help her feel more positive about herself, feel less depressed and might, if she wished, involve talking about worries that she might have about her sexually abusive experiences. Laura agreed to keep a diary of her daily activities and feelings.

Laura attended the second session unaccompanied. She reported feeling much more positive since she had ended her relationship with her boyfriend. She now had a new boyfriend and said she no longer felt depressed. However, she subsequently became very distressed when, reviewing her diary, she reported that she had seen a television programme about sexual abuse and had nightmares the following two nights. The session concluded with the therapist talking about helping Laura learn some skills for coping with the emotional distress caused by her memories. Coping-skills training (Deblinger & Heflin, 1996) was developed to enhance children's ability to be aware and share the feelings, thoughts and sensations that they experience as a result of abuse. The therapist decided that Laura needed to learn gradually the connection between her feelings of depression, the impact of sexual abuse, and problems within her relationship with her mother as a result of this. This all needed to be taken at Laura's pace.

In the following sessions, the therapist talked with Laura about the connections between thoughts, emotions and behaviour. Laura was encouraged to use her diary to demonstrate how thoughts might influence emotions. A low key approach was taken allowing Laura to control the pace at which she disclosed her sexual abuse. Sessions also included some education regarding child sexual abuse – the educational discussions allowing Laura to participate generally, providing a vocabulary for focusing on the details of her own experience. Thus, a model of gradual exposure to anxiety-provoking topics was adopted.

During this period of about three months, Laura missed occasional sessions, and talked of wishing to forget what had happened to her. However, she reliably rearranged failed sessions. The therapist then began to help Laura to identify her depressive assumptions and to devise strategies to deal with them. At about the twelfth session, Laura's mood showed consistent improvement, she began making more arrangements to visit friends and placed less emphasis on her dating activities. There was a gradual shift in the topic of discussions from those relating to abusive experiences to discussion of peer group conflicts and day-to-day activities. The strategy of cognitive restructuring was continued, together with social problem solving in relation to the difficulties within her peer group.

Sessions with the mother

During Laura's individual treatment, her mother had had occasional individual sessions with another therapist, discussing in the first instance her own feelings in relation to Laura's sexual abuse and the likely impact that this would have on Laura. She made some progress in individual sessions and it became clear that general issues between them would now be more amenable to discussion in joint sessions, supported initially by continuing individual work with Laura.

Acknowledgements

The authors wish to acknowledge the support of the MacArthur Foundation Research Network on Psychopathology and Development and the Medical Research Council of Great Britain.

References

Abramson, L., Metalsky, G. & Alloy, L. (1989). Hopelessness depression: a theory-based subtype of depression. *Psychology Reviews*, **96**, 358–72.

Abramson, L., Seligman, M. & Teasdale, J. (1978). Learned helplessness in humans: critique and reformulation. *Journal of Abnormal Psychology*, **87**, 49–74.

American Psychiatric Association (1994). *Diagnostic and statistical manual of mental disorders*, 4th edn. American Psychiatric Association, Washington, DC.

Andrews, G. (1996). Talk that works: the rise of cognitive–behaviour therapy. *British Medical Journal*, **313**, 1501–2.

Angold, A., Costello, E.J., Pickles, A. & Winder, F. (1987). *The development of a questionnaire for use in epidemiological studies of depression in children and adolescents*. Medical Research Council Child Psychiatry Unit, London.

Asarnow, J.R. & Bates, S. (1988). Depression in child psychiatric inpatients: cognitive and attributional patterns. *Journal of Abnormal Child Psychology*, **16**, 601–15.

Asarnow, J.R. & Carlson, G.A. (1988). Childhood depression: Five year outcome following cognitive-behavior therapy and pharmacotherapy. *American Journal of Psychotherapy*, **XLII**, 456–62.

Beardslee, W.R., Salt, P., Porterfield, K., Rothberg, P.C., Velde, P.v.d., Swatling, S., Hoke, L., Moilanen, D.L. & Wheelock, I. (1993). Comparison of preventive interventions for families with parental affective disorder. *Journal of the American Academy of Child and Adolescent Psychiatry*, **32**, 254–63.

Beardslee, W.R., Wright, E., Rothberg, P.C., Salt, P. & Versage, E. (1996). Response of families to two preventive intervention strategies: long-term differences in behavior and attitude change. *Journal of the American Academy of Child and Adolescent Psychiatry*, **35**, 774–82.

Beck, A.T. (1967). *Depression: clinical, experimental and theoretical aspects*. Harper & Row, New York.

Beck, A.T. (1983). Cognitive therapy of depression: new perspectives. In *Treatment of depression: old controversies and new approaches* (ed. P.J. Clayton & J.E. Barrett), pp. 265–84. Raven Press, New York.

Beck, A.T., Brown, G., Steer, R.A., Eidelson, J.I. & Riskind, J.H. (1987). Differentiating anxiety and depression: a test of the cognitive content-specificity hypothesis. *Journal of Abnormal Psychology*, **96**, 179–83.

Beck, A.T., Rush, A.J., Shaw, B.F. & Emery, G. (1979). *Cognitive therapy of depression*, Guilford Press, New York.

Brent, D., Holder, D., Kolko, D., Birmaher, B., Baugher, M., Roth, C., Iyengar, S. & Johnson, B. (submitted). A clinical psychotherapy trial for adolescent depression comparing cognitive, family, and supportive treatments.

Burns, D. (1980). *Feeling good: the new mood therapy*. Signet, New York.

Butler, L., Meizitis, S., Friedman, R. & Cole, E. (1980). The effect of two school-based intervention programs on depressive symptoms in pre-adolescents. *American Education Research Journal*, **17**, 111–19.

Caron, C., Wickramaratne, P., Warner, V., Weissman, M. & Merette, C. (1993). A search for pathways to comorbidity of major depression and conduct disorder. Unpublished manuscript.

Castonguay, L.G., Goldfried, M.R., Wiser, S., Raue, P.J. & Hayes, A.M. (1996). Predicting the effect of cognitive therapy for depression: a study of unique and common factors. *Journal of Consulting and Clinical Psychology*, **64**, 497–504.

Cicchetti, D. & Schneider-Rosen, K. (1986). An organizational approach to childhood depression. In *Depression in young people: developmental and clinical perspectives (ed. M. Rutter, C. Izard & P.B. Read, pp. 71–134. Guilford Press, New York.*

Clarke, G.N., Hawkins, W., Murphy, M., Sheeber, L.B., Lewinsohn, P.M. & Seeley, J.R. (1995). Targeted prevention of unipolar depressive disorder in an at-risk sample of high school adolescents: a randomized trial of a group cognitive intervention. *Journal of the American Academy of Child and Adolescent Psychiatry*, **34**, 312–21.

Clarke, G.N., Hops, H., Lewinsohn, P.M., Andrews, J.A., Seeley, J.R. & Williams, J.A. (1992). Cognitive–behavioral group treatment of adolescent depression: prediction of outcome. *Behavior Therapy*, **23**, 341–54.

Cohen, P., Cohen, J. & Brook, J. (1993a). An epidemiological study of disorders in late childhood and adolescence – II. Persistence of disorders. *Journal of Child Psychology and Psychiatry*, **34**, 869–77.

Cohen, P., Cohen, J., Kasen, S., Velez, C.N., Hartmark, C., Johnson, J., Rojas, M., Brook, J. & Streuning, E.L. (1993b). An epidemiological study of disorders in late childhood and adolescence – I. Age- and gender-specific prevalence. *Journal of Child Psychology and Psychiatry*, **34**, 851–67.

Cole, D.A. & Turner, J.E. (1993). Models of cognitive mediation and moderation in child depression. *Journal of Abnormal Psychology*, **102**, 271–81.

Dadds, M.R., Sanders, M.R., Morrison, M. & Rebgetz, M. (1992). Childhood depression and conduct disorder: II. An analysis of family interaction patterns in the home. *Journal of Abnormal Psychology*, **101**, 505–13.

Deblinger, E. & Heflin, A.H. (1996). *Treating sexually abused children and their non-offending parents: a cognitive–behavioural approach.* Sage, London.

Dweck, C. & Elliot, E. (1983). Achievement motivation. In *Handbook of child psychology*, Vol. 4. *Social and Personality Development* (ed. P. Mussen & M. Hetherington), pp. 643–91. Wiley, New York.

Emslie, G., Rush, A., Weinberg, W., Kowatch, R., Hughes, C. & Rintelmann, J. (1995). *Efficacy of fluoxetine in depressed children and adolescents.* Paper presented at the 42nd Annual Meeting of the American Academy of Child and Adolescent Psychiatry, New Orleans.

Evans, M.D., Hollon, S.D., DeRubeis, R.J., Piasecki, J.M., Grove, W.M., Garvey, M.J. & Tuason, V.B. (1992). Differential relapse following cognitive therapy and pharmacotherapy for depression. *Archives of General Psychiatry*, **49**, 802–8.

Feehan, C.J. & Vostanis, P. (1996). Cognitive–behavioural therapy for depressed children: children's and therapists' impressions. *Behavioural and Cognitive Psychotherapy*, **24**, 171–83.

Fennell, M.J.V. (1989). Depression. In *Cognitive behaviour therapy for psychiatric problems. A practical guide* (ed. K. Hawton, P.M. Salkovskis, J. Kirk & D.M. Clark), pp. 169–234. Oxford University Press, Oxford.

Fine, S., Forth, A., Gilbert, M. & Haley, G. (1991). Group therapy for adolescent depressive disorder: a comparison of social skills and therapeutic support. *Journal of the American Academy of Child Psychiatry*, **30**, 79–85.

Fleming, J.E. & Offord, D.R. (1990). Epidemiology of childhood depressive disorders: a critical review. *Journal of the American Academy of Child Psychiatry*, **29**, 571–80.

Fleming, J.E., Offord, D.R. & Boyle, M.H. (1989). Prevalence of childhood and adolescent depression in the community: Ontario child health study. *British Journal of Psychiatry*, **155**, 647–54.

Frame, C., Matson, J.L., Sonis, W.A., Fialkov, M.J. & Kazdin, A.E. (1982). Behavioral treatment of depression in a prepubertal child. *Journal of Behavior Therapy and Experimental Psychiatry*, **3**, 239–43.

Garber, J., Weiss, B. & Stanley, N. (1993). Cognitions, depressive symptoms, and development in adolescents. *Journal of Abnormal Psychology*, **102**, 47–57.

Goodyer, I.M., Germany, E., Gowrusankur, J. & Altham, P. (1991). Social influences on the course of anxious and depressive disorders in school-age children. *British Journal of Psychiatry*, **158**, 676–84.

Gotlib, I.H., Lewinsohn, P.M., Seeley, J.R., Rohde, P. & Redner, J.E. (1993). Negative cognitions and attributional style in depressed adolescents: An examination of stability and specificity. *Journal of Abnormal Psychology*, **102**, 607–15.

Hammen, C., Adrian, C. & Hiroto, D. (1988). A longitudinal test of the attributional vulnerability model in children at risk for depression. *British Journal of Clinical Psychology*, **27**, 37–46.

Harrington, R.C. (1992). Annotation: the natural history and treatment of child and adolescent affective disorders. *Journal of Child Psychology and Psychiatry*, **33**, 1287–302.

Harrington, R.C. (1993). *Depressive disorder in childhood and adolescence.* Wiley, Chichester.

Harrington, R.C., Bredenkamp, D., Groothues, C., Rutter, M., Fudge, H. & Pickles, A. (1994). Adult outcomes of childhood and adolescent depression. III. Links with suicidal behaviours. *Journal of Child Psychology and Psychiatry*, **35**, 1380–91.

Harrington, R.C., Fudge, H., Rutter, M., Bredenkamp, D., Groothues, C. & Pridham, J. (1993). Child and adult depression: a test of continuities with data from a family study. *British Journal of Psychiatry*, **162**, 627–33.

Harrington, R.C., Fudge, H., Rutter, M., Pickles, A. & Hill, J. (1990). Adult outcomes of childhood and adolescent depression: I. Psychiatric status. *Archives of General Psychiatry*, **47**, 465–73.

Harrington, R.C., Fudge, H., Rutter, M., Pickles, A. & Hill, J. (1991). Adult outcomes of childhood and adolescent depression: II. Risk for anti-social disorders. *Journal of the American Academy of Child Psychiatry*, **30**, 434–9.

Harrington, R.C. & Vostanis, P. (1995). Longitudinal perspectives and affective disorder in children and adolescents. In *The depressed child and adolescent. Developmental and clinical perspectives* (ed. I.M. Goodyer), pp. 311–41. Cambridge University Press, Cambridge.

Harter, S. (1983). Developmental perspectives on the self-system. In *Handbook of child psychology*, Vol. 4. *Social and personality development* (ed. P. Mussen & M. Hetherington), pp. 275–385. Wiley, New York.

Hawton, K. & Catalan, J. (1982). *Attempted suicide*. Oxford Medical Publications, Oxford.

Hazell, P., O'Connell, D., Heathcote, D., Robertson, J. & Henry, D. (1995). Efficacy of tricyclic drugs in treating child and adolescent depression: a meta-analysis. *British Medical Journal*, **310**, 897–901.

Henry, J.A. (1992). Toxicity of antidepressants: comparisons with fluoxetine. *International Clinical Psychopharmacology*, **6** Suppl. 6, 22–7.

Hollon, S.D., Shelton, R.C. & Davis, D.D. (1993). Cognitive therapy for depression: conceptual issues and clinical efficacy. *Journal of Consulting and Clinical Psychology*, **61**, 270–5.

Hops, H. & Lewinsohn, P.M. (1995). A course for the treatment of depression among adolescents. In *Anxiety and depression in adults and children* (ed. K.D. Craig & K.S. Dobson), pp. 230–45. Sage, Thousand Oaks, Calif.

Jacobson, N.J., Dobson, K.S., Truax, P.A., Addis, M. E., Koerner, K., Gollan, J.K., Gortner, E. & Prince, S.E. (1996). A component analysis of cognitive-behavioral treatment for depression. *Journal of Consulting and Clinical Psychology*, **64**, 295–304.

Jacobson, N.S. & Hollon, S.D. (1996). Cognitive-behavior therapy versus pharmacotherapy: now that the jury's returned its verdict, it's time to present the rest of the evidence. *Journal of Consulting and Clinical Psychology*, **64**, 74–80.

Jaycox, L.H., Reivich, K.J., Gillham, J. & Seligman, M.E.P. (1994). Prevention of depressive symptoms in school children. *Behaviour Research and Therapy*, **32**, 801–16.

Jayson, D., Wood, A.J., Kroll, L., Frazer, J. & Harrington, R.C. (in preparation). Predictors of response to cognitive–behaviour therapy in adolescent depressive disorder.

Kagan, J. (1982). The emergence of self. *Journal of Child Psychology and Psychiatry*, **23**, 363–81.

Kahn, J.S., Kehle, T.J., Jenson, W.R. & Clarke, E. (1990). Comparison of cognitive-behavioral, relaxation, and self-modelling interventions for depression among middle-school students. *School Psychology Review*, **19**, 195–210.

Kazdin, A.E. & Bass, D. (1989). Power to detect differences between alternative treatments in comparative psychotherapy outcome research. *Journal of Consulting and Clinical Psychology*, **57**, 138–47.

Keating, D.P. (1990). Adolescent thinking. In *At the threshold. The developing adolescent* (ed. S.S. Feldman & G.R. Elliott), pp. 54–89. Harvard University Press, Cambridge, Mass.

Kendall, P.C. (1991). Guiding theory for therapy with children and adolescents. In *Child and adolescent therapy. Cognitive–behavioural procedures* (ed. P.C. Kendall), pp. 3–22. Guilford Press, New York.

Kerfoot, M., Dyer, E., Harrington, V., Woodham, A. & Harrington, R.C. (1996). Correlates and short-term course of self-poisoning in adolescents. *British Journal of Psychiatry*, **168**, 38–42.

Klein, D.F. (1996). Preventing hung juries about therapy studies. *Journal of Consulting and Clinical Psychology*, **64**, 81–7.

Klein, D.F. & Ross, D.C. (1993). Reanalysis of the National Institute of Mental Health Treatment of Depression Collaborative Research Programme general effectiveness report. *Neuropsychopharmacology*, **8**, 241–51.

Kolvin, I., Barrett, M.L., Bhate, S.R., Berney, T.P., Famuyiwa, O.O., Fundudis, T. & Tyrer, S. (1991). The Newcastle Child Depression Project: diagnosis and classification of depression. *British Journal of Psychiatry*, **159** Suppl. 11, 9–21.

Kovacs, M. (1986). A developmental perspective on methods and measures in the assessment of depressive disorders: the clinical interview. In *Depression in young people: Developmental and clinical perspectives* (ed. M. Rutter, C.E. Izard & R.B. Read), pp. 435–65. Guilford Press, New York.

Kovacs, M., Feinberg, T.L., Crouse-Novak, M., Paulauskas, S.L., Pollock, M. & Finkelstein, R. (1984). Depressive disorders in childhood. II. A longitudinal study of the risk for a subsequent major depression. *Archives of General Psychiatry*, **41**, 643–9.

Kroll, L., Harrington, R.C., Gowers, S., Frazer, J. & Jayson, D. (1996). Continuation of cognitive–behavioural treatment in adolescent patients who have remitted from major depression. Feasibility and comparison with historical controls. *Journal* of the American Academy of Child and Adolescent Psychiatry, 35, 1156–61.

Kuhn, D., Amsel, E. & O'Loughlin, M. (1988). The development of scientific thinking skills. Academic Press, San Diego.

Laurent, J. & Stark, K. (1993). Testing the cognitive content-specificity hypothesis with anxious and depressed youngsters. Journal of Abnormal Psychology, 102, 226–37.

Lazarus, A.A. (1968). Learning theory and the treatment of depression. Behavior Research and Therapy, 6, 83–9.

Lewinsohn, P.M., Clarke, G.N., Hops, H. & Andrews, J. (1990). Cognitive–behavioural treatment for depressed adolescents. Behavior Therapy, 21, 385–401.

Lewinsohn, P.M., Clarke, G.N., Rohde, P., Hops, H. & Seeley, J.R. (1996). A course in coping: a cognitive-behavioral approach to the treatment of adolescent depression. In Psychosocial treatments for child and adolescent disorders. Empirically based strategies for clinical practice (ed. E. Hibbs & P.S. Jensen), pp. 109–35. American Psychological Association, Washington, DC.

Lewinsohn, P.M., Hoberman, H., Teri, L. & Hautzinger, M. (1985). An integrative theory of depression. In Theoretical issues in behavior therapy (ed. S. Reiss & R. Bootzin), pp. 331–59. Academic Press, New York.

Lewinsohn, P.M., Rohde, P. & Seeley, J.R. (1993). Psychosocial characteristics of adolescents with a history of suicide attempt. Journal of the American Academy of Child and Adolescent Psychiatry, 32, 60–68.

Lewinsohn, P.M., Weinstein, M.S. & Alper, T.A. (1970). A behavioral approach to the group treatment of depressed persons: a methodological contribution. Journal of Clinical Psychology, 26, 525–32.

Liddle, B. & Spence, S.H. (1990). Cognitive–behaviour therapy with depressed primary school children: a cautionary note. Behavioural Psychotherapy, 18, 85–102.

Marriage, K., Fine, S., Moretti, M. & Haley, G. (1986). Relationship between depression and conduct disorder in children and adolescents. Journal of the American Academy of Child and Adolescent Psychiatry, 25, 687–91.

Marton, P., Connolley, J., Kutcher, S. & Korenblum, M. (1993). Cognitive social skills and social self-appraisal in depressed adolescents. Journal of the American Academy of Child and Adolescent Psychiatry, 32, 739–44.

McCauley, E., Mitchell, J.R., Burke, P. & Moss, S. (1988). Cognitive attributes of depression in children and adolescents. Journal of Consulting and Clinical Psychology, 56, 903–8.

Mitchell, J., McCauley, E., Burke, P.M. & Moss, S. J. (1988). Phenomenology of depression in children and adolescents. Journal of the American Academy of Child Psychiatry, 27, 12–20.

Mufson, L., Moreau, D., Weissman, M.M. & Klerman, G.L. (1993). Interpersonal psychotherapy for depressed adolescents. Guilford Press, New York.

Nolen-Hoeksema, S., Girgus, J.S. & Seligman, M.E.P. (1992). Predictors and consequences of childhood depressive symptoms: a 5-year longitudinal study. Journal of Abnormal Psychology, 101, 405–22.

Petti, T.A., Bornstein, M., Delamater, A. & Conners, C.K. (1980). Evaluation and multimodality treatment of a depressed prepubertal girl. Journal of the American Academy of Child and Adolescent Psychiatry, 19, 690–702.

Piaget, J. (1970). Piaget's theory. In Carmichael's manual of child psychology (ed. P.H. Mussen), pp. 703–32. Wiley, New York.

Puig-Antich, J. (1982). Major depression and conduct disorder in prepuberty. Journal of the American Academy of Child and Adolescent Psychiatry, 21, 118–28.

Puig-Antich, J., Goetz, D., Davies, M., Kaplan, T., Davies, S., Ostrow, L., Asnis, L., Twomey, J., Iyengar, S. & Ryan, N.D. (1989). A controlled family history study of prepubertal major depressive disorder. Archives of General Psychiatry, 46, 406–18.

Puig-Antich, J., Kaufman, J., Ryan, N.D., Williamson, D.E., Dahl, R.E., Lukens, E., Todak, G., Ambrosini, P., Rabinovich, H. & Nelson, B. (1993). The psychosocial functioning and family environment of depressed adolescents. Journal of the American Academy of Child and Adolescent Psychiatry, 32, 244–53.

Puig-Antich, J., Lukens, E., Davies, M., Goetz, D., Brennan-Quattrock, J. & Todak, G. (1985a). Psychosocial functioning in prepubertal major depressive disorders. II. Interpersonal relationships after sustained recovery from affective episode. Archives of General Psychiatry, 42, 511–17.

Puig-Antich, J., Lukens, E., Davies, M., Goetz, D., Brennan-Quattrock, J. & Todak, G. (1985b). Psychosocial functioning in prepubertal major depressive disorders. I. Interpersonal relationships during the depressive episode. Archives of General Psychiatry, 42, 500–7.

Quinton, D., Rutter, M. & Liddle, C. (1984). Institutional rearing, parenting difficulties and marital support. Psychological Medicine, 14, 107–24.

Rao, U., Weissman, M.M., Martin, J.A. & Hammond, R.W. (1993). Childhood depression and risk of suicide: preliminary report of a longitudinal study. Journal of the American Academy of Child Psychiatry, 32, 21–7.

Rehm, L. (1995). Psychotherapies for depression. In Anxiety and depression in adults and children (ed.

K.D. Craig & K.S. Dobson), pp. 183–208. Sage, Thousand Oaks, Calif.

Rehm, L.P., Kaslow, N.J. & Rabin, A.S. (1987). Cognitive and behavioral targets in a self-control therapy program for depression. *Journal of Consulting and Clinical Psychology*, **55**, 60–7.

Reynolds, W.M. & Coats, K.I. (1986). A comparison of cognitive–behavioural therapy and relaxation training for the treatment of depression in adolescents. *Journal of Consulting and Clinical Psychology*, **54**, 653–60.

Rholes, W., Blackwell, J., Jordan, C. & Walters, C. (1980). A developmental study of learned helplessness. *Developmental Psychology*, **16**, 616–24.

Robins, C.J. & Hinkley, K. (1989). Social-cognitive processing and depressive symptoms in children: a comparison of measures. *Journal of Abnormal Child Psychology*, **17**, 29–36.

Robinson, N.S., Garber, J. & Hilsman, R. (1995). Cognitions and stress: direct and moderating effects on depressive versus externalizing symptoms during the junior high school transition. *Journal of Abnormal Psychology*, **104**, 453–63.

Rutter, M. (1986). The developmental psychopathology of depression: issues and perspectives. In *Depression in young people. Developmental and clinical perspectives* (ed. M. Rutter, C. Izard & P. Read), pp. 3–30. Guilford Press, New York.

Rutter, M. (1991). Age changes in depressive disorders: some developmental considerations. In *The development of emotion regulation and dysregulation* (ed. J. Garber & K.A. Dodge), pp. 273–300. Cambridge University Press, Cambridge.

Ryan, N.D., Puig-Antich, J., Ambrosini, P., Rabinovich, H., Robinson, D., Nelson, B., Iyengar, S. & Twomey, J. (1987). The clinical picture of major depression in children and adolescents. *Archives of General Psychiatry*, **44**, 854–61.

Seligman, M.E.P. & Peterson, C. (1986). A learned helplessness perspective on childhood depression: theory and research. In *Depression in young people: developmental and clinical perspectives* (ed. M. Rutter, C.E. Izard & P.S. Read), pp. 223–50. Guilford Press, New York.

Shaffer, D., Gould, M.S., Brasic, J., Ambrosini, P., Fisher, P., Bird, H. & Aluwahlia, S. (1983). A children's Global Assessment Scale (C-GAS). *Archives of General Psychiatry*, **40**, 1228–31.

Shapiro, D.A., Barkham, M., Rees, A., Hardy, G.E., Reynolds, S. & Startup, M. (1995). Decisions, decisions, decisions: determining the effects of treatment method and duration on the outcome of psychotherapy for depression. In *Research foundations of psychotherapy practice* (ed. M. Aveline & D.A. Shapiro), pp. 151–74. Wiley, Chichester.

Shea, M., Elkin, I., Imber, S.D., Sotsky, S.M., Watkins, J.T., Collins, J.F., Pilkonis, P.A., Beckham, E., Glass, D.R., Dolan, R.T. & Parloff, M.B. (1992). Course of depressive symptoms over follow-up. Findings from the National

Institute of Mental Health treatment of depression collaborative research program. *Archives of General Psychiatry*, **49**, 782–7.

Simons, A.D., Murphy, G.E., Levine, J.L. & Wetzel, R.D. (1986). Cognitive therapy and pharmacotherapy for depression: sustained improvement over one year. *Archives of General Psychiatry*, **43**, 43–8.

Stark, K. D. (1990). *Childhood depression: school-based intervention*. Guilford Press, New York.

Stark, K.D., Reynolds, W.M. & Kaslow, N. (1987). A comparison of the relative efficacy of self-control therapy and a behavioral problem-solving therapy for depression in children. *Journal of Abnormal Child Psychology*, **15**, 91–113.

Stark, K.D., Rouse, L.W. & Livingston, R. (1991). Treatment of depression during childhood and adolescence: cognitive-behavioral procedures for the individual and the family. In *Child and adolescent therapy. Cognitive–behavioural procedures* (ed. P.C. Kendall), pp. 165–206. Guilford Press, New York.

Strober, M., Morrell, W., Burroughs, J., Lampert, C., Danforth, H. & Freeman, R. (1988). A family study of bipolar I disorder in adolescence. Early onset of symptoms linked to increased familial loading and lithium resistance. *Journal of Affective Disorders*, **15**, 255–68.

Teasdale, J.D. (1988). Cognitive vulnerability to persistent depression. *Cognition and Emotion*, **2**, 247–74.

Teasdale, J. & Barnard, P.J. (1993). *Affect, cognition and change: re-modelling depressive thought*. Lawrence Erlbaum, Hillsdale, NJ.

Vostanis, P., Feehan, C., Grattan, E. & Bickerton, W. (1996). Treatment for children and adolescents with depression: lessons from a controlled trial. *Clinical Child Psychology and Psychiatry*, **1**, 199–212.

Vostanis, P. & Harrington, R.C. (1994). Cognitive–behavioural treatment of depressive disorder in child psychiatric patients – rationale and description of a treatment package. *European Child and Adolescent Psychiatry*, **3**, 111–23.

Wilkes, T.C.R., Belsher, G., Rush, A.J. & Frank, E. (Eds.) (1994). *Cognitive therapy for depressed adolescents*. Guilford Press, New York.

Wilkes, T.C.R. & Rush, A.J. (1988). Adaptations of cognitive therapy for depressed adolescents. *Journal of the American Academy of Child and Adolescent Psychiatry*, **27**, 381–6.

Williams, J.M.G. (1992). *The psychological treatment of depression*, 2nd edn. Routledge, London.

Wood, A., Kroll, L., Moore, A. & Harrington, R.C. (1995). Properties of the Mood and Feelings Questionnaire in adolescent psychiatric outpatients: a research note. *Journal of Child Psychology and Psychiatry*, **36**, 327–34.

Wood, A., Moore, A., Harrington, R.C. & Jayson, D. (1996a). Clinical validity of major depression-endogenous subtype in adolescent patients. *European Child and Adolescent Psychiatry*, **5**, 155–66.

Wood, A.J., Harrington, R.C. & Moore, A. (1996b). Controlled trial of a brief cognitive–behavioural intervention in adolescent patients with depressive disorders. *Journal of Child Psychology and Psychiatry*, **37**, 737–46.

11
Adolescent conduct disorders

Martin Herbert

Introduction

Adolescence is a biosocial construct – it begins in puberty and ends in a cultural definition of independence – and, as such, is a movable feast. For the purposes of this chapter, it has been taken to include young people of between 11 and 18 years of age. But adolescence is not a homogeneous stage of development. The differences between 11 and 18 year olds can, depending on individual development, be the difference between someone who, in body and mind, is still a child, and a person who is, in most respects, an adult. Developmental tasks and preoccupations and, indeed, their cognitive maturity, vary to an extent that requires us to consider assessment and treatment in terms of *early* and *late* adolescence.

The conduct disorders

This issue of early as opposed to late adolescence is relevant, because conduct disorders, with their extreme anti-social, aggressive manifestations, have age-related *prognostic* and *treatment* implications. There are two developmental pathways to the fully fledged condition: an early onset in childhood and a later appearance during the years of adolescence, the latter being difficult enough to deal with clinically, but not generally as resistant to change as the early version (Robins & Price, 1991; Farrington, 1992; Herbert, 1994a, 1995).

This consideration gives rise to a conceptual boundary problem. At what stage in childhood-onset conduct disorders does one shift the therapy paradigm from the so-called triadic model, that involves caregivers as primary mediators of change (notably in successful parenting skills programmes), to one that more appropriately deals with an individual in his or her own right (as in dyadic or group-based cognitive–behaviour therapy)? Whatever the answer to this question, the involvement of the family remains crucial, as the conduct disorders have such a devastating impact on family life (Webster-Stratton & Herbert, 1994) as well as on life at school and the wider community.

What are these problems? The ICD-10 (World Health Organization, 1992) classifies a conduct disorder as a 'repetitive and persistent pattern of behaviour, in which either the basic rights of others or major age-appropriate societal norms are violated, lasting at least 6 months' (p.157). Twenty-three symptoms, increasing in severity from tantrums, non-compliance and arguments to acts of cruelty and crimes of arson, vandalism and rape, are classified into four subcategories: (a) conduct disorder confined to the family context; (b) unsocialised conduct disorder; (c) socialised conduct disorder; (d) oppositional defiant disorder.

Serna, Sherman and Sheldon (1996) refer to adolescents who are referred to the juvenile courts but are allowed to remain at home (because the crimes are not serious enough to warrant incarceration), or are referred for professional help by parents or teachers, as individuals *at risk for failure* in the school and community. They may not have committed the more extreme injurious acts, but their behaviour and interactions with family members, peers or others, are highly inappropriate and stressful.

What we are dealing with then, in this chapter, is a substantial group of young people – some nearer to childhood than adulthood – displaying an array of conduct problems, ranging from those that are maladaptive but relatively contained and moderate in frequency and intensity, to those that are extreme and possibly criminal. In terms of their onset, they may have a deeply rooted repertoire of anti-social behaviour of many years duration or the acquisition of conduct problems in recent adolescence. Undercontrolled, aggressive and anti-social activities, notable at their worst for their frighteningly inconsequential 'mindless' quality, are the hallmarks of the conduct disorders. Hyperactivity (attention-deficit hyperactivity disorder) may be a feature in a sizeable proportion of cases, and this makes for a particularly poor long-term outcome (Farrington, 1995). The need for effective preventive and remedial interventions for this personally and socially costly condition could not be more urgent (see Herbert, 1994a, 1995).

Rationale for using cognitive–behavioural therapy

A cognitive-based intervention can be defined as a treatment approach that aims to alter specific perceptions, images, thoughts and beliefs through direct manipulation and restructuring of faulty, maladaptive cognitions. A growing number of practitioners acknowledge the significance of the cognitive representation of events and experiences in the development of the conduct disorders and other anti-social manifestations (e.g. delinquent activities) of children and adolescents. The view taken by cognitive theorists of their uncontrolled, rebellious and aggressive behaviour is that it is characterised by a range of social–cognitive distortions and ineffectual problem-solving skills (e.g. Bright & Robin, 1981; Lochman *et al.*, 1984; Kazdin, 1987, 1994; Hollin, 1990a; Powell & Oei,

1991; Kendall, 1993; Kendall & Hollon, 1994). Adolescents with conduct disorders tend to:

have difficulty anticipating consequences of their behaviour;

recall high rates of hostile cues present in social stimuli;

attend to fear cues when interpreting the meaning of others' behaviour;

attribute others' behaviour in ambiguous situations to their hostile intentions;

under-perceive their own level of aggressiveness;

under-perceive their responsibility for early stages of dyadic conflict;

generate few verbal assertion solutions to social problems;

generate impulsively more action-oriented and aggressive solutions without stopping to think of non-aggressive solutions.

They appear to be hypervigilant in scanning their social environment for hostile cues which encourage them to respond in a non-verbal, action-orientated manner. Aggressive adolescents are likely to believe that aggression will enhance their self-esteem, create a positive image, but not cause suffering to the victims (Slaby & Guerra, 1988). Lochman (1992) has shown how adolescent boys' aggressive solutions to problems involved little or no bargaining.

Therapeutic goals
As aggression and poor control are among their foremost problems, the focus might be:

attributional processes (e.g. misinterpreting others' intentions);

cognitive distortions (e.g. their aggression does not have injurious consequences);

negotiating conflict situations;

labelling affect appropriately;

social-skills deficits;

general problem-solving strategies.

Assessment
Rigorous assessment is the *sine qua non* of an effective cognitive–behavioural inter-vention. A clinical formulation – the 'explanatory story' about the client's problem that bridges the assessment and the treatment plan and implementation – is arrived at by several stages (Table 11.1). The stages set out in Table 11.1 are broadly conceived, and the ways in which they are operationalised are too many and varied to describe

Table 11.1. Stages in cognitive–behavioural assessment for intervention

Stage	Aims and rationale	Procedures
1. Taking an inventory of the client's problems	To compile a comprehensive picture of the client's difficulties	A semi-structured interview to draw up a problem profile
2. Selection of target behaviour(s)	Focusing on problem areas to change	Collaborative negotiation of goals
3. Identification of replacement actions	Emphasis on positive objectives	Operationalising of goals
4. Design of data-recording method	To obtain pre-treatment baseline	Instructing client; charting
5. Identification of problem-controlling conditions	To identify contingencies, attributions, etc., preceding and following the occurrence of problem(s)	Charting (recording) ABCs of behaviours/beliefs indicative of problem(s)
6. Assessment of environmental resources/influences	To identify possible resources/ significant influence in the client's problems	Interview of client and significant others (genogram/social support systems)
7. Formulation of a cognitive–behavioural intervention plan	To select appropriate methods, i.e. the most effective programme for change	Familiarity with the literature. Analysis of the *function* of dysfunctional behaviour (i.e. social learning implications and meaning of the problem)
8. Implementing of programme	To change behaviour/cognitions by means of methods carried out in a collaborative context (e.g. Webster-Stratton & Herbert, 1994)	Applying cognitive–behavioural methods/techniques
9. Monitoring progress and outcomes	To be sensitive to difficulties in the progress of therapy and to obtain information about effectiveness	Gathering appropriate data
10. Planning for generalisation and maintenance of change	To achieve generality of improvements and stabilisation of change	Using the environment for maintenance; planning generalisation strategies (e.g. self-reinforcement)

adequately in this chapter. The main techniques and their rationale can be found in Herbert (1987, 1994b), Kendall (1991), Goldstein (1995) and also in this chapter.

Therapeutic methods

The cognitive–behavioural approaches to interventions for children and adolescents consist usually of techniques which have been adapted from adult work (see Meichenbaum & Burland, 1979; Ollendick & Cerny, 1981; Hollon & Beck, 1994; Kendall & Hollon, 1994). Some have their roots in cognitive therapy (e.g. socratic questioning, persuasion, challenging, debate, hypothesising, cognitive restructuring, verbal self-instruction and internal dialogues). Others are drawn from behaviour therapy (e.g. operant procedures, desensitisation, exposure training, social-skills training, role-play, behaviour rehearsal, modelling, relaxation, exercises, redefinition, self-monitoring).

Given the nature of the problems and the intimate relationship of cognitive–behavioural therapy and social learning theory, there is a strong focus on social influence, social cognitions and relationships (Bandura, 1977; Herbert, 1987, 1991; Webster-Stratton & Herbert, 1994).

Individual programmes
Self-instruction training

'Self-statements', or 'self-talk', are perceived by the individual as plausible and logically related to the situation at hand. For example, a child exhibiting intense aversion to social evaluation might think, 'If I make a mistake, the teacher and the other kids might think I'm stupid, everyone says so anyway'. These self-statements underpin cognitive functions such as self-instruction, self-control, self-evaluation and self-reinforcement. The modification of self-statements to achieve *self-control* through self-instruction training has been attempted successfully with hyperactive aggressive boys (also using modelling) by Goodwin and Mahoney (1975), and with aggressive young offenders by Snyder and White (1979). A case history illustration is provided at the end of the chapter.

Anger-control training (cognitive change)

There are anger-management programmes designed specifically for adolescents (Feindler & Ecton, 1986), many drawing heavily on the research and procedures published by Novaco (1975, 1979). Most of them consist of three stages: cognitive preparation; skill acquisition; and application training. The intention is to lower the likelihood of aggressive behaviour by increasing awareness of the signs of incipient hostile arousal and techniques to encourage self-control. The performance of aggressive, anti-social behaviour may be influenced by antecedent cognitive events such as aversive thoughts (e.g. remembering a past grudge), being unaware of the probable consequences of aggressive actions, or being incapable of solving problems mentally, rather than 'lashing out' automatically. D'Zurrilla and Goldfried (1971) identify the processes which often precede and guide adaptive behaviour in different circumstances as follows:

being able to recognise problematic situations when they occur;

making an attempt to resist the temptation to act impulsively or to do nothing to deal with the situation;

defining the situation in concrete or operational terms and then formulating the major issues to be coped with;

generating a number of possible responses which might be pursued in this situation;

deciding on the course(s) of action most likely to result in positive consequences;

acting upon the final decision and verifying the effectiveness of the behaviour in resolving the problematic situation.

Adolescents with conduct problems are helped to identify their aggressive behaviour and recognise the conditions which provoke and maintain it. The problem situation is analysed, broken down into its component parts, and represented in a manner most likely to lead to a solution. A number of procedures are available for this purpose. They include self-recording by the adolescent of his or her hostile activities, together with observations of the circumstances in which they occurred and their consequences.

Lochman (1992) reported a three-year follow-up of aggressive young adults (males) participating in a school-based anger-control programme. The results were encouraging: the treated group had lower rates of substance abuse and higher levels of self-esteem and social problem-solving skills than untreated controls. There was no evidence, however, that the programme had a significant long-term effect on delinquent behaviour. A study by McDougall *et al.*, (1987) with 18 institutionalised young offenders found that the anger-control programme assisted in lowering the level of institutional offending.

Training in self-governing behaviour

Fixsen, Phillips and Wolf (1973) developed a system of self-government at Achievement Place (described later) in order to teach delinquent youths some of the social skills involved in group decision making and problem solving. The youngsters were taught to establish many of their own rules on a democratic basis. If one of them violated a rule, the others had to determine guilt or innocence and decide on the consequences. These discussions occurred during daily 'family conferences'. In one of the experiments designed to evaluate how well youths participated in this system of self-government, it was clear that more boys took part in the discussion of consequences for a rule violation when they had complete responsibility for setting the consequences. The comparison involved staff determining the consequences for each rule violation before the family conference. An analysis of rule violations revealed that the boys reported more transgressions than were reported by the teaching-parents, school personnel, or natural parents.

Moral reasoning

There is evidence that immature moral reasoning is a general characteristic of juvenile delinquents (Nelson, Smith & Dodd, 1990). Programmes have been designed to develop moral reasoning in young offenders. Gibbs *et al.* (1984) conducted an intervention in the form of small group discussions on a range of socio-moral dilemmas: the young offenders not only gave their views, but were required to justify their opinions and to attempt to reach a consensus on the best solution. On a measure of Kohlberg's moral judgement stages, the intervention led to a significant upward shift in moral-reasoning ability.

Role-taking and perspective-taking

Chandler (1973) described a programme designed to encourage male young offenders to see themselves from the perspective of other people and so to develop their own role-taking abilities. The study was a clear clinical success, enhancing the young offenders' role-taking skills in a manner that enhanced pro-social behaviour. A similarly successful programme in social perspective-taking skills, carried out with female delinquents, has been reported by Chalmers and Townsend (1990).

Problem-solving skill training

Problem-solving skill training (PSST) with children and adolescents suffering from conduct problems has been implemented in schools, clinics, day treatment and inpatient hospital settings (see Kendall & Braswell, 1993; Kendall & Lochman, 1994). Deficits in cognitive problem-solving processing abilities which mediate social interaction may reduce a young person's interpersonal effectiveness. Research has indicated that when presented with interpersonal problem situations, rejected children, those with conduct disorders, find it difficult to consider alternative courses of action. They do not search effectively for clues or facts and generate few appropriate solutions to conflict situations. On the other hand, they display a high proportion of aggressive and incompetent solutions (Hollin, 1990a, 1991).

Given the social impact of the conduct disorders and the fact that, for most young people, the transition to adolescence is marked by impulsiveness, independence-seeking and a dramatic expansion and complexity of their social lives (Mussen *et al.*, 1984; Robin, 1985), important therapeutic agendas are likely to be about self-control, the resolution of conflict and confrontation within the family, in the school and residential settings, and the acquisition of social skills. Furnham (1986), in a review of skill deficits in adolescents, is of the opinion that difficulties in establishing and maintaining relationships with peers and authority figures reduce the quantity and quality of potential and significant learning experiences available to them.

Spivack, Platt and Shure (1976) suggested that several cognitive problem-solving skills are necessary for successful social interaction: sensitivity to interpersonal problems; the ability to choose the desired outcome of a social exchange ('means–end thinking'); considering the likely outcomes of one's actions ('consequential thinking'); and generating different ways to achieve the desired outcome ('alternative thinking').

Overall, PSST has proved an effective remedial and secondary preventive intervention with oppositional defiant and conduct disorders in children and adolescents (e.g. Spivack & Shure, 1974; Feindler & Ecton, 1986; Kendall *et al.*, 1990; Kolko, Loar & Sturnick, 1990). Kazdin and colleagues (1987, 1989) have obtained statistically and clinically significant improvements in 9–13-year-old inpatients with conduct disorders.

Social skills training

Social skills training (SST) has had a number of aims: to encourage related problem-solving skills, to reduce delinquent behaviour, to improve specific skills such as interview skills, and to increase the effectiveness of penal staff–delinquent interaction.

There is a fairly considerable literature on social skills training with young offenders and pre-delinquent youths (Spence & Marzillier, 1981; Herbert, 1986; Hollin, 1990b). Henderson and Hollin (1983) critically reviewed 15 studies on social-skills training with young offenders and concluded that both practitioners and administrators need to recognise the limitations of the technique; it cannot cure the 'causes of crime' and it is naive to assume it can. SST techniques may have a role to play for some aspects of young offenders' development, but considerable experimental investigation is required before any unqualified faith in, or firm commitments for, the intervention can be made.

Residential group programmes

These are programmes which have been designed to take into account several of the methods described earlier and to apply them systematically in planned environments. An outstanding example of such a unit is Achievement Place – a family-style group home for six to eight pre-delinquent or delinquent boys under the direction of teaching parents. The rationale for this work is that the delinquent behaviour of these boys is the product of inadequate social learning experiences. As Phillips *et al.* (1971) explain: the past environment of behaviourally disturbed youths has failed to provide the instructions, examples and feedback necessary to develop appropriate behaviour. This general behavioural failure often forces the youth to become increasingly dependent upon a deviant peer group, which provides inappropriate instructions, models and reinforcement that exacerbate the behaviour problems.

Cognitive–behavioural methods are used in trying to reverse such developments. The most important role of family-style group homes is educational. They teach youths a variety of social, academic, vocational and self-help skills to equip them with alternative, more adaptive behaviours.

The behaviour change system progresses from a Token Economy Programme (TEP) to a 'merit system', with a peer manager organisation. Individually based programmes in social, educational and self-management skills also take place (see Burchard & Lane, 1982). The evaluation of procedures has played a significant part in the development and refinement of the Achievement Place model. The majority of the original research publications evaluating Achievement Place were intra-individual reversal designs (ABAB) or variations on this theme. There are several reviews of the wealth of research output from Achievement Place (e.g. Kirigin *et al.*, 1982; Braukmann & Wolf, 1987). It appears overall that the Achievement Place model is successful in enhancing pro-social behaviour and reducing offending while in operation, but that this success does not always transfer to the community in the longer term.

Residential practice continues to develop. Hagan and King (1992) describe an intensive treatment programme conducted in a correctional facility for young offenders. This programme combined a range of interventions, including individual cognitive and psychotherapy, a residential management programme, education, family therapy and an independent living programme. At a two-year follow-up, there were encouraging findings with regard to the success of the programme in reducing return to further correctional placements. Similar examples of 'successful' residential outcomes, even with the most difficult and disadvantaged young people, are to be found in a succession of studies (e.g. Jesness, 1975; Hobbs & Holt, 1976; Bullock *et al.*, 1990). There are qualifications to these reports that are dealt with later in this chapter.

Eitzen (1975) notes that the dependent variable for behaviour modifiers in group and community programmes has often been limited to overt behaviour. Providing the behaviour of the youngster becomes more socially acceptable, it is of little importance to some therapists whether a concomitant shift in attitude takes place. Eitzen challenges this indifference on two grounds: (1) an attitude change corresponding with a change in behaviour is likely to increase the probability of a lasting effect, and (2) such an eventuality will make the case for behavioural work more compelling to community agencies contemplating the direction to take in their efforts to attack a particular social problem.

In order to assess whether the Achievement Place experience brings the attitudes of delinquent boys in line with non-delinquent boys, controls from a junior high school were selected. The school chosen was sited in the school district in which most families of Achievement Place youngsters lived. A questionnaire was designed which included scales of achievement orientation, internal–external attitudes, machiavellianism, and self-esteem. Upon entering the programme, the delinquent boys, as expected, tended to be externals, but by the time they left the average score had dropped below the mean of the control group in the internal direction. The data on machiavellianism demonstrated that the Achievement Place experience did not lead to greater machiavellian attitudes among the boys (88 per cent of the boys improved in self-concept). The longer the stay at Achievement Place, the greater the improvement in self-concept. Accompanying the behavioural changes of these delinquent boys were positive shifts in attitudes. The greatest shifts in attitudes were from poor to good self-esteem and from externality to internality. The author poses the unsolved problem: are these positive attitudinal changes a function of the treatment model or the result of placing troubled boys in a stable environment with caring 'parents'?

Community-based interventions

The penal system is often naive about the extent to which changes in behaviour in one setting represent fundamental changes (e.g. in personality) and which, therefore, will accompany the youth when he or she returns to society – no matter what its temptations and deprivations.

In the wake of the failure of traditional institutional environments to provide effective amelioration, treatment of pre-delinquent and delinquent youths has shifted increasingly to community-based settings, giving witness to a growing awareness of the potential of local non-professional people in producing beneficial change (Fo & O'Donnell, 1974, 1975).

The problem with most therapeutic interventions is that the anti-social activity may remain available to the youth as a potential response every time he or she is placed in an environment similar to that in which the original response was made; a return to old haunts may ensure that it comes to be strongly entertained again as a source of satisfaction or survival.

The novelty of the work of Tharp and Wetzel (1969) is that they go into the youth's natural environment to counter this difficulty. They have implemented non-residential programmes using not only parents, but also youth counsellors, teachers and friends as mediators of change. A large-scale study was made with a single individual working as a consultant in an Appalachian community (Wahler & Erickson, 1969). Thirteen volunteers were trained to intervene with 66 families. The volunteers treated a wide range of problems; 197 behaviours were tackled. The presenting problems were classified into classroom disruptive behaviour (including shouting, fighting and disobedience); classroom study behaviour (attending to teaching materials or teacher); school absences; home disruptive behaviour (including fighting with siblings, parents or others, destructiveness and disobedience); and home study behaviour. The theory that these were being maintained by the responses of others in the child's environment was emphasised. A general discussion of social learning theory followed. The staff member and volunteer met for supervision once a fortnight, with the focus on the child's progress and the mediators' maintenance of appropriate contingencies.

On average, occurrences of problem behaviours in the classroom-disruptive and home-disruptive categories fell (by termination) to one-third of their baseline levels. Classroom study behaviour was almost twice as frequent per time-period as at baseline, and home study behaviour was four times as frequent. School absences fell to just over a fifth of their baseline level. All of these differences were statistically significant. The authors note that the lack of a control group means that the precise role of the therapeutic techniques and volunteer strategy cannot be asserted with the same confidence, though the results can be treated as tentative evidence for their effectiveness.

The cost in professional time, and the number and duration of cases, were amenable to a direct comparison with more traditional practice. Twice as many cases were seen annually using the triadic model, and the number of weeks between screening and termination averaged 9 as compared with 19 during dyadic practice. The input of professional time per case was halved using the triadic model. Comparison of the effectiveness of the two approaches was not possible since there had been no evaluation of the dyadic practice.

The possession of *vocational skills* is important (as is academic performance) in the long-term adaptation to social living. There are many dangers for young adults faced with long-term unemployment of (if still at school) chronic academic under-achievement. It seems that in some children the very fact of educational failure leads to disillusionment, boredom and resentment, which throws the children into the arms of a deviant peer group. Their search for excitement, adventure and resolution of different tensions and needs leads them into a variety of rebellious, aggressive and delinquent acts, such as truancy, theft and vandalism.

An unusual study of vocational performance was conducted by Schwitzgebel and Kolb (1964). They developed a Boston area street-corner research project. Twenty 15–21-year-old delinquents, each with multiple arrests and court appearances, were recruited from the streets and were paid an hourly wage to participate in taped interviews. The treatment was described to the delinquent youths as an experiment whose purpose was to find out how teenagers feel about things, how they arrive at certain opinions, and how they change. The specific 'job' of the delinquents was to talk into a tape recorder, for which they were paid. These youths had an average of 15.1 months of incarceration and an average of 8.2 arrests. Thirty other delinquents served as matched controls.

The tape-recorder interviews lasted for one hour, two or three times per week. Generally, the experimenter suggested topics to discuss and shared some personal experience with the youth. He reinforced the youth for particular types of verbalisation with praise, small cash bonuses, or unexpected privileges. Advice giving was decidedly avoided. The youngster was encouraged to talk about his own experiences with emotion and in great detail. Through successive approximations and positive reinforcement, these young men were taught social skills such as coming to work on time, being dressed appropriately, and limiting hostile statements in their conversation. In addition, they were taught technical skills before they were helped to find jobs in the community.

Generally, the youths were associated with the project for ten months. On follow-up three years later, the arrest and conviction record of the first 20 subjects was about half of that of the control group. Unfortunately, the *number* of persons returned to prison or a reformatory did not differ. In other words, the project was associated with a reduction but not an elimination of delinquent behaviour. Of note, however, is the fact that the youths who participated in the experimental project seemed to have less serious offences and were arrested less frequently.

Ayala et al. (1973) worked out a set of procedures to improve performance by youths on a part-time job. Training consisted of instructing them in how to carry out tasks, demonstrating appropriate behaviour, and having them practise the appropriate behaviour. Feedback was provided during training and each day on the job. The results showed that training and feedback were effective in producing substantial improvements in the youngsters' behaviour at work. The research team found that with continued training, the improved behaviour generalised to other work settings.

Braukmann et al. (1974) developed an 'instructional package' to teach job interview skills to delinquent boys in a group home. It contained a detailed description of appropriate interview behaviours and a detailed description of a training procedure consisting of instructions, demonstrations of appropriate behaviours, and differential feedback to the youth on his performance while rehearsing these behaviours during training. The authors conducted three experiments and found that the 'instruction package' was effective in achieving appropriate interview behaviour.

School-based interventions

Cognitive–behavioural interventions for issues of academic concern have become increasingly popular in recent years (Wong, Harris & Graham, 1991). Examples of programmes used with schoolchildren and adolescents are the Anger Coping Programme (Lochman et al., 1989), the Problem Solving Skills Training (PSST) Programme (Kazdin et al., 1987), the Programme for Academic Survival Skills (PASS; Greenwood et al., 1977), the Practice Skills Mastery Programme (Erken & Henderson, 1976) and the Good Behaviour Game (Barrish, Saunders & Wolf, 1969).

These interventions provide operational definitions of appropriate and inappropriate behaviour and draw on different combinations of methods for their promising results (see Braswell & Bloomquist, 1991). The main components are those which train young people to use self-talk, adaptive attributions, problem-solving techniques and self-instruction/self-control skills, in order to modify their dysfunctional classroom activities.

A significant approach to classroom disruption involves the triadic model of providing consultations to teachers, on the assumption that they are the persons best placed to bring about behavioural change in students and, indeed, in their own attitudes, behaviour and curricula (see Goldstein (1995) for a review of the literature on classroom interventions).

An example of a programme for treating aggressive adolescents is that of Feindler and Ecton (1986). They provide aggressive adolescents with a rationale for cognitive restructuring that includes the analogy of rebuilding thoughts as a carpenter rebuilds some area of faulty construction. The rationale also emphasises the importance of learning to moderate extreme negative thinking that could trigger actions that might ultimately lead to a loss of personal power. The self-assessment process involves the following steps: (1) identify the tension, (2) identify what triggered the tension, (3) identify the negative thought connected to the tension, (4) challenge or dispute the negative thought, and (5) tone down or rebuild the thought or substitute positive thought in place of a negative one.

The school-based programme of Sarason and Sarason (1981) is an interesting example of a problem-solving intervention at the high school level. Working with students identified as at-risk for continued delinquent actions and possible dropping-out from school, the authors designed an intervention that was presented as a special unit within a required course. The training content emphasised modelling both the overt behaviours and the cognitive antecedents of adaptive problem solving and included many opportunities for classroom behaviour rehearsal. At the end of the programme, the students participating in the intervention class were able to generate more adaptive solutions for addressing problem situations than control subjects, and were able to give improved self-presentations in the context of a job interview for summer employment. The students were unaware of the fact that their interview was being evaluated with regard to the outcome of the intervention. At one-year follow-up, treated students had fewer absences, less tardiness, and fewer referrals for problematic behaviour than controls.

Reid and Borkowski (1987) have attempted to develop appropriate effort-orientated attributions in hyperactive schoolchildren. Such children have been reported as having a highly externalised locus of control. They are thus more likely to view what happens to them as being the result of external influences. The authors paired self-control training following a curriculum like that reported in Kendall and Braswell (1993) with instruction in effort attributions for both success and failure. In this training, failure was presented as the result of not using the treatment strategies, and success was considered to be the result of the child's active commitment to the strategy. The self-control plus attribution training group displayed a more reflective cognitive style than the group receiving self-control training only, and an increased sense of personal causality. At ten-month follow-up, a notably hyperactive subgroup displayed more positive teacher ratings of pro-social actions than previously.

One of the most widely cited programmes in the literature is the Preparation through Responsive Education Programme (PREP), described in several publications in the late 1970s (see Burchard & Lane (1982) for a review). Based in Maryland, USA, PREP was designed for pupils recommended to the programme because of academic, social and offending problems. It consisted of academic tutoring, social-skills training and some family work. The outcome data, from over 600 pupils, showed that the programme had a significant impact on school discipline and academic performance. However, there was little indication that the programme had an effect on offending.

Multi-modal (combined treatments) programmes

The rationale of multi-modal programmes is the inclusion of several therapeutic strategies to address the many-sided problems that are manifested in adolescents with conduct problems. These include: (a) dysfunctional parent–child relationships; (b) verbal abuse; (c) parenting skills deficits; (d) intra-familial communications; (e) negative self-talk; (f) academic difficulties; and (g) coercive interactions of family members.

The Kendall and Braswell (1993) approach is a fairly typical multi-modal programme which includes problem solving, instructional training, behavioural contingencies, modelling, role-play, and training in the identification of feelings about oneself and others. The typical stages in the problem solving are:

1. *Problem identification*: developing the empathy to identify feelings – as an antidote to impulsive, thoughtless reactivity, denial and avoidance strategies;
2. *Alternative thinking*: developing the skill to generate several alternative solutions in the face of a particular interpersonal situation;
3. *Consequential thinking*: encouraging the capacity to foresee immediate and more long-term information in the process of reaching decisions;

4. *Means–end thinking*: developing the ability to elaborate or plan a series of specific actions to attain a given goal, use a realistic time framework in implementing steps toward that goal, and the means to evaluate the outcome.

Therapists have drawn on *communication skills* as one of their primary methods in multi-modal interventions. The treatment package might involve communication training, feedback, positive interruptions, problem-solving and decision-making skills, providing rationales, happy talk, positive requests, non-blaming communication, negotiation-skill training, didactic dialogue and family games. The behavioural methods might include self-correction, over-correction, positive practice, observation and recording behaviour, self-management, cognitive restructuring, positive reinforcement, differential attention, response–cost, time-out, and the use of symbolic rewards (tokens and points).

Some investigations (e.g. Blechman, Olson & Hellman, 1976; Besalel & Azrin, 1981; Alexander & Parsons, 1982) have used such methods along with behavioural contracting to good effect with conduct problems. Others have used various combinations without the application of behavioural contracting (e.g. Bright & Robin, 1981; Foster, Prinz & O'Leary, 1983).

Gross *et al.* (1980) applied a combination of social-skills training, behaviour therapy and self-management training with ten young female offenders with the outcome of greater self-control, and reduced problematic behaviour and absenteeism from school. Slaby and Guerra (1988) using a programme based on their analysis of cognitive mediation of aggression in adolescent offenders, were able to bring about increases in problem-solving skills, a reduction in belief in the legitimacy of aggression, and a lessening of aggressive activity. There were, unfortunately, no long-term gains as evaluated by violations of parole.

Many of the investigations that have been published suffer from design inadequacies, notably the failure to control for extraneous variables that allow a confident linkage between method used and changes in the targeted behaviours. Among the exceptions are the programmes reported by Kifer *et al.* (1974), Schumaker, Hovell and Sherman (1977) and Serna *et al.* (1991) which resulted in improved negotiation skills, better school attainment and conduct, and effective conflict resolution, respectively.

Among the best-known multi-modal cognitive–behavioural programmes is *Aggression Replacement Training* (ART; Glick & Goldstein, 1987), which includes three main approaches to changing behaviour: structured social-skills learning (social skills and social problem solving), anger-control training and moral education. The outcome studies indicated that the programmes have led to improved skills, improved self-control and more acceptable institutional behaviour. A programme based on ART by Leeman, Gibbs and Fuller (1993) was successful in improving conduct and reducing recidivism. The *Reasoning and Rehabilitation Programme* developed by Ross and Fabiano (1985), incorporating as it does several methods, is another example of useful multi-modal work.

While there are encouraging demonstrations from studies like the ones listed above that, on a variety of quantitative and qualitative outcome measures (notably behavioural indices, cognitive functioning, family relationships, and different academic and social skills), short-term changes can be brought about, there is less room for optimism on the issues of temporal generalisation and (in the case of delinquents) generalisation to actual offending behaviour. Whether the conduct problems reviewed above are functionally related to offending such that changing targeted behaviours will modify delinquent activities is a moot point (Hollin & Henderson, 1984). Undoubtedly, at the offending end of the conduct-problem spectrum, the effective role of CBT as reported up to the early 1980s was not securely established (see Burchard & Lane, 1982; Blakely & Davidson, 1984). This was in contrast to a good track record with conduct-disordered children (Webster-Stratton & Herbert, 1994). The literature provides pointers to a moderately encouraging, if short-term, effect for the non-offending conduct problems of adolescence. Much of this evidence accrued from individual therapy studies.

Family-based programmes
Under this rubric come a variety of essentially multi-modal approaches, notably behavioural parent management (skills) training and behavioural (functional) family therapy. These are likely to be more effective with younger adolescents.

Parent management training
Parent management training (PMT), often adopting a collaborative style of working and using cognitive–behavioural methods of change (see Webster-Stratton & Herbert, 1994), typically aims to guide parents to reinforce socially appropriate behaviour, and to use appropriate sanctions for inappropriate behaviour. A study by Kazdin, Siegal and Bass (1992) evaluated the combined effects of problem-solving skills training and PMT targeted at children showing severe anti-social behaviour. They found that the treatments combined were highly effective in ameliorating aggression and anti-social behaviour, as well as parental stress and depression. A study of young offenders (Bank, Patterson & Reid, 1989) demonstrated that PMT had positive effects on family communication and family relationships, with some indication of a reduction in offending.

Behavioural family therapy
Parent management training and behavioural family therapy (BFT) have much in common. However, in BFT the emphasis is much more explicitly systemic and focuses on dysfunctional family interactions. Several studies have used *contingency contracting* as a means of changing such interactions in the case of the families of young offenders, and with a degree of success in reducing offending (e.g. Stumphauzer, 1976).

Other studies have used a broader range of techniques: Henderson (1981) used behavioural, cognitive and BFT methods in a programme that was successful in reducing stealing. Similarly, Alexander and Parsons (1982) have used skills training, contingency contracting and problem solving to good effect with conduct problems.

Case illustrations

A case of proactive aggression and bullying

Mandy, aged 14, was referred to the clinic for her aggressive outbursts and bullying activities. She agreed to keep a simple diary in order to record episodes of aggression, delineated as hitting, punching and hair-pulling (physical aggression), name-calling, obscenities and threats (verbal aggression). She also rated her feelings of anger and noted down other feelings on a special, individually prepared form. Bullying was discussed and subsumed under the same operational criteria.

After an analysis of the circumstances, persons, places, times and situations related to aggressive incidents, her thoughts and feelings at the time, and their frequency and intensity of the interactions, it was formulated that Mandy was interpreting (misinterpreting) many situations as provocative (e.g. teasings, 'put downs'). Apart from these reactions, she was pre-emptively and proactively attacking (bullying) certain youngsters. Her belief was that such dominance gave her a protective 'big-time' status. She agreed she was friendless because of her behaviour, and in several therapeutic conversations indicated her low self-esteem and revealed a family and developmental history that accounted for it. After jointly deciding on goals, the technique of cognitive structuring was used, challenging her negative thoughts about herself by socratic questioning and by an examination of her many (unacknowledged) personal assets. Positive self-talk was encouraged. Social-skills training involved role-play, role reversal and behaviour rehearsal. Vignettes of different 'provocative' social situations gave her an opportunity to play-act at first, and later to perform *in vivo*, explore her interpretation of others' intentions, the meaning of varieties of body and verbal language, and the social meanings of different situations. In graded homework tasks, she tried out various friendly overtures to specified fellow students. Mandy was taught anger-control techniques based on self-talk and relaxation techniques (see Novaco, 1975).

The programme, with a few setbacks, was eventually successful as measured by the reduction in the frequency of her aggression, the making of two friends, and an increase in her positive self-regard. The programme (an AB research design) took ten weeks, involving 15 sessions. A three-month followed by a six-month review at home and at school revealed a robust maintenance of these positive outcomes.

A case of reactive verbal and physical aggression

Ian, aged 12, was referred for his verbally and physically abusive behaviour toward his peers at school. An assessment revealed, inter alia, a basically insecure adolescent, low in self-esteem and high in reactivity to what he perceived (often appropriately, but not always so) to be the mocking of his schoolmates. The focus of the programme was to teach Ian the processing skills to problem-solve in conflictual situations. The first objective was to help him understand how to recognise a genuine (as opposed to imaginary) problem, and then how to think about solutions to the problem. Next, he was encouraged to think of more alternative solutions to problems. The therapist debated with Ian how 'to think ahead' to the consequences of the solutions he put forward. Finally, they discussed how to evaluate the best solutions. In doing this, they discussed his personal difficulties in responding to problems such as teasing, being rejected, hitting, and anger from others. There were six treatment sessions, each covering a different step in the problem-solving process. The process of problem-solving skills training in this case had the following objectives:

to review concepts regarding feelings and self-talk;

to introduce the idea of problem-solving steps and solutions;

to practise thinking of, and evaluating, alternative solutions to problems;

to introduce assertive but non-violent/abusive responses or judicious ignoring.

In order to assess and rehearse these cognitive–behavioural strategies, the methods described by Goodwin and Mahoney (1975) were adapted prior to the first problem-solving training session. Ian was shown a three-minute videotape of a young adolescent boy being teased and taunted by a group of three boys of similar age. His responses were recorded as to what he would have said and done in these circumstances. They were much what he did at school! At the end of the programme training sessions he again viewed the tape, and gave his responses, by now quite significantly modified. At the next post-training session, at which he again viewed the tape, there were some additions to the scenario. In addition to looking at his taunters and remaining in the centre of the circle, the model was portrayed as coping with verbal assaults through a series of covert self-instructions. These thoughts, which were dubbed on the tape, consisted of such statements as 'I'm not going to let them get me down' and 'I won't lose my temper'.

The dubbed thoughts and the overt actions of the model were pointed out, discussed, and verbally emphasised by the therapist. Each coping self-statement was labelled as an effective way to deal with verbal aggression. After viewing the tape, Ian was asked to verbalise as many of these coping responses as he could recall.

He was then given the opportunity to compare his coping strategies with those of the model and to comment on the value or otherwise of his and the boy's management of the provocation. These strategies were practised in homework assignments, which were reviewed over four weeks of 'reporting-in' sessions.

Although there was an improvement in his behaviour at school (teachers' reports), Ian reverted after a few months to aggressive behaviour at school with the advent of a new boy who regularly provoked him and succeeded in penetrating his, as yet, brittle defences. Booster sessions failed to restore the early post-treatment gains in problem solving and self-control.

Evaluation

There have been many attempts over more than 30 years to mitigate the conduct problems using different approaches in a variety of settings: in clinics (e.g. individual and group psychotherapy); within institutions (places of incarceration); in community social programmes (e.g. group homes); in home settings; in prevention projects (e.g. community diversion programmes). Sadly, much of this work has met with limited success in reducing adolescent conduct problems (e.g. Graziano & Mooney, 1984; Trojanowicz & Morash, 1992); many promising-looking results are compromised by research designs which were inadequate for evaluating treatment-specific outcomes. At the offender end of the conduct disorders there is a bewildering contrast of views as to whether rehabilitation is possible. Views range from the pessimistic 'nothing works'

(Martinson, 1974) to the optimistic 'treatment can be successful' (Ross & Gendreau, 1980; Gendreau and Ross, 1987).

Hollin (1991, p.305) has this to say:

> When we consider cognitive–behavioural programmes it quickly becomes apparent that there is little to say regarding their effects on offending. There are very few such studies which have included offending as a measure of the effectiveness of the programme: few cognitive behaviour modification studies have included measures of recidivism. Indeed, as the reviews of behavioural interventions with delinquents note with consistent regularity, the literature is sorely lacking in follow-up data. It appears that cognitive-behavioural programmes are setting off on the same path.

A similar polarisation of opinion emerges from the literature on non-delinquent conduct-disordered youth (see Herbert, 1987). In the age group from around 3 to 10 or 11, the success rates of cognitive–behaviour therapy (in individual or group mode) are undoubtedly positive (see Webster-Stratton & Herbert, 1994), but there is still a significant number of failures. Nevertheless, this is generally recognised as the method of choice with incipient behaviour problems (oppositional defiant disorder) and the conduct disorders which are diagnosed after the age of six.

What, then, are the findings with regard to the conduct disorders (excluding targets concerned with delinquent activities) of adolescents? The outcome evidence with such conduct problems shows that cognitive–behavioural techniques can be effective in changing behaviour, although temporal generalisation remains a contentious and not yet satisfactorily resolved issue. With the use of cognitive (internalising) strategies and of booster sessions, these technical problems should not prove insurmountable.

Maximising success; minimising failure

Hollin (1991, 1995) suggests ways of enhancing the modest success rates achieved so far:

> Good programme design will, of course, include a selection of suitably motivated clients, treatment integrity, rigorous assessment distinguishing between clinical and criminological targets, and appropriate evaluation measures.

> Strategies for increasing the chances of generalisation should be built into the programme (Burchard & Harrington, 1986).

> In the field of clinical work, not all programmes are run by appropriately trained cognitive–behavioural therapists. This issue of programme 'integrity' is critical (see Hollin, 1995). Quay (1987) has commented on this issue of treatment integrity, citing the example of one published study in which the majority of those responsible for carrying out the treatment were not convinced that it would affect recidivism and the group leaders (not professional counsellors) were poorly trained. As might be

expected, this treatment programme was not successful and another 'failure' entered the literature.

It is important to have some knowledge of the strength and integrity of training in order to assess the merits of a study: some researchers are beginning to build such a measure into their evaluations (Davidson *et al.*, 1987).

To be effective, programmes must attend to the sources of resistance. A number of strategies can be used, including clear communication with all concerned about the programme, and good staff training tackling misconceptions and prejudice about cognitive–behavioural work.

Schlichter and Horan (1981) noted that their self-control programme, conducted in a residential establishment, was undermined by staff members who modelled aggressive behaviour in response to anger provocations and encouraged the subjects to experience and express their 'pent-up' anger (p.364).

Influencing policy (see Hollin, Epps & Kendrick, 1995)
Burchard (1987) argues that social and political contingencies have a profound influence on the work of those who seek to design therapeutic contingencies. It is administrators who decide on funding of research projects (including expensive follow-up research), on equipment, on disposal of young offenders, and ultimately on what the therapist can achieve. He makes a distinction between therapeutic contingencies and social and/or political contingencies. The former are designed by therapists; the latter – generally known as rules, regulations, policies or laws – are established by administrators and legislators. For example, policies towards offenders that result in a high proportion being 'locked up' create challenges for therapists far greater than those that emphasise care and treatment in the community. Generalisation of improved behaviour from a residential to a community setting is hard to achieve. Policymakers need to be aware of this problem in formulating their strategies for offenders.

Burchard asserts the urgent need for change. As he puts it: 'Behaviour analysts must broaden their focus. Social/political contingencies should be brought into the realm of behaviour analysis and behaviour therapy' (p.88). As Hollin (1991) comments with appropriate realism, as administrators are unlikely to rush to us for advice, it follows that we should be devising strategies to engage the attention of policymakers in order to make our voice heard. This requires new skills in lobbying, commenting on policy papers, and educating administrators to use psychological expertise properly. It seems unlikely that this can be accomplished on an individual level and it is therefore incumbent on our professional bodies to develop the structures and mechanisms to allow work of this type to develop.

References

Alexander, J. F. & Parsons, B.V. (1982). *Functional family therapy*. Brooks/Cole, Monterey, CA.

Ayala, H.E., Minken, N., Phillips, D.L. & Wolf, M.M. (1973). *Achievement Place: The training and analysis of vocational behaviors*. Paper read to the American Psychological Association, Montreal, Canada.

Bandura, A. (1977). *Social learning theory*. Prentice-Hall, Englewood Cliffs, NJ.

Bank, L., Patterson, G.R. & Reid, J.B. (1989). Delinquency prevention through training parents in family management. *Behavior Analyst*, 75–82.

Barrish, A.H., Saunders, M. & Wolf, M.M. (1969). Good behavior game. *Journal of Applied Behavior Analysis*, 2, 119–24.

Besalel, V.A. & Azrin, N.H. (1981). The reduction of parent–youth problems by reciprocity counseling. *Behavior Research and Therapy*, 19, 297–301.

Blakely, C.H. & Davidson, W.S. (1984). Behavioral approaches to delinquency: a review. In: *Adolescent behavior disorders: foundations and contemporary concerns* (ed. P. Karoly & J.J. Steffan), pp. 33–41. Lexington Books, Lexington, Mass.

Blechman, E.A., Olson, D.H.L. & Hellman, I.D. (1976). Stimulus control over family problem-solving behavior: The family contract game. *Behavior Therapy*, 7, 686–92.

Braswell, L. & Bloomquist, M. (1991). *Cognitive behavioral therapy with ADHD children: child, family and school intervention*. Guilford Press, New York.

Braukmann, C.J., Maloney, D.M., Fixsen, D.L., Phillips, E.L. & Wolf, M.M. (1974). Analysis of a section interview training package. *Criminal Justice and Behaviour*, 1, 30–42.

Braukmann, C.J. & Wolf, M.M. (1987). Behaviourally based group homes for juvenile offenders. In: *Behavioural approaches to crime and delinquency: a handbook of application, research, and concepts* (ed. E.K. Morris & C.J. Braukmann(, pp. 121–41. Plenum Press, New York.

Bright, P.D. & Robin, A.L. (1981). Ameliorating parent–adolescent conflict and problem-solving communication training. *Journal of Behavior Therapy and Experimental Psychiatry*, 12, 275–80.

Bullock, R., Hosie, K., Little, M. & Millham, S. (1990). Secure accommodation for very difficult adolescents: some recent research findings. *Journal of Adolescence*, 13, 205–16.

Burchard, J.D. (1987). Social policy and the role of the behaviour analyst in the prevention of delinquent behaviour. *The Behaviour Analyst*, 10, 83–8.

Burchard, J.D. & Harrington, W.A. (1986). Deinstitutionalization: programmed transition from the institution to the community. *Child and Family Behavior Therapy*, 7, 17–32.

Burchard, J.D. & Lane, T.W. (1982). Crime and delinquency. In: *International handbook of behavior modification and therapy* (ed. A.S. Bellack, M. Hersen & A.E. Kazdin), pp. 71–84. Plenum Press, New York.

Chalmers, J.B. & Townsend, M.A.R. (1990). The effects of training in social perspective taking on socially maladjusted girls. *Child Development*, 61, 178–90.

Chandler, M.J. (1973). Egocentrism and anti-social behavior: the assessment and training of social perspective-taking skills. *Developmental Psychology*, 9, 326–32.

Davidson, W.S., Redner, R., Blakely, C.H., Mitchell, C.M. & Emshoff, J.G. (1987). Diversion of juvenile offenders: an experimental comparison. *Journal of Consulting and Clinical Psychology*, 55, 68–75.

D'Zurrilla, T.J. & Goldfried, M.R. (1971). Problem solving and behavior modification. *Journal of Abnormal Psychology*, 78, 107–26.

Eitzen, D.S. (1975). The effects of behavior modification on the attitudes of delinquents. *Behavior Research and Therapy*, 13, 295–9.

Erken, N. & Henderson, H. (1976). Practice skills mastery program. Mastery Programs, Logan, UT.

Farrington, D.P. (1992). Psychological contributions to the explanation, prevention and treatment of offending. In *Psychology and law: international perspectives* ed. F. Losel, D. Bender & T. Bliesender, pp. 141–52. De Gruyter, Berlin.

Farrington, D.P. (1995). The development of offending and anti-social behaviours from childhood: key findings from the Cambridge study of delinquent development. *Journal of Child Psychology and Psychiatry*, 360, 929–64.

Feindler, E.L. & Ecton, R.B. (1986). *Adolescent anger control: cognitive–behavioral techniques*. Pergamon Press, New York.

Fixsen, D.L., Phillips, E.L. & Wolf, M.M. (1973). Achievement Place: experiments in self-government with pre-delinquents. *Journal of Applied Behavior Analysis*, 6, 31–47.

Fo, W.S.O. & O'Donnell, C.R. (1974). The buddy system: relationship and contingency conditions in a community intervention program for youth and non-professionals as behavior change agents. *Journal of Consulting and Clinical Psychology*, 42, 163–8.

Fo, W.S.O. & O'Donnell, C.R. (1975). The buddy system: effect of community intervention on delinquent offences. *Behavior Therapy*, 6, 522–4.

Foster, S.L., Prinz, R.J. & O'Leary, K.D. (1983). Impact of problem-solving communication training and generalization procedures on family conflict. *Child and Family Behavior Therapy*, 5, 1–23.

Furnham, C. (1986). Social skill training with adolescents. In *Handbook of Social Skills Training*, Vol. 1 (ed. C.R. Hollin & P.Trower), pp. 33–58. Pergamon Press, Oxford.

Gendreau, P. & Ross, R.R. (1987). Revivification of rehabilitation: evidence from the 1980s. *Justice Quarterly*, **4**, 349–407.

Gibbs, J.C., Arnold, K.D., Chessman, F.L. & Ahlborn, H.H. (1984). Facilitation of sociomoral reasoning in delinquents. *Journal of Consulting and Clinical Psychology*, **52**, 37–45.

Glick, B. & Goldstein, A.P. (1987). Aggression replacement training. *Journal of Counseling and Development*, **65**, 356–67.

Goldstein, S. (Ed.) (1995). *Understanding and managing children's classroom behavior*. John Wiley, New York.

Goodwin, S.E. & Mahoney, M.J. (1975). Modification of aggression through modelling: an experimental probe. *Journal of Behavior Therapy and Experimental Psychiatry*, **6**, 200–2.

Graziano, A.M. & Mooney, K.C. (1984). *Children and behavior therapy*. Aldine Publishing, New York.

Greenwood, C., Hops, H., Dolquadri, J. & Walker, H.M. (1977). *PASS Consultant Manual*. Center at Oregon for Research in the Behavioral Education of the Handicapped, Eugene.

Gross, A.M., Brigham, T.A., Hopper, C. & Bologna, N.C. (1980). Self-management and social skills training: a study with pre-delinquent and delinquent youths. *Criminal Justice and Behavior*, **7**, 161–84.

Hagan, M. & King, R.P. (1992). Recidivism rates of youths completing an intensive treatment program in a juvenile correctional facility. *International Journal of Offender Therapy and Comparative Criminology*, **36**, 349–58.

Henderson, J.Q. (1981). A behavioral approach to stealing: a proposal for treatment based on ten cases. *Journal of Behavior Therapy and Experimental Psychiatry*, **12**, 231–6.

Henderson, M. & Hollin, C.R. (1983). A critical review of social skills training with young offenders. *Criminal Justice and Behavior*, **10**, 316–41.

Herbert, M. (1986). Social skills training with children. In *Handbook of Social Skills Training*, Vol. 1 (ed. C.R. Hollin & P. Trower), pp. 11–32. Pergamon Press, Oxford.

Herbert, M. (1987). *Conduct disorders of childhood and adolescence*. Wiley, Chichester.

Herbert, M. (1991). *Clinical child psychology: social learning, development and behaviour*. Wiley, Chichester.

Herbert, M. (1994a). Etiological considerations. In *International handbook of anxiety disorder in children and adolescents* (ed. T.H. Ollendick, N.J. King & W. Yule), pp. 3–20. Plenum Press, New York.

Herbert, M. (1994b). Behavioural methods. In *Child and adolescent psychiatry: a modern approach* (ed. M. Rutter, E. Taylor & L. Hersov), pp. 858–79. Blackwell Scientific, Oxford.

Herbert M. (1995). A collaborative model of training for parents of children with disruptive behavior disorders. *British Journal of Clinical Psychology*, **34**, 325–42.

Hobbs, T.R. & Holt, M.H. (1976). The effects of token reinforcement on the behavior of delinquents in cottage settings. *Journal of Applied Behavior Analysis*, **9**, 189–98.

Hollin, C.R. (1990a) *Cognitive–behavioural interventions with young offenders*. Pergamon, Elmsford, NY.

Hollin, C.R. (1990b) Social skills training with delinquents: a look at the evidence and some recommendations for practice. *British Journal of Social Work*, **20**, 483–93.

Hollin, C.R. (1991). Cognitive–behaviour modification with delinquents. In *Clinical child psychology: social learning, development and behaviour* (ed. M. Herbert), pp. 293–308. Wiley, Chichester.

Hollin, C.R. (1995). The meaning and implications of 'programme integrity'. In *What works: effective methods to reduce reoffending* (ed. J. McGuire), pp. 4–23. Wiley, Chichester.

Hollin, C.R. & Henderson, M. (1984). Social skills training with young offenders: false expectations and the 'failure of treatment'. *Behavioural Psychotherapy*, **12**, 331–41.

Hollin, C.R., Epps, K.J. & Kendrick D.J. (1995). *Managing behavioural treatment: policy and practice with delinquent adolescents*. Routledge, London.

Hollon, S.D. & Beck, A.T. (1994). Cognitive and cognitive–behavioural therapies. In *Handbook of psychotherapy and behavior change* 4th edn, (ed. A.E. Bergin & S.L. Garfield), pp. 428–66. Wiley, New York.

Jesness, C.F. (1975). Comparative effectiveness of behaviour modification and transactional analysis programs for delinquents. *Journal of Clinical and Consulting Psychology*, **43**, 758–79.

Kazdin, A.E. (1987). Treatment of anti-social behaviour in children: current status and future directions. *Psychological Bulletin*, **102**, 187–203.

Kazdin, A.E. (1994). Psychotherapy for children and adolescents. In *Handbook of psychotherapy and behaviour change*, 4th edn, (ed. A.E. Bergin & S.L. Garfield), pp. 543–94. Wiley, New York.

Kazdin, A.E., Bass, D., Siegel T. & Thomas C. (1989). Cognitive behavioural therapy in the treatment of children referred for anti-social behaviour. *Journal of Clinical and Consulting Psychology*, **57**, 522–35.

Kazdin, A.E., Esveldt-Dawson, K., French, N.H. & Unis, A.S. (1987). Problem solving skills training and relationship therapy in the treatment of anti-social child behavior. *Journal of Consulting and Clinical Psychology*, **55**, 76–85.

Kazdin, A.E., Siegel, T.C. & Bass, D. (1992). Cognitive problem-solving skills training and parent management training in the treatment of anti-social behaviour in children. *Journal of Consulting and Clinical Psychology*, **60**, 733–47.

Kendall, P.C. (ed.) (1991). *Child and adolescent therapy: cognitive–behavioral procedures*. Guilford Press, New York.

Kendall, P.C. (1993). Cognitive-behavioral therapies with youth: Guiding theory, current status, and emerging developments. *Journal of Consulting and Clinical Psychology*, **61**, 235–47.

Kendall P. & Braswell L. (1993). *Cognitive–behavioural therapy for impulsive children*. 2nd edn. Guilford Press, New York.

Kendall, P.C. & Hollon, S.D. (eds.) (1994). Cognitive–behavioural interventions: theory, research and procedures. Academic Press, New York.

Kendall, P.C. & Lochman, J. (1994). Cognitive–behavioural therapies. In *Child and adolescent psychiatry: modern approaches* (ed. M. Rutter, E. Taylor & L. Hersov), pp. 844–57. Blackwell Scientific Publications, Oxford.

Kendall, P.C., Reber, M., McLeer, S., Epps, J. & Ronan, K.R. (1990). Cognitive-behavioral treatment of conduct-disordered children. *Cognitive Therapy and Research*, **14**, 279–97.

Kifer, R.E., Lewis, M.A., Green, D.R. & Phillips, E.L. (1974). Training predelinquent youths and their parents to negotiate conflict situations. *Journal of Applied Behavior and Analysis*, **7**, 357–64.

Kirigin, K.A., Braukmann, C.J., Atwater J. & Wolf, M.M. (1982). An evaluation of Achievement Place (Teaching-Family) group homes for juvenile offenders. *Journal of Applied Behavior Analyst*, **15**, 1–16.

Kolko, D.J., Loar, L.L. & Sturnick, D. (1990). Inpatient social–cognitive skills training groups with conduct-disordered children. *Journal of Child Psychology and Psychiatry*, **31**, 737–48.

Leeman, L.W., Gibbs, J.C. & Fuller, D. (1993). Evaluation of a multi-component group treatment programme for juvenile delinquents. *Aggressive Behavior*, **19**, 281–92.

Lochman, J.E. (1992). Cognitive–behavioral intervention with aggressive boys: three-year follow-up and preventive effects. *Journal of Consulting and Clinical Psychology*, **60**, 426–32.

Lochman, J.E., Burch, P.P., Curry, J.F. & Lampron, L.B. (1984). Treatment and generalization effects of cognitive–behavioural and goal-setting interventions with aggressive boys. *Journal of Consulting and Clinical Psychology*, **52**, 915–16.

Lochman, J.E., Lampron, L., Gemmer, R.C., Harris, S. Wycroff, G. (1989). Teacher consultation and cognitive–behavioral interventions with aggressive boys. *Psychology in the Schools*, **26**, 179–88.

Martinson, R. (1974). What works? Questions and answers about prison reform. *The Public Interest*, **35**, 22–54.

McDougall, C., Barnett, R.M., Ashurst, B. & Willis, B. (1987). Cognitive control of anger. In *Applying psychology to imprisonment: theory and practice* (ed. B.J. McGurk, D.M. Thornton & M. Williams), pp. 120–43. HMSO, London.

Meichenbaum, D.H., Bream, L.A. & Cohen, J.S. (1985). A cognitive–behavioural perspective of child psychopathology: implications for assessment and training. In *Childhood disorders: behavioural developmental approaches* (ed. R.J. McMahon & R. Peters), pp. 36–52, Bruner/Mazel, New York.

Meichenbaum, D.H. & Burland, S. (1979). Cognitive behavior modification with children. *School Psychology Digest*, **8**, 426–33.

Mussen, P.H., Conger J.J., Kagan, J. & Huston, A.C. (1984). *Child development and personality*. Harper and Row, New York.

Nelson, J.R., Smith, D.J. & Dodd, J. (1990). The moral reasoning of juvenile delinquents: a meta-analysis. *Journal of Abnormal Child Psychology*, **18**, 231–9.

Novaco, R.W. (1975). *Anger control: the development and evaluation of an experimental treatment*. D.C. Heath, Lexington, Mass.

Novaco, R.W. (1979). The cognitive regulation of anger and stress. In *Cognitive–behavioural interventions: theory, research and practice* (ed. P.C. Kendall & S.E. Hollon), pp. 241–85. Academic Press, New York.

Ollendick, T.H. & Cerny, J.A. (1981). *Clinical behaviour therapy with children*. Plenum Press, New York.

Phillips, E.L., Phillips, E.A., Fixsen, D.L. & Wolf, M.M. (1971). Achievement place: modification of the behaviours of pre-delinquent boys with a token economy. *Journal of Applied Behavior Analysis*, **4**, 45–59.

Powell, M.B. & Oei, T.P.S. (1991). Cognitive processes underlying the behaviour change in cognitive–behaviour therapy with childhood disorders: a review of experimental evidence. *Behavioural Psychotherapy*, **19**, 247–265.

Quay, C. (ed.) (1987). *Handbook of juvenile delinquency*. Wiley, New York.

Reid, M.K. & Borkowski, J.G. (1987). Causal attributions of hyperactive children: implications for teaching strategies and self-control. *Journal of Educational Psychology*, **79**, 296–307.

Robin, A.L. (1985). Parent adolescent conflict: a developmental problem of families. In *Childhood disorders: behavioural developmental approaches* (ed. R.J. McMahon & R.D. Peters), pp. 38–62. Bruner/Mazel, New York.

Robins, L.N. & Price, R.K. (1991). Adult disorders predicted by child epidemiologic catchment area project. *Psychiatry*, **54**, 116–32.

Ross, R.R. & Fabiano, E.A. (1985). *Time to think: a cognitive model of delinquency prevention and offen-*

der rehabilitation. Institute of Social Sciences and Arts, Johnson City, Tenn.

Ross, R.R. & Gendreau, P. (1980). *Effective correctional treatment*. Butterworths, Toronto.

Sarason, I.G. & Sarason, B.R. (1981). Teaching cognitive and social skills to high school students. *Journal of Consulting and Clinical Psychology*, **49**, 908–18.

Schlichter K.J. & Horan J.J. (1981). Effects of stress inoculation on the anger and aggression management skills of institutionalized young offenders. *Cognitive Therapy and Research*, **5**, 359–65.

Schumaker, J.B., Hovell, M.F. & Sherman, J.A. (1977). An analysis of daily report cards and parent-managed privileges in the improvement of adolescent classroom performance. *Journal of Applied Behaviour Analysis*, **10**, 449–64.

Schwitzgebel, R.L. & Kolb D.A. (1964). Inducing behaviour change in adolescent delinquents. *Behaviour research and therapy*, **1**, 297–304.

Serna, L.A., Schumaker, J.B., Sherman, J.A. & Sheldon, J.B. (1991). In-home generalization of social interactions in families of adolescents in behavior problems. *Journal of Applied Behavior Analysis*, **24**(4), 733–46.

Serna, L.A., Sherman, J.A. & Sheldon, J.B. (1996). Empirically based behavioural treatment programmes for families with adolescents who are at risk of failure. In *Clinical approaches to working with offenders* (ed. C.R. Hollin & K.Howells), pp. 165–79. Wiley, Chichester.

Slaby, R.G. & Guerra, N.G. (1988). Cognitive mediators of aggression in adolescent offenders: 1. Assessment. *Developmental Psychology*, **24**, 580–8.

Snyder, J.J. & White, M.J. (1979). The use of cognitive self-instruction in the treatment of behaviourally disturbed adolescents. *Behavior Therapy*, **10**, 227–35.

Spence, S.H. & Marzillier, J.S. (1981). Social skills training with adolescent male offenders: 1. Short-term effects. *Behaviour Research and Therapy*, **17**, 7–16.

Spivack, G., Platt, J.J. & Shure, M.B. (1976). *The problem-solving approach to adjustment: a guide to research and intervention*. Jossey-Bass, San Francisco.

Spivack, G. & Shure, M.B. (1974). *Social adjustment of young children: a cognitive approach to solving real-life problems*. Jossey-Bass, San Francisco.

Stumphauzer, J.S. (1976). Elimination of stealing by self-reinforcement of alternative behavior and family contracting. *Journal of Behavior Therapy and Experimental Psychiatry*, **7**, 265–8.

Tharp, R.G. & Wetzel, R.J. (1969). *Behavior modification in the natural environment*. Academic Press, New York.

Trojanowicz, R.C. & Morash, M. (1992). *Juvenile delinquency: concepts and control*. Prentice Hall, Englewood Cliffs.

Wahler, R.G. & Erickson, M. (1969). Child behavior therapy: a community programme in Appalachia. *Behavior Research and Therapy*, **7**, 71–8.

Webster-Stratton, C. & Herbert, M. (1994). *Troubled families: problem children. Working with parents – a collaborative approach*. Wiley, Chichester.

World Health Organisation (1992). *The ICD-10 classification of mental and behavioural disorders. Clinical descriptions and diagnostic guidelines*. WHO, Geneva.

Wong, B.Y.L., Harris, K. & Graham, S. (1991). Academic applications of cognitive-behavioral programmes with learning disabled students. In: *Child and adolescent therapy: cognitive–behavioral procedures* (ed. P.C. Kendall), pp. 41–50. Guilford Press, New York.

12
Interpersonal problems

Susan H. Spence and Caroline Donovan

The nature and causes of interpersonal problems

Interpersonal problems during childhood are associated with many forms of psycho-pathology. For example, poor relationships with peers are predictive of a range of emotional and behavioural problems during adolescence (Van Hasselt et al., 1979; Coie et al., 1995). Furthermore, many families will seek professional help for children's problems relating to relationship difficulties, such as parent–adolescent conflict, peer rejection at school, social isolation, loneliness and extreme shyness. Thus, cognitive–behavioural approaches to the enhancement of children's social competence play an important part in the prevention and treatment of child psychopathology.

Social competence, as defined here, refers to the ability to obtain successful outcomes from relationships with others. For children, social competence is reflected in outcomes such as number, quality and durability of friendships, receiving invitations to partici-pate in social activities, general quality of relationships with parents, teachers and peers, and feelings about one's ability to be liked by others. There are many reasons why a young person may or may not be successful in their interactions with others. The major focus of this chapter concerns the importance of social skills and methods of improving social skills performance. However, there are many factors that play an important part in determining the success of children's relationships. For some children, the expecta-tions of parents or teachers may be inappropriate for their developmental level. For others, there may be some disability or unusual characteristic that makes them different from their peers, and that influences the reaction of other children towards them. Thus, before a social skills training (SST) approach is decided upon, it is important to con-sider a wide range of alternative explanations that could account for the child's inter-personal difficulties. These factors should then be dealt with as a component of therapy.

Social–cognitive skills

A multitude of cognitive processes determine the actual behaviour of children in social situations (McFall, 1982). These processes involve a complex interplay between social perception and social problem-solving skills. Problems in any one of these skills may lead to inappropriate behaviour. Social perception skills include:

receiving information from others and the social environment;

attention to relevant social cues;

knowledge of social rules;

knowledge of the meaning of social cues;

correct interpretation of information received;

ability to take the perspective of others;

ability to monitor one's own behaviour and its outcome and alter it when necessary.

Social problem-solving skills include:

identifying the nature and existence of a social problem;

determining the goals for the situation;

generating ideas for possible alternative responses;

predicting the likely consequences of alternatives;

deciding upon a response likely to lead to a successful outcome;

planning the chosen response.

Thus, children need to process social information, problem solve and plan their own behaviour in a way that selects a response that is most likely to lead to a successful outcome. Research has demonstrated that deficits in social cognitive skills are associated with a range of behavioural problems. For example, aggressive children tend to interpret social cues as indicating high levels of threat and negative intent by others and are more likely to generate and select aggressive solutions to interpersonal dilemmas (Dodge, 1986). Anxious children are more likely to interpret ambiguous social situations as indicating social threat, and will pick avoidant solutions (Bell-Dolan, 1995). Thus, deficits or biases in social cognition may be manifest in children's actual behaviour, such as aggression or anxious avoidance.

Behavioural social skills

Although social–cognitive skills are important in determining the way in which children choose to behave, there is also a great deal of skill involved in performing the selected response in a competent manner. There are a large number of behavioural components that influence the impression that our behaviour has upon others. These 'micro-skills' concern the elements of social behaviour that must be carefully integrated and sequenced in the performance of a social response. There is a myriad of behavioural social skills, deficits in which may have a considerable impact upon the way in which social behaviour is judged by others. Many of these micro-skills involve non-verbal behaviours, such as eye contact, posture, facial expression, and social distance. Variations in these responses can have a marked impact on the impression that we make upon others. These non-verbal behaviours also play an important role as listening skills. For example, facial expression, eye contact, posture and head nods are important in demonstrating to the other person that you are interested and listening to the conversation. Other micro-skills are of a verbal nature, such as tone of voice, latency of response, clarity, rate, fluency and volume of speech. Again, variations in these areas of skill may have a marked impact on the way in which other people regard our behaviour.

There are many other important social skills, but space does not permit a complete discussion of them all. However, micro-skills can be regarded as the elements or building blocks which underpin more complex social behaviours. There is an enormous number of complex social responses that children are required to make each day. These include tasks such as starting, maintaining and ending conversations, asking to join in with a peer group activity, offering and asking for help, offering and accepting compliments, and dealing with teasing. Each of these tasks require the integration and sequencing of a myriad of micro-skills, in addition to a strategy for dealing with the specific social situation of concern. Thus, deficits in micro-skills or social strategies may result in unsuccessful outcomes from social situations.

Other factors that determine social competence

There are many other factors that determine why children behave in a particular way in social situations. Social behaviour is determined by the same principles of learning that apply to any other form of human behaviour. Thus, factors such as modelling by others, and reinforcement or punishment contingencies will have a significant impact upon social responding.

Children's thoughts, attitudes and beliefs relating to social interactions also influence their social behaviour. In many instances, children are capable of behaving in a socially appropriate manner, and yet select an inappropriate response as the result of maladaptive thoughts or beliefs. For example, aggressive children have been shown to make attributions about events and the behaviour of others in a way that increases the chance that they will behave in an aggressive manner (Lochman & Dodge, 1994). Our recent research with socially phobic children suggests that their thoughts during social-evaluative situations are characterised by negative expectancies and highly critical self-evaluations. They expect bad things to happen to them in social situations and expect to perform badly. These thoughts are likely to trigger avoidance behaviour and to generate high levels of anxiety. Similarly, the pessimistic cognitive style of depressed children is associated with poor social competence (Garber, Weiss & Shanley, 1993).

Thus, social behaviour may be influenced by interfering anxious and depressed thinking. Even if children technically know what to do, and can perform a social task satisfactorily under low levels of anxiety, their performance is likely to be altered significantly if they are experiencing very high levels of anxiety.

To summarise so far, there are many explanations why a particular child is unsuccessful in social relationships. Although one explanation may be poor social skills, there are many alternative causal factors that need to be considered. These include deficits in social cognition (e.g. poor social problem solving, lack of social knowledge or deficits in social perception), and a learning history or interfering thoughts, beliefs or emotions (e.g. anxiety) that promote inappropriate social behaviour. Furthermore, children do not behave in isolation, and we need to consider whether the problems may reflect the behaviour, attitudes and expectancies of others, rather than problems of the children themselves.

The assessment process

The assessment of children's interpersonal problems begins with evaluation of social competence in order to determine whether social difficulties exist. If social problems are established, then the assessment proceeds to determine which factors are responsible. As mentioned above, there are many reasons why children may experience interpersonal difficulties, including deficits in social–cognitive and behavioural social skills, social anxiety, maladaptive thoughts and beliefs and the behaviour of others.

Assessment of social competence and social skills

A variety of methods is available for the assessment of social competence, social skills and causal variables. These include interviews, questionnaires (completed by the child, parents and/or teachers), and direct behavioural observation undertaken in real-life or role-play situations. Assessment needs to examine social behaviour across a wide range of settings (e.g. home, school, recreation) and with different individuals (e.g. parents, teachers, peers). A detailed outline of measures and processes relating to the assessment of social competence and social skills is provided by Spence (1995). What follows here is a brief summary.

Interviews with parents, teachers and the young person can provide important information about the quality and quantity of the child's social relationships, friendships and social activities. Information can be provided about the type of situations in which the young person has problems, details about what he or she does in each situation, and how other people respond. The child interview also provides a good opportunity for the therapist to observe the child's social skills, albeit in a rather unnatural situation.

Questionnaires and checklists may also provide useful details about social competence and social skills. Sociometry is a useful method of identifying children who are disliked by their peer group or who have few friendships. Two main forms of sociometry are used, the first being a nomination approach in which peers are asked to nominate a set number of individuals with whom they would most like to engage in some specified activity. Negative nominations may also be asked for in which children nominate those peers with whom they would not like to participate in the activity. A second method of sociometry involves each child rating each of his or her peers on some dimension related to popularity, such as a rating of how much he or she likes each classmate. Sociometric methods such as these have been widely used in the research literature to identify children with peer relationship difficulties. However, the method is of limited utility in clinical practice, where children tend to be identified by parents or teachers as experiencing interpersonal problems or some clinical disorder. It is generally impractical and of questionable ethical practice to assess all children in the referred child's classroom in order to obtain a sociometric assessment.

An alternative method for assessing the quality of relationships with peers is the Social Competence with Peers Questionnaire (Spence, 1995), for which child, parent and teacher versions are available. An evaluation of social-skills performance may then be conducted using the parent, teacher and pupil versions of the Social Skills Questionnaire (Spence, 1995). Each questionnaire includes 30 items; the respondent rates the degree to which each item best describes the child over the preceding four weeks. Items cover a wide range of social skills such as the ability to deal with situations requiring an assertive response, to handle conflict situations, and peer and family relationship skills. These measures have well-researched psychometric properties and have been shown to have good reliability and validity.

Most other questionnaires have confounded the assessment of social skills and social competence. However, some useful measures include the Matson Evaluation of Social Skills for Youngsters (Matson, Rotatori & Helsel, 1983), and the Social Skills Rating System (Gresham & Elliott, 1990). Other authors have focused more specifically on children's ability to behave in an assertive rather than aggressive or submissive manner. For example, the Children's Assertive Behaviour Scale (Michelson & Wood, 1982), the Children's Assertiveness Inventory (Ollendick, 1983) and the Children's Action Tendency Scale (Deluty, 1979, 1984) are all useful measures of assertive behaviour in children.

Direct behavioural observation provides important validation of the assessment process. Observations of children's behaviour may be conducted from role-play scenarios in the clinic setting or, preferably, from real-life situations. Measurements of specific micro-skills, such as eye contact, facial expression and tone of voice, are best obtained from videotapes of role-played scenarios. In research settings, careful measures may be taken of specific behaviours performed during structured role-plays such as the Behavioural Assertiveness for Children–Revised (Ollendick, Hart & Francis, 1985). These are very time consuming and require considerable training of observers in order to obtain reliable measurements. In clinical practice, videotaped role-plays may be replayed and behaviours rated on a simple rating system, as outlined by Spence (1995).

Ideally, assessment of social skills and social competence should include observation in real life settings such as the family, school playground or classroom. However, there are many practical difficulties here. Several hours of training of observers is required in order to obtain reliable measurements. Our own experience has shown problems of remaining unobtrusive, children vanishing into the toilet block in the middle of the observation, and difficulty in hearing and seeing exactly what children are doing from a distance. In routine clinical practice, therefore, it may be preferable to conduct informal observations, recording specific behaviours of relevance to the particular child. For example, the clinician may want to know answers to questions such as 'Does the child spend free time with other children?'; 'Does he or she eat lunch alone or with others?'; 'Does he or she start conversations with other children and if so, how do peers respond to his or her initiations?'; 'Does the child answer questions in class or volunteer information?'; 'How does he or she respond when criticised in class'; and 'What happens at home if a parent gives a direct instruction?'. Thus, direct behavioural observation may provide an enormous amount of information about what is actually happening in real-life situations.

Assessment of social–cognitive skills

As part of the assessment, it is important to determine whether children's inappropriate social behaviour reflects a lack of knowledge about how they are expected to behave and/or misinterpretation of the social cues around them. There are several research measures for assessing interpersonal problem-solving skills, although they tend to be complicated to score and lack norms to determine what is 'normal' for children of a particular age. These measures include the Open-Middle Interview (OMI; Polifka *et al.*, 1981) and the Means–Ends Problem Solving Test (MEPS; Platt & Spivack, 1975). The OMI presents children with hypothetical social problems in a cartoon format and asks them to generate as many solutions to the problem as possible. Scores can be produced for the number of different types of solution and their effectiveness. The MEPS assesses children's ability to produce step-by-step methods for reaching solutions to interpersonal problems. Each story presents a beginning and an end to an interpersonal problem, for which children are asked to fill in the middle to indicate various ways that the problem could have been solved. Measures such as these are useful in determining whether children know at a cognitive level how to behave in such a way as to obtain successful outcomes. Some children will report stereotyped, ineffective solutions, such as aggressive or avoidant ways of responding. Deficits may be reflected in either the quantity or quality of solutions proposed. If deficits in social problem-solving skills are found, then social problem-solving training may form an important part of the intervention.

The assessment of social perception skills should also be considered if children are noted to respond inappropriately during social interactions. This area has not been well researched and there are few assessment measures available. However, Spence (1995) provides a screen for children's social perception skills. Photographs depicting a range of adult and child facial expressions and posture cues are provided, each of which depicts a specific emotional state. These materials are useful in identifying children who show biases in the perception of social stimuli. For example, some children may incorrectly interpret a wide range of emotional expressions as depicting anger in another person, and this increases the chance that their subsequent behaviour will be aggressive or defensive. Other children may have great difficulty interpreting the emotional cues of others more generally, with no particular bias but a large number of incorrect responses. In both instances, training in the correct interpretation of social cues would be justified.

Assessment of interfering attitudes and thoughts

Various methods are available to help children to identify thoughts and attitudes that steer their social behaviour in a particular direction. In terms of interfering attitudes, the type of assessment will depend on the nature of the presenting problem. For example, if problems of aggression towards adults are identified, then assessment of anti-authoritarian attitudes may be relevant. For other children, assessment of locus of control may be relevant, if the therapist regards the issues of internal–external control as important. Negative thinking styles along the lines proposed by Beck (1976) can be evaluated using methods such as the Children's Cognitive Error Questionnaire (Leitenberg, Yost & Carroll-Wilson, 1986). This measure provides an indication of children's tendency to overgeneralise predictions of negative outcomes, catastrophise the consequences of events, incorrectly take personal responsibility for negative outcomes, and selectively attend to the negative features of situations.

In clinical practice, cartoons can be useful to assess children's maladaptive thoughts and beliefs. A cartoon is drawn of a social situation of relevance to the child. For example, this might depict a child sitting in the school playground watching a group of peers playing. A blank cartoon bubble is then drawn and the child is asked to imagine himself or herself as the person in the cartoon and to fill in the thoughts in the cartoon bubble. This process may provide some useful insights into the young person's thoughts, such as 'I want to play with them, but I know that I will say something stupid and they will all laugh at me'. The interview with the child also provides an opportunity for the therapist to explore specific thoughts related to relevant social situations.

Assessment of social anxiety

Many of the interfering cognitions that are described above relate to anxious anticipation of negative outcomes. As mentioned above, social anxiety plays an important part in disrupting the social relationships of many children. It has been proposed that social anxiety leads to withdrawal from and avoidance of interactions and also produces performance decrements, such that when socially anxious children do try to use their social skills and attempt to interact in an appropriate way, the high levels of anxiety impair their performance. Thus, it is important that social anxiety is considered as a routine part of the assessment of social functioning. In addition to the identification of anxious thoughts as described in the previous section, several questionnaires can be used for the assessment of children's social anxiety. These include the Social Worries Questionnaire (Spence, 1995) and the Social Anxiety Scale for Children (La Greca & Stone, 1993). The Social Anxiety Scale for Children is particularly useful in that it provides an indication of children's fears of negative evaluation, in addition to their tendency to avoid social situations. In contrast, the Social Worries Questionnaire identifies a range of social-evaluative situations that children avoid or become worried about. This latter measure does have the advantage of parent, child and teacher versions.

Assessment of other relevant features

It is important to note that the assessment of social competence and social skills takes place within the context of other presenting problems, such as child depression, conduct disorders, and so on. There may also be issues in the family, such as parental psychopathology or marital discord, that require attention. Similarly, at school the young person may have learning difficulties or other problems that need to be considered. A wide range of non-social factors may also be influencing the child's success in social interactions. Thus, assessment should also examine factors such as ethnic and cultural differences from the peer group, sensory and physical handicaps, physical attractiveness, personal hygiene, and grooming, all of which may potentially influence the response of others towards the young person. These variables need to be taken into account in designing interventions. For example, improvements in social relationships could involve altering the behaviour of peers towards a child with a particular disability, in addition to or instead of training social skills with the target child.

Techniques for enhancing social competence

Given the many determinants of interpersonal difficulties, it is not surprising that a wide variety of techniques may be required in order to enhance children's social competence. The methods involved in intervention will depend on the outcome of the assessment. In this way, intervention is tailored to the specific needs of each child. Thus, depending on the factors that are responsible for a particular child's social difficulties, intervention could include one or more of the following components:

behavioural social skills training;

social perception skills training;

training in the use of self-instructions to guide behaviour;

social problem-solving skills training;

replacement of unhelpful thoughts with positive, helpful thinking;

relaxation skills and exposure for management of social anxiety;

integration and application of these skills to dealing with specific social problems, e.g. making friends, dealing with teasing, or dealing with disagreements.

There is an enormous number of programmes that have been developed for enhancing children's social competence. Some of these approaches are multimodal and incorporate all or most of the components outlined here (e.g. Cartledge & Milburn, 1986; Spence, 1995). Others are more specific in focus, for example focusing on behavioural-social-skills training (e.g. Goldstein *et al.*, 1986; Matson & Ollendick, 1988) or social problem-solving skills (e.g. Spivack & Shure, 1974; Camp & Bash, 1981; Petersen & Gannoni, 1992). There is some evidence to suggest superior results from multi-modal rather than monomodal approaches (Beelmann, Pfingset & Losel, 1994). What follows is an outline of the multi-component programme developed by Spence (1995) for children and adolescents.

In most multi-component social enhancement programmes, the sessions begin with a behavioural skills training approach to the teaching of specific micro-skills, such as eye contact, facial expression, loudness of speech and posture. The early stages of training also include segments relating to social perception and relaxation skills. Once these prerequisite skills are established, training proceeds to more complex social tasks such as conversations, asking to join in, offering and asking for help, dealing with criticism, offering invitations, and dealing with teasing or bullying. In programmes that incorporate cognitive and behavioural SST, these more complex social tasks are typically taught within the context of a social problem-solving framework.

Behavioural social skills training

A variety of methods may be used to teach behavioural social skills to children. These include verbal instructions, discussion, demonstration of appropriate responding (modelling), behaviour rehearsal, prompting and feedback.

Instructions and discussion

It is important that children play an active part in learning that particular social behaviours are important, rather than just being told to do something. This phase of the learning process should encourage children to identify what behaviours are important in their interactions with others and why this is the case. Pictures, videotapes and role-plays may be used to illustrate important social skills and to provide material for children to discuss.

Modelling

Observation of other people is an important source of learning. Modelling refers to the demonstration by others of the skill to be learned and may take place in situ or may involve pre-prepared videotapes or audiotapes. Videotapes are relatively easy for the therapist to produce, but commercial materials may be purchased (e.g. audiotapes from the Structured Learning Therapy programme of Goldstein *et al.*, 1986). An alternative is to use other children from the group or the group trainers as models. There is some evidence, however, that children learn most from certain types of modelling (Bandura, 1977). It has been suggested that the model should ideally be of similar age to the child, should be shown to receive some positive outcome after performing the target skill, and should be competent but not extremely skilled. This latter point is important as children appear to learn best from models whom they see struggling slightly and who show how they coped with the situation, rather than those who show a super-confident, extremely competent performance.

It is also important that modelling is made as vivid and realistic as possible. As much information as possible should be obtained from the group about the characteristics of the situations with which children have to deal, and these details should be woven into the modelled demonstration. Props may be used to create a situation that is as realistic as possible for the trainees. Once the model has been shown, the content is discussed by the trainees in order to identify component skills and the strategies being used.

Behaviour rehearsal

Behaviour rehearsal refers to the opportunity for the trainees to practise the skills that they have observed or in which they have received instruction. Role-playing provides an opportunity for children to practise these skills within the training session before they attempt to use them in real-life situations. The aim of role-play is to act out the situation as it would occur in real life. Thus, it is important for the group leader to try to make the cues and content of the role-play as realistic as possible. Children are asked to think of a real-life example, relevant to their own situation, in which the target skill or social problem would occur. They are then asked to describe where it would occur, who would be present, and what the other people involved would be likely to say and do. The trainer then selects other group members to play the roles of other people in the interaction and tries to create as much realism as possible by using props and rearranging furniture. Ideally, the co-actors should be selected so that they resemble the real people involved in the situation. Prior to the role-play, the trainer reviews the steps and skills that the trainee will try to use in the interaction. The trainee and others involved in the role-play then act out the situation, with the trainee attempting to use the skills discussed. Role-plays of this type provide the opportunity to practise new skills in a relatively non-threatening environment in which feedback about performance can be given in a constructive manner.

Feedback about performance

Feedback about the quality of performance and suggestions for improvement are important in enhancing skill development. As with any type of skill, children learn in steps and gradually become more proficient at a task. It is important, therefore, to break social skills down into steps and try to produce gradual improvements in target skills. Feedback should be given immediately after a performance, and should be clear and specific, highlighting the exact behaviours that were good and those that need improvement. In addition, feedback should be positive and constructive, and accompanied by praise for effort as well as for successful performance. If peers are involved in providing feedback, it is important that the focus is on the positive aspects of the trainee's performance. Thus, although feedback about performance is important, the trainer needs to maintain a non-threatening training environment. Finally, feedback may also be obtained from self-evaluation during which the trainees observe and comment on their own performance during videotaped replay.

Home tasks

A feature of behavioural social skills training is the use of home-tasks to encourage skill development between sessions. In addition to increasing the amount of practice time, home tasks also provide a chance for children to practise their new skills in real-life situations. Successful skill performance in naturalistic settings is suggested to increase the generalisation of skills into everyday situations once the training programme ends. These tasks are generally a continuation of those that were rehearsed within the training sessions. Home-task instructions should be clear and specific and recorded on cards that can be taken home. Tasks should be selected that are within the trainee's ability and that are likely to lead to a successful outcome. Trainees are asked to record when they complete each task and to note any difficulties that they encountered. Training sessions usually begin with a review of the previous sessions' home tasks, with a strong emphasis being placed on the importance of home practice of skills.

Social perception skills training

There have been few attempts to evaluate the effectiveness of social perception skills training, and this approach is not recommended in isolation from other interventions to enhance social competence (Milne & Spence, 1987). However, Milne and Spence describe the elements of a programme to teach social perception skills that included the ability to: (i) recognise and discriminate one's own emotions or feelings, (ii) recognise and discriminate other people's emotions or feelings from their verbal and non-verbal cues, (iii) identify the characteristics of social situations, such as the social rules and the aims of those involved, (iv) understand how others may interpret or view social situations, and (v) be aware that a social problem exists. Pictures, videotapes, audio-tapes and role-play depicting a range of non-verbal cues of emotional expression and social dilemmas were used as stimuli to teach these five social perception skills.

Self-instructional training

The concept of self-instructional training stems from the work of Vygotsky (1962) and Luria (1961), who noted that much of our behaviour is under the control of our thoughts or internal speech. When children begin to learn control over their behaviour, this is initially the result of external influences, such as parents who reward and punish behaviour and provide instructions as to what behaviours should and should not occur. As children become older, they begin to control their behaviour through their own verbal instructions, and can be observed to talk out loud as they guide their own behaviour. Gradually this control shifts to silent, inner speech, until a level is reached when the response is automatic.

Meichenbaum and Goodman (1971) were among the first therapists to make use of this approach for teaching children to gain better control over their behaviour. They used a series of steps that mirrored the normal pattern through which children develop behavioural control. The first step involved an adult model who performed the target task while talking out loud. In the second step, the child was asked to perform the same task under the direction of the adult's instructions. The third step required the child to perform the task while instructing himself or herself aloud. In the fourth step, the child was asked to whisper the instructions to himself or herself while performing the task. Finally, the child performed the task while using silent, inner speech to guide his or her performance.

This approach has been used successfully to teach children to control their own behaviour and to practise new skills. Thus, self-instructional training provides a valuable tool for teaching children to use social problem-solving methods, and to use the social skills that they have learned.

Social problem solving

Several authors have adapted social-problem-solving training for use with children (Spivack & Shure, 1976; Camp & Bash, 1981). These approaches aim to teach children to use a series of steps in their thinking in order to respond in an appropriate way to social problems. These steps include:

1. identifying the existence and nature of a social problem;
2. thinking before acting, rather than being impulsive;
3. thinking of possible alternative ways of behaving to solve the problem;
4. predicting the likely consequences of these alternative solutions;
5. selecting and performing the best solution.

The training of social problem-solving skills involves instruction and discussion of the problem-solving steps and practice with a range of hypothetical social dilemmas. Once the steps have been learned at an academic level, self-instructional methods can be used to guide children through the steps. Initially, children listen to the instructions for each problem-solving step as modelled by an instructor. Then they are asked to talk aloud as they give themselves the instructions for each problem-solving step. After practice out loud, children are taught to talk to themselves silently as they instruct themselves through the problem-solving sequence. Initially, non-social tasks, such as solving mazes and colouring exercises, may be used, followed by a series of interpersonal tasks. For example, the Think Aloud Programme (Camp & Bash, 1981) teaches children to ask four questions whenever they are presented with a problem:

1. What is the problem?
2. What can I do about it?
3. Is it working?
4. How did I do?

Teaching positive, helpful thinking

There are many types of thoughts that might prevent us from behaving in a socially skilled way. For example, thoughts that anticipate a negative outcome, are excessively self-critical, or dismiss the rights of others are likely to influence the way that children behave. It is possible to make children aware of such unhelpful thoughts and to replace them with more positive, helpful thinking. This area of work has been called cognitive restructuring. What is presented here is a very simple form, as children have difficulty with some of the more complicated methods of cognitive restructuring that are used with adults. Three components are involved, the first being an educational process that teaches children what negative or unhelpful thoughts are and why they are problematic. The second step teaches youngsters to identify when they have unhelpful thoughts. Finally, children are taught to replace negative or unhelpful thoughts with more positive and helpful ways of thinking.

In the first step, trainees are provided with examples of negative, unhelpful thoughts and given a rationale as to why such thoughts are unhelpful. Vignettes are presented that show a particular event, such as not being invited to a party. Examples are used to illustrate the various thoughts that different people might have and how these thoughts might influence what they are likely to feel and do. Ellis's (1958) ABC model can be used with children to show the link between events, thoughts, feelings and actions (see also Chapter 6). Children as young as 8 years can understand that the way in which we feel and behave in response to a particular event is dependent upon our thoughts about the event, rather than on the event per se. It is also possible to teach children about common patterns of negative and unhelpful thinking. In clinical practice, it is helpful to teach children to label certain types of thoughts using nicknames, such as 'hot' (versus 'cool') thoughts, or 'black', 'mad, bad and sad' thoughts. Different children may select their own names for anxious, aggressive or depressive thinking.

In the second step, trainees are taught to identify where and when their own unhelpful thoughts occur. This may be done partly in the group by asking participants to recall a time when they had to face a difficult interpersonal situation in which they felt really bad. They are then asked to remember the types of things that they were thinking at the time and how these influenced their behaviour. Also, home-tasks can be used to identify current examples.

The third step involves a simplified version of cognitive challenging in which trainees are taught to replace irrational or maladaptive thinking with more realistic and positive thinking.

Cognitive therapy with adults typically involves a complicated process of demonstrating that certain thoughts are irrational or incorrect and identifying more rational, logical interpretations of events based on interpretation of the evidence. Many children have great difficulty with true cognitive therapy and the approach suggested here is easier for children to follow. Once children are able to identify thoughts in response to particular events that make them feel bad, they are asked to think of alternative ways of thinking about the situation that would make them feel more positive emotions. This process begins with examples of potential situations in which unhelpful thoughts are likely to occur. Examples of unhelpful thoughts are provided and the group is asked to suggest alternative, more helpful thoughts. Once this process has been learned, it is then applied during subsequent training related to a wide range of social dilemmas and during home tasks.

Relaxation training

Emotions such as anger, guilt and fear often prevent children from using their social skills. Relaxation is a state that is incompatible with such emotions. Thus, if we can teach children to relax when social problems occur, this is likely to reduce negative emotions and increase the chance that they will respond in a skilful manner. There are many types of relaxation exercises that can be taught to children and adolescents, including meditation, self-hypnosis, imagery, progressive muscular relaxation and rapid, cue-controlled relaxation. Irrespective of the method used, relaxation training will require several sessions, with home practice in between sessions. Spence (1995) provides a series of relaxation and imagery scripts suitable for use with young clients. The scripts are relatively short, to allow for brief attention spans, and include interesting content relevant to children and adolescents. Once relaxation skills have been established, the training aims to teach a more rapid approach to relaxation that can be used immediately in response to stressful life situations. Trainees are taught how to identify situations that trigger negative emotions and to use rapid relaxation methods in response to these cues.

Integrating the components of social enhancement programmes

If children are to be taught to use the various skills that are needed for effective social interaction, it is important that intervention programmes find a way of integrating the use of behavioural social skills, social perception, social problem solving, relaxation and cognitive restructuring. Spence (1995) makes use of a self-instruction approach to integrate the use of these skills to deal with a wide range of child-relevant interpersonal problems. The self-instruction method is used to teach the use of three main steps for dealing with social problems. The steps are tailored into a game called the Social Detective in order to cue the use of the skills taught in previous sessions. Children are taught to investigate and solve. Each step triggers a series of instructions that are important for solving social problems. Table 12.1 summarises the steps of the Social Detective.

Table 12.1. The Social Detective model

Step 1: Detect
Stop.
What is the problem?

Step 2: Investigate
Relax
What could I do?
What would happen next?
Which of these would be best?

Step 3: Solve
Make a plan
Remember social skills
Do it
How did I do?

Step 1: Detect

This step cues trainees to use their social perception skills to look for clues by watching, listening and feeling in order to detect social problems. If a social problem is detected, youngsters are taught to STOP before acting further and to work out exactly what the problem is. This aims to reduce impulsive and emotionally cued responding and to give the child a chance to work out an appropriate way of dealing with the situation. In working out what the problem is, the feelings of each person in the situation need to be examined.

Stop.

What is the problem?

Step 2: Investigate

In the second step, children are taught to investigate ways of dealing with the problem. The first skill is to relax in order to reduce feelings of anxiety or anger which might interfere with sensible problem solving. The next component is to bring in social problem-solving strategies in an attempt to think of alternative ways of responding, to work out what is likely to happen with each of these actions, and to select a solution that is likely to produce a successful outcome. Older adolescents may also be asked to look for negative, unhelpful thoughts that might inhibit a response or make them feel bad. The aim is then to replace unhelpful thoughts with more helpful alternatives. A series of self-instructions may be used, including:

Relax.

What could I do?

What would happen next?

Which of these would be best?

Watch for unhelpful thoughts (with adolescents).

Step 3: Solve

Having formed a plan, children are then asked to perform their chosen strategy, making sure that they use their micro-social skills and that they monitor the outcome. Most importantly, children are encouraged to praise themselves for trying. Even if the plan does not succeed in producing their desired outcome, it is important that trainees reward themselves for having gone through the steps and attempted a solution.

Make a plan.

Remember social skills.

Do it.

How did I do?

The steps of the Social Detective are taught through a series of interpersonal dilemmas, which are selected according to the needs of the participants. Although each group may vary slightly, some common themes are usually found, such as dealing with criticism, making assertive requests, asking to join in with peer activities, and friendship-making skills (e.g. sharing, invitations, offering help). Self-instruction methods are used to teach the steps of the Social Detective. Initially, the trainer talks out loud through each of the steps in an attempt to solve a social problem. In our clinic, we use a large poster that illustrates the Social Detective steps. Trainees then themselves talk aloud through the steps, as they practise solving a range of interpersonal dilemmas. Home tasks are set to practise the steps in real-life situations, using silent self-instruction.

Practical aspects of intervention

There are many questions that are frequently asked about the practical aspects of running programmes to enhance children's social competence. There are no hard and fast rules here, but there a few comments that we would like to make on the basis of clinical experience. It is certainly an advantage if training can be performed on a small-group basis so that other children are available to participate in role-plays and increase the opportunities for incidental training opportunities within the group. If one-to-one sessions are necessary, then it is helpful to invite a couple of children along to some of the sessions to provide peer modelling and practice.

The group size and duration of sessions will depend upon the characteristics of the group members. Disruptive and very young children may require small groups and short session duration. Similarly, children with very severe social-skills deficits may require a small group in which an adequate level of individual attention can be provided.

It is particularly important to keep the sessions as interesting as possible. A wide range of miming, role-play games and puzzles can be used to maintain trainee attention and enthusiasm for the sessions (see Spence (1995) for some examples). Trainers need to be well prepared prior to each session in terms of session plans and materials. Effective skills-training requires careful adherence to the skills training methods within sessions, and this requires considerable structure and organisation on the part of the trainer. In addition to maintaining the interest and direction of the sessions, the trainer must also ensure that the sessions remain non-threatening and positive in focus. A further task concerns the management of disruptive behaviour that may emerge in some groups with children with conduct problems. Reward systems and token economies may be helpful here to encourage on-task behaviour and skill rehearsal. At the commencement of the sessions, strict rules should be set, through negotiation with all group members, concerning issues such as confidentiality, participation and restrictions on hurtful behaviour towards other participants.

Finally, one of the hardest issues that we face in enhancing children's social competence is the transfer of new skills from the clinic or classroom situation to everyday life. Wherever possible, it is helpful to involve parents and teachers in the programme so that they are able to model, prompt and reward the use of skills outside the training sessions. In some of our groups, parents observe the training sessions through a one-way screen and have written instructions for participation in the home-tasks. We also provide written handouts for teachers to keep them informed about the particular skills being taught and ways that they can help in boosting the effects of training. However, perhaps the greatest benefits have been observed from the 30-minute free-time sessions that we hold at the end of each training session. Age-appropriate games are provided that facilitate interpersonal communication and the use of social skills. No direct skills training is conducted during these free-time sessions which are popular amongst trainees of all age groups, as is the graduation party at the end of each course.

The effectiveness of programmes to enhance children's social competence

There have been many attempts to evaluate the effectiveness of programmes to enhance children's social competence. Some of these have focused on the evaluation of mono-modal approaches, such as social problem-solving skills training or behavioural social skills training. Others have assessed the outcome of multicomponent interventions that combine cognitive and behavioural methods. A recent meta-analysis reported by Beelmann et al. (1994) demonstrated that social competence training was moderately effective in general. The strongest effects were found upon outcome measures relating to social interaction skills and social cognitive skills. Thus, training was certainly effective in teaching the skills that the programmes were designed to teach. However, these authors noted that the long-term effects of interventions tended to be weak. Furthermore, the impact of social competence training on broad constructs such as social adjustment, emotional and behavioural disorders was also weak. Interestingly, Beelmann et al., (1994) noted that only multi-modal programmes that combined cognitive and behavioural SST produced significant effects upon the broader aspects of behavioural and social adjustment. When used separately, behavioural and cognitive social skills training produced significant effects upon the targeted skills, but not upon more global indices of emotional and behavioural adjustment. There was some evidence of an age difference here, with younger children responding well to mono-modal methods and older children responding better to multi-modal approaches. However, the effects of social competence methods in general tended to be superior with younger children in the 3–5-year-old group compared to older children. Outcome also tended to be better for children classed as 'at risk' (e.g. children from economically disadvantaged groups) and worse for children presenting with externalising behaviour problems.

The meta-analysis reported by Beelmann *et al.* (1994) confirms the conclusions drawn from several reviews of the literature regarding the effectiveness of social competence training programmes. Generally, it has been concluded that behavioural and social cognitive skills training methods are effective in enhancing the skills trained within the intervention. However, most literature reviews have emphasised the difficulty of obtaining long-term benefits, transfer of newly acquired skills into real-life situations, and improvements in the broader aspects of behavioural and emotional problems. Thus, the challenge for researchers is to find methods of enhancing generalisation and training benefits.

The following discussion of social skills studies is not intended to be comprehensive, as space does not permit a detailed review. Rather, studies have been selected to illustrate particular points.

Selection of children for intervention

One of the major issues in determining the success of social competence training has been whether the trainees actually showed deficits in the target skills in the first place. Many of the studies that failed to find significant benefits from SST failed to ensure that the participants actually experienced social skills deficits. Rather, the children were selected on the basis of some presenting problem such as low peer popularity, depression, or conduct disorder (e.g. Spence & Marzillier, 1981; Tiffen & Spence, 1986; Reed, 1994). These studies assumed that the empirically demonstrated association between the presenting problem (e.g. depression or conduct problems) and social skills deficits was sufficient justification to warrant SST with the children concerned. However, this assumption is questionable when it comes to the skill level of the particular individuals in the training programmes. Thus, it is important that studies ensure that children in SST programmes actually do have social skills deficits if training is to be expected to produce significant benefits.

Studies that have ensured skills deficits have typically produced positive outcomes from training. For example, Ladd (1981) reported positive results from a SST programme with third graders who were low in peer acceptance and were identified as having deficits in specific friendship skills in a natural play situation. The study compared eight sessions of behavioural SST with a procedure designed to control for non-specific aspects of therapy (e.g. attention from the therapist). This control procedure involved no intervention, but taught children to play games according to rules. The SST and non-specific condition produced improvements in sociometric status and general social behaviour, but these benefits were not maintained for the non-specific conditions. As expected, the SST method was the only condition to produce improvements in specific friendship skills. Children who did not receive either intervention did not improve on any measure. This study was particularly encouraging because it demonstrated that the benefits of SST can be sufficiently strong as to produce improvements in social competence as reflected by peer acceptance. The success of SST for children selected on the basis of the dual criteria of low levels of peer popularity and observed behavioural deficits in social skills has also been demonstrated by Mize and Ladd (1990) and Bierman and Furman (1984).

Peer-mediated interventions

One of the major difficulties in SST programmes has been the failure to maintain skill improvements within everyday situations (Lovejoy & Routh, 1988). It was traditionally assumed that skill improvements would lead to more successful outcomes from social interactions, thereby maintaining the use of social skills. Unfortunately, there is some evidence to suggests that children's efforts to use their new skills in real-life settings, particularly with peers, do not necessarily lead to positive responses from others. For example, when unpopular children who have been through a SST programme begin to try out their new skills with their peers, there is a tendency for the peer group to continue to ignore or punish the efforts of the unpopular peers (Lovejoy & Routh, 1988). It is as if the negative attitudes towards the children continue even though their behaviour may have changed. Thus, we need to make active efforts to ensure that attempts to use newly acquired social skills lead to a successful response from the peer group, and indeed from interactions with significant others such as parents, teachers and siblings. However, attempts to change the behaviour of the peer group towards previously unpopular children have met with mixed results.

For example, Hepler and Rose (1988) reported a study in which low social status elementary schoolchildren attended a small-group SST programme along with their more popular peers. The intervention aimed to teach social skills to lower-status children, to help higher-status peers to accept and include lower-status classmates, and to train all children in effective strategies for resolving social problems. In addition to the SST components, the programme made use of activities that promoted interactions between high-status and low-status children. The five low status children in the sample all improved on role-play measures of target skills and showed a reduction in negative peer nominations. However, no changes in peer sociometric ratings or positive nominations were found.

In contrast, Guevremont et al. (1989) made use of peers as behaviour-change agents to initiate and reinforce positive social behaviour of young children. Guevremont and colleagues used a single case design methodology to assess the benefits of peer mediation with two socially isolated girls. Two or three helpers, who did not have interpersonal difficulties, were appointed for each girl and were taught to use four interaction skills, namely initiating interactions, responding to refusals, maintaining interactions and responding. The helpers could earn stickers and back-up rewards for playing with their target child. The results demonstrated an extremely positive outcome. The low-interaction target girls showed an increase in the frequency of interactions with the helpers but, more interestingly, they also showed an increase in interaction frequency with other children in the peer group. When the contingencies were withdrawn, so that the helpers were no longer rewarded for playing with the target child, the two socially isolated girls showed a decrease in interactions with the helpers, but continued to interact more often with the other children. The improvements also generalised to a situation in which the helpers were not reinforced, and interactions with other peers also increased here too. At follow-up, the target girls continued to interact more often with other children. Decreases in self-reported depression and loneliness scores were also found. Overall, this study suggests that attempts to change the response patterns of the peer group towards socially isolated classmates can be effective in bringing about long-term benefits in social interaction patterns. Certainly, studies of this type indicate the potential value of ensuring that newly acquired skills lead to positive outcomes in the peer group.

Enhancing social–cognitive skills

The meta-analysis reported by Beerman *et al.* (1994) demonstrated the greater benefits of social cognitive skills amongst pre-school children compared to older age groups, these effects being particularly marked for 'at-risk' children from low socio-economic backgrounds. This finding can be illustrated by examining some of the studies. The social-problem-solving curriculum developed by Spivack and Shure (1974, 1976) for use with preschoolers was particularly effective in preventing the onset of behavioural difficulties with 'at-risk' populations. During this ten-week intervention, a wide range of social conflict situations was enacted using stories, games, puppets and role-plays to teach children to identify problems, generate alternative solutions and predict likely consequences. The children were then encouraged to practise appropriate solutions and were given feedback about their performance. Spivack and Shure reported this approach to be more effective than control conditions in improving performance on tests of social problem-solving ability and increasing teacher ratings of adjustment. These benefits were found to be maintained at one- and two-year follow-ups. Of particular interest were the findings that improvements in social cognitive skills were associated with improvements in behavioural adjustment, and that children who were rated initially as most maladjusted showed the most benefit from the programme. Weissberg *et al.* (1981) also reported positive results with a similar programme for third grade children (around 7–8 years old).

However, not all studies have found social problem-solving skills training to be as beneficial as Spivack and Shure. Although children typically show improvements on tests of social cognitive skills following training in such skills, these benefits have not always resulted in behavioural changes or improved sociometric status (Allen *et al.*, 1976; Nelson & Carson, 1988; Erwin & Ruane, 1993). Overall, the evidence suggests that more complex interventions are needed with older children who have already developed behavioural or emotional difficulties. This proposal is reflected in the results of Beelmann *et al.*'s (1994) meta-analysis that suggest that multi-modal interventions, combining behavioural and cognitive SST, are more effective than mono-modal approaches with older children.

Children with disabilities

There is considerable evidence to show that many children with physical, sensory or intellectual disabilities experience difficulties in their interpersonal relationships. The reasons for this are varied. In some instances, the interpersonal problems may reflect deficits in behavioural or cognitive social skills; in others it may reflect the unfavourable attitudes and behaviours of the peer group. A detailed review of studies and programmes for enhancing social functioning of children with disabilities is provided by Spence (1995). This review noted that social competence training for children with disabilities has focused on five main areas, including (1) teaching behavioural and cognitive social skills to disabled children who have deficits in these skills; (2) increasing the opportunities for disabled children to interact with disabled and non-disabled peers; (3) changing the attitudes of non-disabled children towards their disabled peers; (4) teaching non-disabled children to initiate interactions with their disabled peers; and (5) training non-disabled children to respond positively when disabled children interact in a socially skilled manner.

Clearly, the most appropriate approach to intervention will depend on the nature and severity of each child's disability and the setting in which he or she lives. For example, the focus of training is very different for children with severe intellectual impairments compared to those with mild intellectual disabilities. Interventions with children with severe intellectual handicaps tend to focus on simple, specific social skills, with very frequent but brief skills training sessions backed up with ongoing reinforcement of skill usage (Stokes *et al.*, 1974; Bradlyn *et al.*, 1983). Various approaches have been used with children with mild and moderate disabilities. Some programmes have used traditional social skills training sessions in which an adult trainer conducts training in specific skills within individual or small-group settings. One interesting variation was reported by Staub and Hunt (1993) in which peer tutors were trained to teach specific communication skills to schoolmates with mild or moderate intellectual disabilities. This approach successfully increased interactions between pupils with and without disabilities and enhanced specific targeted skills in the disabled participants.

Social enhancement training has also been effective in improving the social competence of children with sensory and physical handicaps. Certainly there is considerable evidence of improvements in the use of specific social skills, although the effects have not always been beneficial in terms of interactions with non-disabled peers (Sisson, Babeo & Van Hasselt, 1988). However, peer tutoring has been found to be a valuable method of enhancing social competence with children with sensory handicaps (Sacks & Gaylord-Ross, 1989). This approach appears to increase the chance that peers will respond positively to children with disabilities when they do try to use their newly acquired social skills, thereby enhancing the generalisation and maintenance of the training effects.

Case illustrations

The Kids' Coping Project, currently being conducted within the Psychology Department at the University of Queensland, incorporates the use of SST in the treatment of social phobia. Two case examples from this project can be used to illustrate both the success and failure of SST with this population of children.

Case 1

David, a 13-year-old boy, was referred to The Kids' Coping Project by his parents due to their concern about his inability to make friends and his fear of social situations. A family history interview suggested that David's social concerns were prevalent at an early age and had been exacerbated recently due to his entry into a large high school. David, an only child, had a very close relationship with both his parents and performed well academically. The family's income was comfortable although not affluent, with David's father working as a sales consultant and David's mother performing household duties.

An initial assessment was conducted with David and both parents, using a revised version of the Anxiety Disorders Interview Schedule for Children–Parent Version (ADIS-P; Silverman & Nelles 1988). A number of questionnaires was also completed by both David and his parents. The interview confirmed the diagnosis of social phobia, with a moderate clinical severity rating of 5 out of 8, in addition to less clinically significant phobias of dogs, injections, the dark and spiders.

Information gained through the interview and questionnaires highlighted both David's social anxiety and his social skills deficits. David's scores on the Social Worries (Spence, 1995), Social Competence (Spence, 1995), and Social Skills Questionnaires (Spence,1995) as reported by David and his parents, suggested that he had a number of social worries, had a low social competence and had problems in a number of social skills areas (Table 12.2). In addition, David's internalising score on the Achenbach Child Behaviour Checklist (Achenbach, 1991), by parent report, was in the clinical range (Table 12.2).

The assessment revealed a number of specific social skills problem areas for David. David's parents reported a withdrawal from social situations, and avoidance of both eye contact and verbal contact. He tended to avoid parties, clubs and sports activities, and was anxious about meeting new people. He was reticent to join in activities with other children, was anxious about entering a room full of people, and was fearful of speaking in front of others. David's parents reported that he experienced severe problems coping with teasing and reacted inappropriately when assertion was called for. In addition, he experienced problems with sharing, controlling his temper and inviting others to join games and activities. David himself reported great difficulty in making friends and was painfully aware that he was not popular with others. It upset him greatly that he was rarely invited to other children's homes or to social activities. A school observation of David at school confirmed his reports of being unpopular, with David making little contact with peers during class, and being alone throughout the lunch hour.

Table 12.2. Pre-treatment and post-treatment measures for David

Measure	Pre-treatment measures	Post-treatment measures	Population mean	Standard deviation	Direction of change
Social Competence (Pupil)	5	12	15.53	3.17	Improved
Social Skills (Pupil)	41	56	47.15	6.59	Improved
Social Worries (Pupil)	18	7	8.44	5.30	Improved
Social Competence (Parent)	0	4	14.82	3.12	Improved
Social Skills (Parent)	41	50	46.11	9.03	Improved
Social Worries (Parent)	15	10	6.42	6.17	Improved
Child Behaviour Checklist (Parent)	64	60	–	–	Improved

Given David's severe social anxiety and social skills deficits, SST was deemed appropriate, and David was placed in a group of seven other 13–14 year olds for SST. Therapy consisted of twelve, 90-minute sessions conducted over 12 consecutive weeks. The children's parents were informed of the group proceeding by means of a summary sheet provided at the end of each session.

Social skills training progressed from refinement of micro-skills such as eye contact, posture, facial expression and tone/volume of voice, through to more complex social behaviour. Children were given instruction on conversation and listening skills such as asking questions, adhering to the conversation topic, and demonstrating to others that they were attending and interested in what they had to say. Friendly behaviours such as giving invitations, asking to join in, sharing, helping, giving compliments and turn taking were also covered. In addition, a small amount of assertiveness training was conducted, focusing primarily on teaching children to say 'no', and to cope with teasing, bullying, arguments and disagreements.

For all skills, instruction began with an explanation of the skill followed by group discussion. The therapist then modelled the appropriate behaviour, and each child practised the particular skill in a role-play situation. Prompting was used when necessary, and feedback was given by both the therapist and other group members. For many of the skills, the Social Detective (as described above) was introduced to the children as a way to identify social problems and subsequently to choose the most appropriate course of action. Therefore, modelling and role-play of the skills also included self-instruction through the steps of the Social Detective model.

In order to provide children with a greater number of situations in which to practise the various skills, a half-hour session of 'games' as well as session-relevant homework tasks were conducted each week. At the end of each session, group members were allowed to play a variety of games, during which the therapist provided positive reinforcement for the demonstration of appropriate social skills. Homework tasks were then given in line with the level of difficulty of the session. For example, the first session's task was to ensure eye contact while talking to another person, while the last session's task was to join a social, sporting or recreational club. These homework tasks not only provided children with further opportunities to practise their newly acquired skills, but also allowed generalisation of these skills beyond the 'safe' confines of the group.

The members of the particular group of which David was a part worked well together and were very supportive and helpful of one another. David was very eager to improve and, despite living a considerable distance from the University, missed only one session due to illness. He enjoyed the group immensely and quickly emerged as one of its most active members. He frequently offered answers and suggestions, and enjoyed providing positive feedback to other group members. While the homework tasks were anxiety provoking for him, he pushed himself to complete them. This resulted in David managing to perform many previously feared social activities such as asking a peer to his house, sharing and joining in. While David had previously tended to respond inappropriately to bullying, teasing, arguments and disagreements, he learned more appropriate ways of coping with such situations and was able to use them proficiently.

Upon completion of the 12 sessions, a second assessment session revealed that while David still met criteria for social phobia according to the ADIS-P, the severity of the disorder was significantly lower, dropping to a non-clinical severity of 3 on an 8-point scale. In addition, David's parents rated improvement in terms of his overall functioning, anxiety and avoidant behaviours, as well as a marked improvement in his ability to deal with previously feared or avoided situations. As illustrated in Table 12.2, David's scores on the social competence, social worries and social skills questionnaires improved after treatment, and his internalising score fell slightly so that it was no longer in the clinical range. A school observation of David conducted after termination of treatment revealed that he now interacted more with his peers during class and played with newly acquired friends during lunch time.

In order to maintain the improvements gained through treatment, booster sessions are scheduled three months and six months after treatment completion. During these sessions, the skills taught throughout the course are revised and social problems encountered by the children since termination of treatment are discussed and role-played. David's three-month booster session will be conducted shortly and it is expected that the many benefits evident from SST at completion of his treatment will still be evident.

Successful results from a single case study cannot be taken as conclusive evidence of a successful treatment programme. However, given the long-term nature of David's social skills deficits and social anxiety, spontaneous recovery seems highly unlikely. In addition, the reduction of social worries and the improvements in social skills and competence, according to David and his parents, provide encouraging support for the efficacy of the SST programme.

The above case example illustrates a successful SST outcome. Unfortunately, not all attempts at social skills training are so beneficial. The next case example illustrates the detrimental effects of extraneous variables on SST.

Case 2

Phillip, a 13-year-old boy, was referred by his older, adult brother due to concerns about school-refusal behaviour. According to Phillip's older brother, Phillip rarely attended school or engaged in social interaction. A family history assessment conducted with Phillip's father revealed that Phillip's mother suffered from schizophrenia and over the years had often refused to take her medication. This had resulted in severe marital strain and, although Phillip's father had often suggested marital separation to his wife, her threats of suicide had prevented him from leaving. The family's socio-economic status was under strain, with Phillip's father working only part-time as a massage therapist and Phillip's mother being unable to work.

Previous help for Phillip had been sought through community health services, resulting in a psychologist visiting the home. On arrival, a brief conversation resulted in Phillip physically assaulting the psychologist, who attempted to restrain Phillip and place him in 'time-out'. Outraged at the psychologist's attempt to restrain his child without explanation, Phillip's father ordered the psychologist from the home and had never attempted to seek outside help for his son again. Phillip's father then took it upon himself to encourage Phillip to attend his new high school by visiting it at week-ends and during holidays and allowing Phillip to become familiar with the new surroundings. While successful for a short time, Phillip again began school refusing, attending school only one out of every three days. It was at this point that Phillip's older brother contacted the Kids' Coping Project and persuaded his father to seek help for Phillip.

Phillip's father was interviewed using the revised version of the ADIS-P (Silverman & Nelles, 1988) and both father and son received the Social Worries (Spence, 1995), Social Competence (Spence, 1995), and Social Skills (Spence, 1995) Questionnaires. According to the ADIS-P, Phillip met criteria for social phobia, receiving an extremely high clinical severity rating of 8 on an 8-point scale. However, there was no evidence of separation anxiety disorder or other diagnosable conditions.

The questionnaire and interview information highlighted the extent of Phillip's social phobia and revealed an extreme lack of social skills, low social competence, and high levels of social worries (Table 12.3). According to Phillip himself, he did not engage in conversations with his peers, and rarely did kind things for people or gave them compliments. He rarely used appropriate facial expression, rarely said sorry, and rarely joined in family activities. In addition, he did not invite other children to join in games of activities, and did not tell a parent or teacher when he had a problem or needed help. Furthermore, Phillip avoided and was worried about meeting new people, speaking in front of others, entering a room full of people and eating in public. Parental report also revealed that Phillip was not popular amongst others his age, was rarely invited to parties or social events, and found it extremely difficult to make friends. A school observation of Phillip conducted prior to treatment suggested minimal contact with peers and teachers during both class and play time.

Given Phillip's social skills deficits and social anxiety, it was decided that he would benefit from SST, and he was subsequently placed in the same treatment group as David. Thus the skills taught and procedures employed were identical to those described in Case 1 above and will not be repeated here.

Phillip's social anxiety and social skills deficits were the most severe of the group. Initially he curled himself up, refused to make eye-contact and rarely spoke. He was compliant during therapy, participating in the role-plays and providing feedback when asked. The group therapist felt that Phillip was gradually improving as he was maintaining eye-contact for longer periods and beginning to speak in an audible voice. Phillip also began attending school more often, due partly to therapy and partly to a guidance officer at the school who had taken a special interest in the case. Considering the severity of Phillip's social anxiety and social skills deficits, the therapist believed him to be making progress, albeit rather small in comparison to the other group members.

Despite identical treatment, however, circumstances and subsequent treatment outcome were very different for David and Phillip. First, clinical severity differed for the two boys. Whereas David's social anxiety and social skills deficits were moderate, Phillip's were extremely severe. There was also some suggestion that more disturbing psychological problems may have been present or at least developing for Phillip. He had a tendency to walk around in circles, stand while other group members were sitting, and express irrelevant remarks during conversation. In addition, contact by the school guidance officer during week seven of therapy revealed that Phillip

Table 12.3. Pre-treatment and post-treatment measures for Phillip

Measure	Pre-treatment measures	Post-treatment measures	Population mean	Standard deviation	Direction of change
Social Competence (Child)	12	7	15.53	3.17	Worsened
Social Skills (Child)	23	18	47.15	6.59	Worsened
Social Worries (Child)	15	19	8.44	5.30	Worsened
Social Competence (Parent)	9	4	14.82	3.12	Worsened
Social Skills (Parent)	28	25	46.11	9.03	Worsened
Social Worries (Parent)	17	12	6.42	6.17	Improved

was consistently writing stories of a violent and macabre nature and that he expressed enjoyment of the scenes depicted in his essays.

Second, the two boys differed in terms of their commitment to therapy. While David enjoyed the sessions and completed his homework diligently, Phillip rarely completed his homework tasks and made it very clear that his attendance was due only to the promise of his brother's stereo if he attended the sessions regularly.

Finally, and most significantly, the end of the 12-session programme coincided with the departure of the guidance officer with whom Phillip had developed a strong relationship. This in combination with the severity of Phillip's problems and his lack of commitment to treatment, appeared to result in a relapse of severe school-refusal behaviour and an increase in Phillip's social anxiety and social skills deficits. An ADIS-P interview with Phillip's father after termination of treatment revealed that Phillip had retained his clinical severity of 8 on an 8-point scale for social phobia. Phillip's scores on the social worries, social competence and social-skills questionnaires (see Table 12.3) taken after treatment completion are evidence of this relapse and illustrate the failure of SST for this child.

It was clearly unrealistic to expect SST alone to be beneficial when a multitude of concurrent problems existed. Had some of these other problems been addressed first, perhaps the outcome would have been more positive. Unfortunately for Phillip, therapy was of little benefit and his school refusal, social anxiety and social skills deficits are now stronger than ever. The guidance officer is so concerned about Phillip that Family Services have now been called in, and Phillip is likely to be taken from the family home and placed in either hospital or foster care.

Phillip's case highlights the need to address family problems and higher-order psychiatric and psychological disorders first before attempting to employ SST. When the family situation is positive, other psychological disorders are not present, and the child demonstrates a conscientious approach to treatment (as in David's case), SST may be highly effective. However, when these factors are not present (as in Phillip's case), SST may be less beneficial and should take a lower priority to other psychological treatment.

Conclusions

Relationship problems, particularly with peers, are associated with a variety of negative long-term consequences. Thus, it is important that children with interpersonal difficulties are identified as early as possible and provided with interventions to enhance their social competence. This chapter emphasises the many reasons why children may experience difficulties in their relationships with others. A detailed assessment is needed in order to identify the likely causes of interpersonal difficulties. These causal variables can then be dealt with in an individually tailored intervention programme. Deficits in behavioural and cognitive social skills represent just some of the causal factors that may need to be remedied during treatment.

There is some evidence to suggest that multicomponent interventions that train behavioural and cognitive social skills are more effective than mono-modal approaches with older children, and this chapter describes a range of intervention components. These approaches have been found to be helpful for children and adolescents across a wide age range and who present with a variety of behavioural and emotional difficulties. For example, social competence training has been helpful with young people presenting with problems relating to aggression, social anxiety, and unpopularity with their peers. Such approaches have also been helpful in enhancing the social competence of children presenting with a range of physical, intellectual and sensory handicaps.

A key point to emerge from the treatment outcome literature is the need to ensure that behavioural and cognitive SST is targeted to those children who have deficits in the skills concerned. Failure to find significant benefits is not surprising if children did not show deficits in the target skills in the first place.

The future challenge for therapists is to identify methods of ensuring that skill improvements carry over into real-life situations and are maintained over time. Peer-mediated training appears to offer promise as a method of increasing the chance that peers will positively reinforce newly acquired social skill usage in school settings. The involvement of parents and teachers in training programmes may also be a valuable method of enhancing generalisation and maintenance of training effects.

References

Achenbach, T.M. (1991). *Manual for the child behaviour checklist/4–18 and 1991 profile*. University of Vermont, Department of Psychiatry, Psychiatry.

Allen, G.J., Chinsky, J.M., Larcen, S.W., Lockman, J.E. & Selinger, H.V. (1976). *Community psychology and the schools: A behaviorally oriented multilevel preventative approach*. Erlbaum, Hillsdale, NJ.

Bandura, A. (1977). *Social learning theory*. Prentice Hall, London.

Beck, A.T. (1976). *Cognitive therapy and the emotional disorders*. International Universities Press, New York.

Beelmann, A., Pfingset, U. & Losel, F. (1994). Effects of training social competence in children: A meta-analysis of recent evaluation studies. *Journal of Clinical Child Psychology*, **23**, 260–71.

Bell-Dolan, D.J. (1995). Social cue interpretation of anxious children. *Journal of Clinical Child Psychology*, **24**, 1–10.

Bierman, K.L. & Furman, W. (1984). The effects of social skills training and peer involvement on the social adjustment of preadolescents. *Child Development*, **55**, 151–62.

Bradlyn, A.S., Himadi, W.G., Crimmins, D.B., Christoff, K.A., Graves, K.G. & Kelly, J A. (1983). Conversation skills training for retarded adolescents. *Behavior Therapy*, **14**, 314–25.

Camp, B.W. & Bash, M.A. (1981). *Think aloud.* Research Press, Champaign, Ill.

Cartledge, G. & Milburn, J.F. (1986). *Teaching social skills to children.* Pergamon Press, New York.

Coie, J., Terry, R., Lenox, K. & Lochman, J. (1995). Childhood peer rejection and aggression as predictors of stable patterns of adolescent disorder. *Development and Psychopathology*, **7**, 697–713.

Deluty, R.H. (1979). Children's Action Tendency Scale: a self report measure of aggressiveness, assertiveness and submissiveness in children. *Journal of Consulting and Clinical Psychology*,**47**, 1061–71.

Deluty, R.H. (1984). Behavioural validation of the Children's Action Tendency Scale. *Journal of Behavioural Assessment*, **6**, 115–30.

Dodge, K.A. (1986). A social information processing model of social competence in children. In *Cognitive perspectives on children's social and behavioral development. The Minnesota Symposia on Child Psychology* (ed. M.Perlmutter), pp. 77–125. Lawrence Erlbaum, New Jersey.

Ellis, A. (1958). Rational psychotherapy. *Journal of General Psychology*, **59**, 35–49.

Erwin, P.G., & Ruane, G.E. (1993). The effects of a short-term social problem solving programme with children. *Counselling Psychology Quarterly*, **6**, 317–23.

Garber, J., Weiss, B. & Shanley, N. (1993). Cognitions, depressive symptoms and development in adolescents. *Journal of Abnormal Psychology*, **102**, 47–57.

Goldstein, A.P., Sprafkin, R.P., Gershaw, N.J. & Klein, P. (1986). The adolescent: Social skills training through structured learning. In *Teaching social skills to children: Innovative approaches*, 2nd edn. (ed. G. Cartledge & J.F. Milburn), pp. 249–80. Pergamon Press, New York.

Gresham, F.M. & Elliott, S.N. (1990). *Social Skills Rating System.* American Guidance Service, Circle Pines, Minn.

Guevremont, D.C., MacMillan, V.M., Shawchuck, C.R. & Hansen, D.J. (1989). A peer-mediated intervention with clinic referred socially isolated girls. *Behavior Modification*, **13**, 32–50.

Hepler, J.B. & Rose, S.F. (1988). Evaluation of a multi-component approach to improving social skills of elementary school children. *Journal of Social Service Research*, **11**, 1–17.

Ladd, G.W. (1981). Effectiveness of a social learning method for enhancing children's social interactions and peer acceptance. *Child Development*, **52**, 171–8.

La Greca, A.M. & Stone, W.L. (1993). Social Anxiety Scale for Children–Revised: Factor structure and concurrent validity. *Journal of Clinical Child Psychology*, **22**, 17–27.

Leitenberg, H., Yost., L.W. & Carroll-Wilson, M. (1986). Negative cognitive errors in children: Questionnaire development, normative data, and comparisons between children with and without self-reported symptoms of depression, low self-esteem, and evaluation anxiety. *Journal of Consulting and Clinical Psychology*, **54**, 528–36.

Lochman, J.E. & Dodge, K.A. (1994). Social-cognitive processes of severely violent, moderately aggressive and nonaggressive boys. *Journal of Consulting and Clinical Psychology*, **62**, 366–74.

Lovejoy, M.C. & Routh, D.K. (1988). Behavior disordered children's social skills: Increased by training, but not sustained or reciprocated. *Child and Family Behavior Therapy*, **10**, 15–27.

Luria, A. (1961). *The role of speech in the regulation of normal and abnormal behaviours.* Liveright, New York.

Matson, J.L. & Ollendick, T. H. (1988). *Enhancing children's social skills: Assessment and training.* Pergamon Press, New York.

Matson, J.L., Rotatori, A. & Helsel, W. J. (1983). Development of a rating scale to measure social skills in children: The Matson Evaluation of Social Skills with Youngsters (MESSY). *Behavior Research and Therapy*, **21**, 335–40.

McFall, R. M. (1982). A review and reformulation of the concept of social skills. *Behavioural Assessment*, **4**, 1–33.

Meichenbaum, D. & Goodman, J. (1971). Training impulsive children to talk to themselves: A means of developing self-control. *Journal of Abnormal Psychology*, **77**, 115–26.

Michelson, L. & Wood, R. (1982). Development and psychometric properties of the Children's Assertive Scale. *Journal of Behavior Assessment*, **4**, 3–13.

Milne, J. & Spence, S. H. (1987). Training social perception skills with primary school children: A cautionary note. *Behavioural Psychotherapy*, **15**, 144–57.

Mize, J. & Ladd, G. W. (1990). A cognitive–social learning approach to social skill training with low-status preschool children. *Developmental Psychology*, **26**, 388–97.

Nelson, G. & Carson, P. (1988). Evaluation of a social problem solving skills program for third- and fourth-grade students. *American Journal of Community Psychology*, **16**, 79–99.

Ollendick, T.H. (1983). Development and validation of the Children's Assertiveness Inventory. *Child and Family Behavior Therapy*, **5**, 1–15.

Ollendick, T.H., Hart, K. J. & Francis, G. (1985). Social validation of the Revised Behavioral Assertiveness Test for Children (BAT-CR). *Child and Family Behavior Therapy*, **7**, 17–33.

Petersen, L. & Gannoni, A.F. (1992). *Stop Think Do: Teachers' manual for training social skills while managing student behaviour.* Vic: ACER, Hawthorn, Victoria.

Platt, J.J. & Spivack, G. (1975). *Manual for the Means-Ends Problem-Solving Procedures (MEPS).* DMHS, Philadelphia.

Polifka, J.A., Weissberg, R.P., Gesten, E.L., de Apodaca, R.F. & Picoli, L. (1981). *The Open-Middle Interview manual.* (Available from R. P. Weissberg, Department of Psychology, Yale University, New Haven, CT.)

Reed, M.K. (1994). Social skills training to reduce depression in adolescents. *Adolescence*, **29**, 293–302.

Sacks, S. & Gaylord-Ross, R. (1989). Peer-mediated and teacher-directed social skills training for visually impaired students. *Behavior Therapy*, **20**, 619–38.

Silverman, W.K. & Nelles, W.B. (1988). The Anxiety Disorders Interview Schedule for Children. *Journal of the American Academy of Child and Adolescent Psychiatry*, **27**, 772–8.

Sisson, L.H., Babeo, T.J. & Van Hasselt, V. B. (1988). Group training to increase social behaviors in young multihandicapped children. *Behavior Modification*, **12**, 497–524.

Spence, S.H. (1995). *Social skills training: Enhancing social competence with children and adolescents.* NFER-Nelson, Windsor.

Spence, S.H. & Marzillier, J. S. (1981). Social skills training with adolescent, male offenders: II Short term, long term and generalized effects. *Behaviour Research and Therapy*, **19**, 349–68.

Spivack, G. & Shure, M.B. (1974). *Social adjustment of young children.* Jossey Bass, San Francisco.

Spivack, G. & Shure, M.B. (1976). *Social adjustment of young children. A cognitive approach to solving real life problems.* Jossey Bass, London.

Staub, D. & Hunt, P. (1993) The effects of social interaction training on high school peer tutors of schoolmates with severe disabilities. *Exceptional Children*, **60**, 41–57.

Stokes, T.F., Baer, D.M. & Jackson, R.L. (1974). Programming the generalisation of a greeting response in four retarded children. *Journal of Applied Behaviour Analysis*, **7**(4), 599–610.

Tiffen, K. & Spence, S.H. (1986). Responsiveness of isolated versus rejected children to social skills training. *Journal of Child Psychology and Psychiatry*, **27**, 343–55.

Van Hasselt, V.B., Hersen, M., Whitehill, M.B. & Bellack, A.S. (1979). Social skills training and evaluation for children: An evaluative review. *Behaviour Research and Therapy*, **17**, 413–37.

Vygotsky, L. (1962). *Thought and language.* Wiley, New York.

Weissberg, R.P., Gesten, E.L., Rapkin, B.D., Cowen, E.L., Davidson, E., Apadoca, R. & McKim, B.J. (1981). Evaluation of a social problem solving training programme for suburban and inner city third grade children. *Journal of Consulting and Clinical Psychology*, **49**, 251–61.

13

Drug and alcohol abuse in young people

Henck van Bilsen and Miriana Wilke

Introduction

During the past 30 years, the general public and health professionals have become increasingly aware of, and concerned about, the level of drug involvement among adolescents. These young people are in the process of change in every area of life. They are individuals in no-man's land, commuting between the relative safety of their childhood and the unfamiliar complexities and expectations of adulthood. While undergoing a myriad of physical transformations and experiencing rapid changes in their psychological, social and cultural roles, they strive for independence and seek to establish their own identity. They are often inconsistent, uncertain and rebellious, alternating between being 'childish' and mature. Adolescents experiment with many different roles, philosophies, values, standards and beliefs. They are particularly attracted to a number of adult activities that have been and/or are still 'forbidden territory' for them: sex, drug use, smoking and drinking alcohol.

Why do adolescents take drugs? Reasons for use may be extremely complex or very simple – there is no single reason or list of reasons that will apply to all adolescents. Drug use is usually the result of a complex interaction of different social, biological and psychological determinants, motives, behaviour patterns and influences.

When talking about adolescent substance use, we refer to the use of many different types of drugs by young people between 12 and 18 years of age, each of which is associated with a different pattern of behaviours and has a different relevance to different users and to society as a whole. Research has confirmed that substance abuse in adolescents is correlated with higher rates of suicide, homicide, violence, accidental death, unprotected sex, arrest, school failure, teen pregnancy and elevated infant mortality, poor physical and mental health, reduced potential earnings and unstable relationships (Donovan, Jessor & Costa, 1988; Colton, Gore & Aseltine, 1991; Wallace & Bachman, 1991)

It is important to differentiate between adolescent substance use (ASU) and adolescent psychoactive substance use disorder (APSUD). ASU refers to the non-pathological use of, experimentation with, or occasional irregular use of psychoactive substances, i.e. use that does not meet the criteria in the *Diagnostic and Statistical Manual of Mental Disorders*, 4th edition (DSM-IV), for substance-related disorders (American Psychiatric Association, 1994). The term APSUD refers to a pathological use of drugs that has become a regular feature of the adolescent lifestyle. Such use includes abuse and dependence, according to DSM-IV.

Although the increased probability of problems with the law and school remains for adolescents using any illegal substances, it is also true that some experimentation with drugs and alcohol is 'normal' by the age of 18 years (Pagliaro & Pagliaro, 1996). A pitfall as a helping professional is to treat ASU as if it were APSUD. In doing so the professional may even become a factor in paving the path from ASU to APSUD.

Kandel (1975) introduced the 'gateway' theory, which suggests that there are at least four distinct developmental stages in the initiation of legal and illegal drug use by children and adolescents, such use progressing through (1) beer or wine, (2) cigarettes or hard liquor, (3) marijuana and (4) other illicit drugs. A further stage, problem drinking, may take place between marijuana and other illicit drug use (Kandel, 1982). Kandel suggested focusing on the following types of transitions, which reflect different dimensions of drug use and abuse:

initiation: the transition from being a non-user to being a user;

continuation: a transition which may lead from adolescent substance use (ASU) to adolescent problematic substance use disorder (APSUD);

maintenance and progression within drug classes, which need to be understood within the norms of a peer group or subculture; for example, college students are particularly at risk for excessive consumption of alcohol and problematic drinking.

Based on these theories, it is possible to conceptualise several levels of adolescent involvement with drugs, each of which requires a different type of intervention.

The first level is of initial use. Adolescence is the phase of life in which experimentation with life, feelings and behaviour is prominent. The adolescent experiments with dating, studying, working, sexual relationships and also with alcohol and drug use. In this phase alcohol or drug use has an appeal for the young person as something new, as a way of broadening life experiences, and as a strategy to identify with a peer group. The qualities of the substances themselves are secondary.

The second level is social use. The adolescent has decided that the consequences of continued moderate use outweigh the consequences of disengagement from use. The drinking or drug use is moderate and does not interfere with other aspects of life. The adolescent has made a conscious choice with respect to which type of substance he or she prefers. The specific qualities of the substance are important. However, if there are certain elements in the psychological and environmental make-up of the adolescent, social use might develop into habitual use, and even into abuse and compulsive use. The relevant element in the psychological make-up of adolescents is a lack of 'normal' skills (assertiveness, social skills, mood management, self-esteem etc.), which the adolescent perceives he or she possesses when under the influence of alcohol or drugs. If this is combined with certain environmental elements, such as models of, and reinforcement for, alcohol or drug abuse, it then becomes an easy step to move from social use into habitual use, abuse and compulsive use.

Interventions for adolescent substance abuse

It may be clear that the interventions for adolescents in the phases of initial use and social use (ASU) should be different from those for adolescents engaging in habitual use, abuse and compulsive use (APSUD).

Few prevention and intervention programmes focusing on adolescents engaged in initial and social use of alcohol and drugs have proven to be effective. If anything, there are indications that focusing the adolescent's mind on the substances has more of a promoting effect then a disengaging effect (Botvin & Botvin, 1992). Therefore, such interventions should not be substance focused or presented as treatment, but should be skills based and preferably incorporated in a school curriculum (van Bilsen, Kendall & Slavenburg, 1995). They should be focused on the psychological and environmental elements that promote progression from ASU to APSUD, and on acquiring the skills that, when lacking, encourage this transition. Skills training should also focus on dealing with an environment that promotes drug use (for examples of skills training programmes, see Chapter 12 in this book).

Case illustration

Susan was 16 when she first saw a therapist. She was 'doing' drugs in a big way: heroin, cocaine, crack. She came from a reasonably well-to-do family. She was an only child, and both her parents were very hard working, and stressed the virtues of hard work and success. Susan's parents described her as someone who, from a very young age, wanted to do things differently; she wanted to be 'her own person'.

All went well until Susan went to secondary school, the most popular school in the area for the children of well-to do parents. The school had strict rules and regulations, and a good life-skills and drug education programme. Susan rebelled against the school and, when she was caught smoking near the school, the strict punishment she received made her identify more and more with the other children who received punishment, who seemed to become role models for her. Susan's parents found it increasingly difficult to support her: the school stood for values they believed in and Susan was 'sinning' against these values. The school and Susan's parents co-operated in a strict regime to try to control Susan and make her toe the line, but this resulted in more 'out-of-control' behaviour: drinking alcohol near the school, bragging in school about smoking cannabis, and actually smoking cannabis. The end-result was that Susan was expelled from the school and had to go to another school where she mixed with children who were also interested in drugs. The therapist became involved when Susan was about to be expelled from her second school as well, and was using a wide range of drugs, mainly at the weekends.

Although both schools had 'good' drug and life-skills education programme, they both focused only on knowledge, providing the adolescents with an enormous amount of information about drugs and alcohol. However, because the use of drugs and the abuse of alcohol were so far removed from the realm of the schools, the information was presented in a way that portrayed users of drugs as bad and evil people. Much of the information was contradicted by the young people's own personal experience. In Susan's words:

the message is drugs are bad, while the experience is drugs gave me a good time;

the message is drugs will kill you, but I have never felt so alive;

the message is that only bad people use drugs, but I like my friends and they are not bad.

In Susan's situation, her personal make-up seemed to combine with the 'organisation' of her environment to produce a compulsive drug user. The preventative actions taken by her school and parents had exactly the opposite effect on her to that desired: the habit of using drugs became more and more entrenched.

Interventions for drug users like Susan should centre on the psychological and/or behavioural elements of the individual that promote substance abuse as well as on specific substance intervention. In Susan's case, an alcohol and drug education pro-gramme offered during the early stages of her involvement with drugs and focusing on learning to deal with the conflicting expectations of herself, her parents and the school, a less uncompromising attitude from her parents and school, and focusing on the positives instead of enlarging the negatives, could have prevented much suffering for both Susan and her parents.

As noted by Catalano *et al.* (1990–91, p. 1086): 'A review of controlled evaluations of adolescent and other drug abuse treatment programs concludes that some treatment is better than no treatment, that few comparisons of treatment method have consistently demonstrated the superiority of one method over another, that post-treatment relapse rates are high, and that more controlled studies of adolescent treatment which allow evaluation of the elements of treatment are needed.' Thus, the focus of the next section is to provide a framework of a cognitive–behavioural approach found to be effective for the treatment of various adolescent mental health problems such as depression (Wilkes *et al.*, 1994).

The most important ground rule when working with adolescents is to create commit-ment for change before anything else. Motivational interviewing (Miller & Rollnick, 1991; van Bilsen, 1996) is a therapeutic approach that aims to increase the client's motivation for change. It is based on the notion that motivation for change is a circular (revolving door) process, which can be conceptualised in six stages (Prochaska &

DiClemente, 1984). It starts with the stage of precontemplation ('I do not have a problem') and moves to contemplation ('Perhaps there is a problem'). The next stage is deciding what to do ('Do I need to change or not?'). The fourth stage is action, in which the clients actively change their behaviour. After action follow maintenance and possibly relapse.

Specific interviewing techniques have been developed to deal with specific problems during each stage. Only an overview of the motivational interviewing techniques is given here (for a more extensive review, see Miller & Rollnick, 1991).

Motivational interviewing is a counselling approach designed to increase commitment for change when clients are ambivalent about the necessity for change. This non-confrontational method uses a combination of person-centred techniques (unconditional positive regard and expressed empathy) with effective listening techniques (repeating, summarising, reflecting, feeling reflections and conflict reflections) and cognitive–behavioural interventions (selective active listening, overshooting, undershooting and positive restructuring). Within this approach, the client is guided through a decision making process whereby the therapist focuses more on the process of decision making (making sure the client does not forget certain elements) and less on the content of the decisions. This approach has been found to be effective with various addictive behaviours (Miller & Rollnick, 1991) and young people (van Bilsen et al., 1995).

Some motivational interviewing techniques

Selective active listening

This technique consists of two components, the first being active listening. By repeating key words used by their clients, and making use of reflections and summaries, therapists make sure that they understand what their clients are trying to tell them (and that the client can see how the therapists listen). The second component is selective listening. The therapist reinforces signs of motivation more than signs of non-motivation. By repeating certain words, incorporating certain words in reflections and summaries, nodding, smiling and giving more attention to motivational elements in their summaries, therapists gradually create an atmosphere in which signs of being motivated for change are reinforced and signs of lacking motivation receive much less attention.

Example

Susan I don't want to be here, my parents keep nagging about drugs but I can't get through to them that I just want to lead my own life. Why are they all against me?

Therapist You really don't want to be here, your parents are making life difficult for you and everyone seems to be against you, while you want to be able to make your own mistakes, lead your own life and discover for yourself what you like and don't like. You really seem fed up with having to do battle all the time. Could you tell me a bit more about that?

Positive restructuring
The basic principle of positive restructuring is to consider aspects of the client's life that were perceived negatively in a positive context. Functions of positive restructuring are: increasing the client's self-esteem and feeling of competence, and strengthening the therapeutic relationship.

Example
Susan This is the second school that is about to throw me out. Not because I am stupid; I am not. Whatever I do they are only interested in their stupid rules and drugs. They are not interested in me, however hard I work.
Therapist You seem to be an individualist; you want to be a unique person, not one of the grey mob, and if that leads to trouble and conflicts you are willing to accept that. Where do you find the courage and strength to fight for your beliefs?

Overshooting versus undershooting
Overshooting the feeling (making it stronger than the client has presented it as being) has the effect of making the person deny the feeling, or at least deny that it is so strong. Undershooting, by understating the intensity of the feeling, results in the client saying something like, 'A little angry! You bet I'm angry and more than a little.' The client then goes on to talk about the feeling.

Example
Susan I hate school, I really do. It makes me sick to think that I have to stay on for another two years.
Therapist You really are completely disgusted with every second you spend in school. All the teachers, all the other kids, they are all morons and idiots according to you. Now you seem to have made up your mind to stop going to school completely and to see what life has got in store for you.
Susan Well, not exactly, I mean, some kids are okay and I really like English and French literature. Oh and there is music. But why do they have to have so many stupid rules?

Reflections of feeling
With feeling reflections, the therapist reflects to the client the feelings behind the spoken words, making an educated guess about how the client is feeling. If the client disagrees, the therapist goes along with that opinion. Feeling reflections are a powerful tool in building up rapport.

Reflections of conflict
It is very important to reflect to clients both sides of a conflict they are thinking about. Is drinking causing me trouble, yes or no? Do I want to change my life, yes or no? If a

therapist hears a client stating a conflict or concludes from reading between the lines that a client is in conflict, then it is important to reflect this back to the client.

The motivational interviewing process

The motivational interviewing process which describes the task of the therapist in three phases is very helpful in providing a framework for interventions. The first phase is the eliciting phase. Here, the therapist establishes an initial therapeutic relationship with the client: the client must become motivated to come back to this therapist, become interested in talking again with this therapist, and become interested in looking into his or her situation in order to decide whether or not there is a problem. In the second phase – the information phase – the therapist and client go on a quest for information to obtain the facts about the client's situation. These facts are structured in a comprehensive, specific package by the therapist and are presented back to the client. The therapist does not draw any conclusions, but helps the client to make sense of the facts and reach a decision about whether or not change is needed.

Example

Therapist Well, Susan, we have talked three times now, about you, the school and your parents. What you have told me is that you really would like to achieve things in your life, you do not want to be a grey person, part of the mob. You hate rules and regulations in school, but like French, English and music very much and would like to continue your studies in these. You feel so angry and pushed out at times that you simply avoid going to school, and hang out with mates who are heavily into drugs. At those moments you feel your use of drugs is really over the top. Looking back now, you have done things to pay for those drugs that make you ashamed. You are happy with your cannabis use during the weekends and the odd school day. We looked at this and found that during the last two months you used cannabis only on Saturdays and Sundays and once or twice a month on a school day. You do not see that as a problem, since you do not drink alcohol and do not smoke otherwise. Your parents and the school have criticised you and you really would like to find ways of avoiding all the flak you are getting from them. Well, what do you think, what do you conclude from this?

Susan Yes, I really would like to continue studying French, English and music, but it is so very difficult with all those rules, I just have to fight them. I wish I could learn to control myself and really show them what I can do.

The negotiating phase is third, and in this phase the client and therapist negotiate on goals and treatment strategies to achieve those goals. This is based on the client's preference, the above-mentioned facts and the available interventions.

Both for the professional and for the adolescent, it is very important to know the facts surrounding the substance use and/or abuse. Guidelines regarding the impact of substance use on the lives of adolescents can be found in Jessor and Jessor (1977).

By using alcohol and/or drugs, adolescents can regain control over their lives when they perceive them as out of control.

1. Drug use may represent an initial attempt to achieve some degree of internal control over perceptions of helplessness. . .[and] may be a relatively quick and effective means of obtaining such control, especially when other control measures are unavailable.
2. If a drug is used for control and is found effective, then its use will probably escalate, as the individual may develop a relatively predictable and controllable method of coping.
3. Dependency may develop if there are no other effective coping mechanisms available.
4. Depending upon the addictive liability of the drug, addiction may occur with continued use, as the physiological consequences of the drug (e.g. withdrawal symptoms) may eventually establish control over the user.

The adolescent likely to engage in problem behaviour shows a concern with personal autonomy, a relative lack of interest in the conventional institutions (such as school and church), a jaundiced view of society as a whole, and a more tolerant attitude about transgression. What is important here is that APSUD-prone youngsters are less parent oriented and more peer oriented. Some of the aspects mentioned above (such as a concern with personal autonomy) are not 'bad' in themselves. Therefore, the therapist has to conduct a detailed inquiry and provide a comprehensive analysis incorporating aspects such as (Jessor & Jessor, 1977, p. 237):

problem-prone aspects of the environment;

level of perceived (in)compatibility between the expectations that the clients' parents and friends hold for them;

level of influence of friends relative to parents;

level of perceived support for problem behaviour among the client's friends; and

the number of friends who provide models for engaging in problem behaviour.

In understanding adolescent drug/alcohol users or abusers it is important to analyse their use with the above-mentioned aspects in mind and to share these findings in an objective and non-confrontational way with the adolescents.

Cognitive–behavioural therapy for adolescents

Wilkes *et al*. (1994) propose the following ground rules for CBT with adolescents (Table 13.1).

Acknowledge the adolescents' concentration on themselves

Adolescents can be somewhat self-centred in their interests and goals, often with little regard for the wishes of others and little ability to accept others' points of view. The greater tendency of adolescents to focus on 'self' relative to many adults is viewed as developmentally appropriate. The therapist accepts this self-centredness and does not insist that the adolescent give it up entirely. If this position is not acknowledged, the therapist risks pushing the adolescents into argumentation, where they may feel obliged to defend their views strongly and thereby prematurely veto discussion on various issues, and as a result of this become more and more entrenched in further oppositional and unmotivated behaviour.

Communication of the therapist's understanding of adolescents' greater concern with themselves is best achieved by using motivational interviewing techniques (Miller & Rollnick, 1991) such as selective active listening. This indicates that the therapist is interested in the details of the adolescent's life and 'feeds' the narcissism in a way that is useful both for understanding the substance abuse and for designing appropriate interventions.

The adolescent's desire for self-determination may also be acknowledged and enhanced by offering choices, which is also a motivational interviewing technique. The cognitive therapist should make a special effort to provide adolescent clients with a menu of choices. For example, when designing homework tasks, the therapist can offer various alternatives. Although the therapist may have a particular technique in mind, two or three 'versions' of it, differing in detail, can be presented to the client. For example, one use of record keeping is to make clients aware of the relationship between environmental stimulus events, their own emotions, their own thoughts and their alcohol/drug use at the time of the events. Adolescents could be asked to keep a three-column record of events, emotion, and thoughts in the usual 'adult' way. Alternatively, they may be more inclined to keep a personal diary that records a narrative story from which the therapist can identify the components of the three columns with them. For some adolescents, the format of a calendar with large, empty squares in which to record daily events, feelings and thoughts is appealing. Homework designed to accomplish the same therapeutic ends could be handwritten in various formats; alternatively, some adolescents we have seen would only do the homework on their computers; others might like to dictate the information using a small tape recorder.

Table 13.1. Summary of guidelines for the cognitive–behavioural treatment of children and adolescents with alcohol and/or drug problems

---

Conduct an assessment regarding the level of the adolescent's involvement in alcohol or drugs prior to initiating interventions

Match interventions to levels of involvement: school/community-based integrated skills training for initial and social users; cognitive–behavioural individualised interventions for habitual users

Conduct a motivational assessment prior to initiating treatment

Conduct a functional assessment before initiating specific treatment interventions

Be non-judgemental in approaching treatment

Create an empathic therapeutic atmosphere

Focus on increasing self-esteem and competence

Roll with resistance

Individualise treatment approaches

Present the adolescent with a menu of options: recognise that different types of treatment may be required – the type of treatment that works best for one child or adolescent may not necessarily work best for another

Remember that success or failure is ultimately the child's or adolescent's responsibility – do not become co-dependent

Respect children and adolescents; do not treat them in a condescending manner

Provide education in a straightforward, non-biased, informative way that is appropriately tailored to the developmental, learning and social needs and cognitive abilities of the child or adolescent

Work towards realistic and achievable goals that have been mutually agreed upon

Remember that reasons for substance use may differ from one child or adolescent to another, and even for the same child or adolescent over time

Appropriately address underlying problems (e.g. lack of self-esteem or poor coping skills)

Involve family, friends and others as appropriate in confrontation, treatment planning, and programme implementation

Use peer groups (group children and adolescents according to age and gender)

Create an atmosphere of collaboration

The term 'collaborative' means co-operating with the adolescents, joining with them to treat the substance abuse. In this co-operation, factual data are the basis for changing cognitions or behaviours that play a role in the substance abuse. Although the principle of collaboration is central to cognitive therapy with any age group, observing this principle with adolescents requires that therapists make some adjustments relative to they way they would treat adult patients.

Adolescents will usually enter therapy with the perception that they are in a 'one-down' position relative to the therapist. Therapists and adolescent clients are 'less equal' in many objective ways than are therapists and adult clients. This is especially the case when adolescents are brought to therapy against their wishes by concerned adults. Because of the hierarchical status difference between therapists and their adolescent clients, it is particularly important that therapists consciously work to build and maintain a collaborative relationship. Their goal is to convey a willingness to co-operate in finding ways to ameliorate the substance abuse.

Motivational interviewing techniques will be helpful in achieving effective collaboration with these clients: selective active listening, reflections of conflict, feeling reflections and actively engaging the client in making choices.

Adopt a non-moralising attitude

A therapist who has adopted a non-moralising attitude is one whose position is non-judgemental with regard to the adolescent's substance abuse. This does not mean that therapists are uninterested or uncommitted, but that they focus on establishing a therapeutic working relationship with their clients instead of demanding that they agree with the concept of right and wrong as perceived by the therapist. Although an objective stance is crucial to cognitive therapy regardless of the patient's age, it is sometimes harder to maintain contact with adolescents because they themselves are less able to suspend their self-centred tendencies in order to consider themselves and their lives from any perspective other than the one to which they currently subscribe. Because adolescents generally adhere so strongly to their views, the therapist may feel a large amount of (covert) pressure to agree with the client's or parent's highly subjective point of view.

Objectivity is enhanced by avoiding the adoption of a 'problem solver' or 'saviour' role in which the therapist prescribes solutions. Rather, the therapist focuses on increasing motivation for change or on teaching adolescents how to develop skills for coping or resolving problems themselves. The therapist does not get entangled in the details of any particular problem, but takes a more detached position, enabling the adolescent to identify and address skill deficiencies or maladaptive cognitions that are common to a variety of situations.

Include members of the social system

The social system of adolescents comprises not only their immediate family members but also their extended family, school personnel, friends, and sometimes other professionals such as child welfare workers or non-parental guardians. Because adolescents are not independent of parental figures and are often not in a position to make certain decisions or changes that affect them, the therapist must sometimes act as a mediator or provider of information to these members of the social system. Sometimes helping to change the environment of the adolescent (for example, as in Susan's case, when her parents and school were motivated to change in their responses to Susan's behaviour) can be a helpful step in decreasing the often massive and overwhelming focus on alcohol and drug abuse. Therapy is sometimes about teaching those with whom the adolescent comes into contact that he or she is more than a person who uses drugs.

Use the adolescents' emotions to reach their cognitions

Regardless of the client's age, most models of psychotherapy and all cognitive therapists will be concerned with displays of emotion. The rationale for attending closely to affect is that it is often the window to cognition. Relative to their adult counterparts, adolescent clients generally have less ability to 'think about thinking', and will need more help to engage in observation of their own thought processes. Fortunately for therapy, adolescents are also often less emotionally controlled than adults and this give the therapist clues to cognitive domains that are particularly relevant to the substance abuse.

Since the relationship between affect and cognition is central to cognitive therapy, it is essential that the therapist investigates affect with feeling reflections, conflict reflections, paraphrasing and focused questions.

In addition to the difficulty of making associations between emotions and thoughts, some adolescents will be unable to give a name to what they feel. Therapists may need to provide education in this regard by providing adolescent clients with a set of affective labels and instructing them in the recognition of emotional states. With particularly young adolescents, such instruction may require the use of cartoons or vignettes.

Use Socratic questioning

'Socratic questioning' refers to the process of asking a series of questions intended to lead clients to challenge their own adherence to assumptions, beliefs or behaviours that are contributing to the substance abuse. The use of direct questions or interrogative statements is central to all cognitive therapy. Questions are used not only to collect information, but also to convey information, to raise topics, or even to offer suggestions.

More than is usually the case with adults, adolescents will be unfamiliar with the role of participating in focused discussion or meaningful inquiry. Adolescents more often come to therapy expecting to be told what to do or with the belief that their opinions are unimportant or unwelcome. Therefore, although the practice of Socratic questioning may be liberating to some adolescents, for others it may initially be threatening. Furthermore, adolescents will assume that there is a 'correct' answer to questions being asked, and will generally have had less experience in exploring a variety of responses, all of which might be quite tenable. Cognitive therapists working with adolescents can do much to dispel the misconception of the therapist as 'prosecutor' and the client as 'witness' by asking questions of themselves, leaving questions unanswered, or even prefacing questions with comments such as 'I'm not sure there is an answer to this question. . .' or 'Different people will probably have different answers to this question. . . .' Also effective in disarming the initial defensiveness about questioning is the adoption of a 'Columbo' style of 'innocent' questioning or 'playing dumb' (van Bilsen, 1991). This style of 'being confused' about something is particularly useful when the therapist wants to draw attention to some discrepancy in factual information or some inconsistency in logic. For example, suppose a therapist wants to draw attention to the cognitive distortion 'disqualifying the positive' that seems to be operative whenever a client evaluates his or her own achievements. Rather than stating that the client's thinking about the issue is in error, a better way would be to ask (confusedly): 'Will you help me understand how your parents can tell me you are a very capable daughter, your sister tells me she wishes she could do all the things you can, you tell me yourself that your friends admire your abilities, but somehow you think you're stupid, to the point of being nearly worthless? How does all that fit together?'

Although some adolescents will welcome the invitation to participate actively in therapy sessions guided by the therapist's use of questions, other, more reluctant clients, perhaps forced to attend sessions by their parents, will resist the invitation to partici-pate either with silence or the ubiquitous 'I don't know' response. Therapists need not be deterred by such initial reluctance, which can usually be addressed by wondering aloud about potential answers the adolescent could have offered, or by using more provocative techniques like overshooting or undershooting. Especially with adolescents who seem reluctant to answer questions, the therapist must be careful not to use seem-ingly 'rapid-fire' questions in sequence in order to avoid unintentionally activating a 'cross-examination' schema. It is best to keep a basic motivational interviewing stance of unconditional positive regard and selective active listening as a basic technique. Most adolescents are extremely sensitive filters of innuendo in content or tone of speech, and therapists should remember that questions can be asked in a wide variety of tones of voice, expressing either approval or disapproval.

Beware of 'black and white' thinking

Adolescents often think in 'all–none' or 'black–white' terms. Although they will often engage in dichotomous thinking that contributes to their substance abuse, the perva-siveness of this thinking style may be greater with younger patients. Binary categories simplify the world, so this way of conceptualising things would seem to be developmen-tally appropriate, at least initially in life. For very young children, the oversimplifica-tion is probably adaptive and contributes to learning. Furthermore, adults may protect young children from potentially confusing exceptions to their largely dichotomous world view. But adolescents begin to experience problems with the oversimplification engendered by dichotomous thought because they increasingly become victims of an unrealistic world view that clashes with reality, causing cognitive dissonance or emo-tional upheaval, which are antecedents to drug and/or alcohol abuse.

This can also result in very strong mood swings. For example, one week an adoles-cent may describe himself as 'depressed' and identify a variety of presumed causal agents. The next week, the same adolescent may report some positive occurrences and describe himself as 'happy'. The rapid substitution of a new emotional state for the former one is not viewed as anything unusual by the adolescent client, who may desc.ibe his emotional life as a roller coaster between these two extremes.

Especially with younger adolescents, it may be necessary to provide some form of an 'emotional thermometer' with gradations for all affective states. Some clients may even need to work with their therapists to generate numbered divisions and 'anchors' from experiences in their own lives to convey the concept of graded emotional response. For example, the therapist could ask for an event that would correspond to a '1', '5', and '9' on a '0-to-10' scale of 'sadness'. Alternatively, the therapist could provide examples of upsetting events from the client's life and ask the adolescent to rate them on a '0-to-10' scale. For example, the therapist could ask, 'What would losing your favourite book be?' or 'What was the rating when your dog died?' The binary motif of affective experience may also be effectively challenged by developing a vocabulary of emotional terminology to correspond to numbered points on the continuum. For example, an event rated as '1 might be 'annoying', whereas one rated a '5' might be 'maddening', and one rated a '9' might be 'infuriating'.

Make it specific and concrete

The specification of what is meant by abstract terms such as 'substance abuse' or 'happiness' or 'caring', for example, is necessary in all cognitive therapy, but especially so with adolescents because the connotative meaning of abstract concepts is often highly idiosyncratic to members of this younger age group. Adolescents are not 'little adults' who use language in the same way with the same intent as adults. A common error of less-experienced cognitive therapists is to assume what adolescents mean. Therapists working with this younger population must use motivational interviewing listening skills to help adolescents to express what they mean. Questions such as 'How would you know...?' or 'How would you notice...?' or 'How would someone else be able to tell...?' or 'What would be going on differently...?' help to convey to adolescents the therapist's request for operationalisation of the abstract.

More so than is the case with adult clients, adolescents may have difficulty specifying in observable terms what something means. The therapist will often need to assist them by offering a list of alternatives or a menu from which to choose the appropriate interpretation.

Once a common ground of shared knowledge has been established, the therapist is in a position to collaborate with the adolescent to examine empirical data relevant to the substance abuse. Once the abstract has been made more specific, cognitive distortions often become apparent and unfounded assumptions are more easily changed.

Conclusions

In essence, CBT for adolescents with alcohol and/or drug abuse problems is not different from CBT for other client groups. As with all other client populations, the therapist has to learn to speak the 'language' of the specific group. However, clients' use and abuse of alcohol or drugs is often shocking for professionals, who tend to 'forget' normal therapeutic skills and become over-focused on the substances (van Bilsen, 1996), which leads to all kinds of pitfalls. Cognitive therapy, in this context, is based on the assumption that problematic patterns of substance use are reflective of maladaptive coping, that the child or adolescent has not learned other ways to cope with his or her problems or to meet certain individual needs. Cognitive therapy is, therefore, directed at the correction or modification of irrational belief systems, maladaptive or deficient coping skills, and faulty thinking patterns or styles.

Training in self-observation, the sharing of thoughts and emotions with the therapist, the systematic analysis of the validity of negative and irrational self-statements, and the gradual substitution of positive logical thinking patterns based on rational belief systems are attempted as part of the cognitive therapy process. Through this process, children and adolescents are gradually made more aware of their problems, which may have been denied or avoided, and are helped to develop the strategies, skills and abilities they need to deal effectively with them.

The development, or strengthening, of specific intrapersonal and interpersonal skills, including anger control, leisure-time management, problem solving, and resistance training, is an integral component of cognitive therapy (see Chapter 12 in this book).

Implications for the future

Implications for the future centre on two aspects. The first is the enormous need for research into effective interventions for adolescents using too much alcohol and/or drugs. Randomised, controlled trials with various subgroups of adolescents have to be conducted in order that clinicians no longer need to rely on adaptations of approaches based on successful interventions with other clinical problems of adolescents.

Further research is also needed into the building up of protective factors against problematic drinking and drug abuse. What can we teach young people about life that will enable them to make informed and responsible choices regarding their alcohol and drug use? Is it possible to make the theories presented in this chapter regarding pathways to addiction practical? Is it possible to develop training programmes for adolescents that will empower them to become responsible in regard to alcohol and drugs?

References

American Psychiatric Association (1994). *Diagnostic and statistical manual of mental disorders*, 4th edn. American Psychiatric Association, Washington, DC.

Botvin, G.J. & Botvin, E.M. (1992). Adolescent tobacco, alcohol and drug abuse: Prevention strategies, empirical findings and assessment issues. *Developmental and Behavioural Pediatrics*, **13**, 290–301.

Catalano, R.F., Hawkins, J.D., Wells, E.A. & Miller, J. (1990-91). Evaluation of the effectiveness of adolescent drug abuse treatment, assessment of risks for relapse and promising approaches for relapse prevention. *International Journal of the Addictions*, **25**, 1085–140.

Colton, M.E., Gore, S. & Aseltine, R.H. (1991). The patterning of distress and disorder in a community sample of high school aged youth. In *Adolescent stress: causes and consequences* (ed. M.E. Colton & S. Gore), pp. 157–80. Aldine de Gruyter, Hawthorne, N.Y.

Donovan, J.E., Jessor, R. & Costa, F.M. (1988). Syndrome of problem behavior in adolescence: a replication. *Journal of Consulting and Clinical Psychology*, **56**, 762–5.

Jessor, R. & Jessor, S.L. (1977). *Problem behaviour and psychosocial development: a longitudinal study of youth*. Academic Press, San Diego.

Kandel, D.B. (1975). Stages in adolescent involvement in drug use. *Science*, **190**, 912–14.

Kandel, D.B. (1982). Epidemiological and psychological perspectives on adolescent drug use. *Journal of the American Academy of Child Psychiatry*, **21**, 328–47.

Miller, W. R. & Rollnick, S. (1991) *Motivational interviewing*. Plenum Press, New York.

Pagliaro, A.M. & Pagliaro, L.A. (1996) *Substance use among children and adolescents; its nature, extent and effects from conception to adulthood*. New York: Wiley.

Prochaska, J.O. & DiClemente, C.C. (1984). *The transtheoretical approach: crossing traditional boundaries of therapy*. Dow Jones-Irwin, Homewood, Ill.

van Bilsen, H.P.J.G. (1991). Perspectives from the Netherlands. In *Motivational interviewing* (ed. W.R. Miller & S. Rollnick). Plenum Press, New York.

van Bilsen, H.P.J.G. (1996). Focusing the mind: effective interventions for addictive behaviours. Public Lecture, June, Central Institute of Technology, Auckland & Wellington.

van Bilsen, H.P.J.G., Kendall, P.C. & Slavenburg, J.H. (1995). *Behavioural approaches for children and adolescents: challenges for the next century*, Plenum Press, New York.

Wallace, J.M. & Bachman, J.G. (1991) Explaining racial/ethnic differences in adolescent drug use: The impact of background and lifestyle. *Social Problems*, **38**, 333–57.

Wilkes, T.C.R., Belsher, G., Rush, A.J., Frank, E. *et al.* (1994). *Cognitive therapy for depressed adolescents*. Guilford Press, New York.

14
Eating disorders and obesity

Ulrike Schmidt

Introduction

Given the obsession with slimness amongst modern Western women, it is not surprising that the dieting craze is increasingly affecting children. A significant proportion of pre-adolescent girls between the ages of 7 and 12 years are weight conscious and diet (Davies & Furnham, 1986; Maloney et al., 1989; Wardle & Marsland, 1990; Collins, 1991; Hill, Oliver & Rogers, 1992; Childress et al., 1993). Those with a higher body weight (Wardle & Beales, 1986; Hill, Rogers & Blundell, 1989; Hill et al., 1992) and those perceiving themselves as overweight (Wadden et al., 1989; Hill et al., 1992) are more likely to diet. Other factors associated with dieting in pre-adolescence and early adolescence include the onset of menarche and dating (Brooks-Gunn & Warren, 1988; Gralen et al., 1990). Maternal and peer influences are also important (Attie & Brooks-Gunn, 1989; Hill, Weaver & Blundell, 1990). The preoccupation with weight and dieting in increasingly younger children has been thought to lead to an increase of eating disorders (anorexia nervosa, bulimia nervosa) in this group (Lask & Bryant-Waugh, 1992), as dieting is a well-known risk factor for the development of these disorders (Patton et al., 1990).

At the other end of the spectrum, childhood obesity is also on the increase. This is probably due to the increasingly sedentary lifestyle of adults and children in our society, the widespread availability of high-calorie snack foods and sugary drinks, and a lessening emphasis on family meals. Those with a genetic vulnerability for obesity are at the greatest risk.

The cognitive model of eating disorders

Cognitive models for both anorexia nervosa (Garner & Bemis, 1985; De Silva, 1995; Freeman, 1995) and bulimia nervosa (Fairburn, 1981; Fairburn *et al.*, 1993b) have been described. There is considerable overlap between the two. The cognitive model of bulimia nervosa (Fairburn, 1981; Fairburn *et al.*, 1993b) holds that extreme concerns about shape and weight are both causative and maintaining factors in this disorder. It is thought that underlying these shape and weight concerns are often long-standing feelings of ineffectiveness and worthlessness. In this model, weight and shape concerns are thought to trigger dieting, which then triggers bingeing, which in turn leads to compensatory vomiting or purging in a cascade of interlocking vicious circles. Treatment attempts to tackle both the behavioural aspects of the disorder as well as the characteristic cognitive distortions.

The cognitive–behavioural model of bulimia nervosa has had a much greater clinical and research impact than that of anorexia nervosa and has been translated into a number of treatment studies based on this approach. Therefore, a detailed description of CBT in bulimia nervosa forms the core of what follows. However, additional sections describe how to adapt the approach for anorexia nervosa and for obesity.

Assessment of patients with eating disorders

Gathering information about the diverse physical and psychological symptoms of the eating disorder and their time course is an important aspect of the assessment. Table 14.1 gives an assessment checklist, which can be used as an aide-memoire. (For reviews of physical symptoms and medical complications, also see Bhanji & Mattingly, 1988; Kaplan & Garfinkel, 1993; Sharpe & Freeman, 1993; Treasure & Szmukler, 1995).

Assessing the patient's motivation for treatment and readiness to change is another important aspect of initial assessment, as eating disorder sufferers are notoriously ambivalent about treatment (Ward *et al.*, 1996). In anorexia nervosa, there is often outright denial that there is anything wrong, whereas in bulimia nervosa there is often a wish that treatment may be able to abolish binges magically, without the sufferer having to make any other changes with regard to eating and weight. In obesity treatment programmes, too, it is often the parents – rather than the obese child – who are highly motivated for their child to have treatment (Duffy & Spence, 1993).

Thus, many younger patients who are brought by their parents and are not themselves ready to accept help will appear silent, withdrawn and rebellious. Alternatively, they may appear superficially pleasing and compliant, without ever really becoming involved in the treatment. It is very important to pay attention to this and not to push patients into therapeutic action for which they are not ready. The self-help manual for bulimic disorders by Schmidt and Treasure (1993) and the associated *Clinician's guide* (Treasure & Schmidt, 1997) address issues of how to motivate patients. Important

Table 14.1. Assessment checklist

Weight history: premorbid, lowest, highest, and ideal weight

Bingeing: types of food eaten, amounts, time spent eating, money spent, when, where, triggers

Methods of weight control: fasting, dieting, vomiting/spitting food (frequency, how soon after eating), laxatives, diuretics, appetite suppressants (brands, quantities, patterns of consumption), exercise (time spent, other methods, e.g. thyroxine, amphetamines)

Eating pattern: calorie counting, weighing

Menstrual history

Associated problems: depression, deliberate self-harm, alcohol and drug abuse, shop-lifting

Past treatments for eating disorders: what has worked, what has failed

Family history of eating disorders/obesity

History of childhood abuse and neglect

Physical assessment: weight, height, check teeth, parotids, Russell's sign, serum haematology and chemistry

---

factors are an emphasis on a collaborative approach, but additionally patients need to be given ample opportunity to express their concerns about change. Exercises like decision-balance charts that allow the expression of ambivalence can be helpful.

Cognitive–behavioural therapy for bulimia nervosa

Number and timing of treatment sessions

Cognitive–behavioural therapy in bulimia nervosa is usually given as a package of approximately 16 to 20 treatment sessions. Fairburn (1981) suggested that early on in treatment, patients should be seen two to three times weekly, and there does seem to be empirical support for this. Mitchell *et al.* (1993) found that a high-intensity treatment approach, an approach with early emphasis on abstinence, or a combination of the two were more effective in inducing remission in patients than once-weekly CBT.

Interrupting the binge–vomit cycle and re-establishing a regular eating pattern

Early on in treatment (sessions 1 to 8), the main emphasis is on helping the sufferer to regain some control over chaotic eating habits and to re-establish regular meals.

The self-monitoring of food intake, binge–purge episodes and associated thoughts and feelings is one of the mainstays of all CBT packages for bulimic patients and will usually be commenced at the beginning of treatment. Self-monitoring on its own leads to some symptom reduction, though not as much as a full CBT package (Agras *et al.*, 1989; Thackwray *et al.*, 1993). An example of a typical food diary is given in Table 14.2.

It is often suggested that, ideally, patients should keep their diaries with them wherever they go. In practice, it can be difficult to persuade patients to comply with detailed regular self-monitoring. This may be particularly true for adolescents, who may loathe the idea of having to do 'homework'.

Common objections patients have to self-monitoring are that:

Table 14.2. A sample food diary

Date	Time	What eaten	B	V	L	Antecedents & consequences

B = binges, V = vomiting, L = laxatives.

they are worried that their diary could fall into the wrong hands;

to write down (and to show to a therapist) what they ate during a binge makes them depressed, humiliated or ashamed;

they have not got the time to keep a diary.

It thus requires a great deal of tact and sensitivity from the therapist to introduce the task. It may help to emphasise the following:

that writing down things will help the patient and therapist to remember the patient's situation at the start of treatment and generally how she is getting on;

that the patient does not have to write a lengthy 'novel';

that the diary does not have to be 'perfect';

that even if the patient can only keep the diary every two to three days out of seven, it will still be better than nothing.

Therapists need to help their patients to be creative with what counts as a diary. For example, if patients decide that the only kind of monitoring they are prepared to do is to put ticks in their calendar whenever they had a binge, it may be advisable for the therapist to go along with this.

Psycho-education (Table 14.3), practical advice on how to establish a regular eating pattern (Table 14.4), and stimulus-control measures (Table 14.5) will also be useful in this phase of treatment.

Table 14.3. Psycho-education

A large range of weights is healthy at a certain height (not everyone can look like Kate Moss or Jody Kidd)

Weight and shape are largely genetically determined

Weight fluctuations of 2–3 kg are normal in young women

Diets do not work as the body adapts to dieting by reducing the metabolic rate

Long intervals between meals and a main meal in the evening foster storage of calories

Starvation can lead to a large number of physical (tiredness; irregular periods; cessation of periods; sleep disturbance; poor circulation, slow pulse, fainting spells; osteoporosis; constipation; anaemia; liver damage; raised cholesterol) and psycholological problems (e.g. low mood, preoccupation with food and cravings to binge; poor concentration; problems with decision making and complex thinking tasks)

Hunger and satiety are disrupted by an eating disorder

Dieting triggers bingeing

Table 14.4. How to establish a regular eating pattern

Eat the majority of food before the evening

Eat small amounts regularly throughout the day (three meals and three snacks); do not allow gaps longer than three hours between eating

Restrict fat, but ensure adequate protein and carbohydrate intake

Avoid artificial sweeteners

Do not skip meals

Gradually expand the variety of food eaten and begin to include 'forbidden' foods

Weigh yourself only once a week

Exercise regularly but not excessively

In helping patients overcome self-induced vomiting and laxative or diuretic abuse, it will be important to educate them about the dubious effects of these measures on weight loss. For example, vomiting only leads to 30 per cent to 50 per cent of calories ingested being lost, depending on how soon after eating it occurs. Laxatives and diuretics do not lead to any loss of calories. For additional measures about how to help patients reduce self-induced vomiting and laxative abuse, see Table 14.6.

The physiological pressure to binge usually lessens once the size and regularity of meals are increased. However, many patients also binge for psychological reasons, to ward off unpleasant feelings like loneliness, boredom or distress. The food diary may be a help in identifying psychological triggers for binges.

At this stage (session 8 onwards), it may be useful to teach patients coping and problem solving strategies to identify alternative and more adaptive ways of dealing with urges to binge (Table 14.7). Planned or programmed binges (Loro, 1984; Steel, Farag & Blaszczynski, 1995) can also be a useful strategy for getting bingeing under

Table 14.5. Stimulus control and allied measures

Eat in a room separate from where food is stored and prepared
Emphasise the visual impact of the meal
Make the place setting as attractive as possible
Do not engage in other activities whilst eating
Look at your food before you begin eating
Eat slowly, putting down your knife and fork between each mouthful
Savour your food
Limit the amount of liquid consumed with your meal
Limit the supply of food available whilst eating
Practise leaving food on the plate
Throw away left-overs
Leave your place once you have finished eating
Limit the amount of 'dangerous' foods in the house
Plan shopping and stick to shopping lists
Avoid shops which have been used to buy food for binges
Shop only after having eaten
Buy food which needs preparation
Judge portion size by looking at other people's portions
Buy individual portions

Table 14.6. Dealing with self-induced vomiting, laxatives and diuretics

Educate your patient about the health risks of vomiting: dental problems; parotid swelling; electrolyte disturbance resulting in tiredness, weakness, inability to concentrate, dizziness, headaches, palpitations; fits; cardiac arrhythmias; kidney damage; abdominal pain, vomiting blood, regurgitation; paralytic ileus, rectal prolapse

If the patient induces vomiting:
   ≤ 2–3 times per week, or
   often several hours after bingeing, or
   sometimes not at all after bingeing,
get her (or him) to cut down the number of times of vomiting per week gradually

If the patient induces vomiting:
   most days, or
   after snacks, meals and binges, or
   immediately after eating,
get her (or him) to delay vomiting gradually (start with 5 or 10 minutes), or do response prevention of vomiting in the clinic (very time consuming!)

Laxatives/diuretics:
   get the patient to cut down gradually,
   warn about oedema and constipation.

Table 14.7. Dealing with bingeing

If regular meals and consequences of bingeing are dealt with, bingeing will greatly improve
Identify triggers of binges, and function of binges
Increase the sense of control: only binge at certain times, or in certain places
Anticipate 'danger' zones (e.g. weekends) with lots of unstructured time
Distract from urges to binge by doing something else pleasurable
Use a problem-solving approach

control. By asking patients to bring on deliberately what they fear most, the therapist forces them to think about their problem behaviour in a new way, which may help them gain a sense of control over it. Bingeing under the therapist's instruction also frees the client from making negative self-attributions about engaging in bingeing.

Cognitive restructuring

Several layers of distorted thinking have been postulated (see Freeman, 1995). At the most superficial level there are automatic dysfunctional cognitions about eating, weight and shape which are abundant in bulimia nervosa and both underlie and maintain dysfunctional eating behaviour. Typical examples of weight-related and shape-related automatic thoughts include the following:

'Even if I only eat a small amount of chocolate I will immediately put on a pound in weight.' (selective abstraction).

'My thighs are so fat. That's probably the only thing people notice about me when I walk into a room full of strangers.' (selective abstraction).

'Either I control my eating perfectly or I am in a total mess.' (all-or-nothing type thinking).

'I failed again with my attempts to diet. I am a useless, hopeless human being.' (over-generalisation).

'I cannot allow myself to have any nice new clothes until my weight and shape are right.' (all-or-nothing type thinking).

'I spoilt the whole week by having a binge on Friday night.' (magnification).

'My weight is up by half a pound today. Everybody will notice how fat I have become.' (magnification).

'When I walked past the building site the workers started to laugh. There must be something weird about how I look.' (personalisation).

The categories for these distorted cognitions are overlapping and it is probably not particularly helpful to be too precise about categorising them. Patients usually have no difficulties in identifying them as they often experience these weight-related and shape-related distorted cognitions at times when they have difficulties with controlling their eating. Whilst the cognitive model will have been explained to the patient right from the beginning, the best time to introduce cognitive restructuring is in the second half of treatment when patients are beginning to get their disordered eating under some control. At this stage of treatment it will be easier for them to begin to challenge their distorted thinking and to generate adaptive alternative ways of thinking.

Underlying the weight-related and shape-related cognitions are often more deep-seated, basic beliefs, which constitute the general assumptions ruling the person's thoughts and behaviour (see Freeman, 1995). These are often conditional (e.g. 'If anything good happens, it will immediately be taken away from me'; 'If I am not the best at everything, people will despise me'). Even more deeply buried are so-called early maladaptive schemata. These may be linked to early traumatic experiences and are usually absolute and unconditional (e.g. 'I am a bad person'; 'I am stupid'; 'I am totally unlikeable and disgusting'; 'I am boring'). Basic assumptions and early maladaptive schemata are more difficult and time consuming to identify and treat than automatic thoughts.

Relapse prevention

Relapse is common in bulimia nervosa (Olmsted, Kaplan & Rockert, 1994) and it is important to warn patients to expect this and to set aside some time at the end of treatment to address this issue. Much will depend on whether they catastrophically interpret this as 'being back to square one' or can see it as a 'lapse' from which they can recover. They need to be aware that at times of stress their eating disorder may threaten to 'raise its ugly head again', and it might be helpful to get them to think of their eating disorder as their particular 'Achilles' heel' or weak spot, in other words a vulnerability that is likely to stay with them for quite a while or possibly even throughout their adult life. However, treatment should have equipped them to cope with any lapses. Helpful strategies include getting them to write out a plan on how they will cope if a lapse should occur. Planned binges may also be helpful in preventing relapse. Additionally, it will be important to reinforce the importance of not dieting.

Special problems: bulimia nervosa in adolescents with insulin-dependent diabetes

Peveler and Fairburn (1992) describe the use of CBT in diabetics with bulimia nervosa. Treatment of this patient group proves more problematic than that of uncomplicated bulimia nervosa. Some diabetic bulimics may perceive self-monitoring as required by CBT as an additional burden, given that they already have to keep records of their blood glucose. In those cases, interpersonal therapy may be an effective alternative. A further problem is that the dietary advice given to diabetics focuses on total avoidance of sugary foods and a strict observance of carbohydrate allowances, whereas CBT attempts to enable patients to relax rigid dietary rules. Therapists will need to help patients to steer a middle course.

The use of cognitive-restructuring techniques to modify concerns about shape and weight and low self-esteem has to be extended in patients with diabetes to include diabetes-related thoughts. For example, some patients may have 'catastrophic' thoughts about the risks of hypoglycaemia and may interpret a high blood glucose value as evidence of incompetence in managing their diabetes. The techniques used for dealing with such dysfunctional thoughts are no different from those used in other forms of cognitive therapy.

Case illustration

Lucy was an academically and musically very gifted student who was sent to boarding school at the age of 13. Within eight months, she developed severe anorexia nervosa necessitating inpatient refeeding over a period of several months, during which her weight was restored. During her inpatient stay, family therapy was commenced and Lucy and her family decided that she would not return to boarding school. By the age of 15, Lucy was referred for CBT as she was suffering from marked bulimic symptoms with large binges up to three times a day, massive laxative abuse (taking up to 30 or 40 laxative tablets a day), and self-induced vomiting after practically everything she had eaten. Her weight, though no longer in the anorexic range, was on the low normal side. She exercised fanatically for at least one to two hours per day. During the assessment, it became clear that Lucy was very ambivalent about changing her behaviour as she was terrified of gaining weight. She commented on how painful her laxative abuse was and how she hated the stomach cramps and diarrhoea that this caused. Lucy was asked to keep a food diary, which showed that she essentially ate no normal meals at all. Upon learning that laxatives did not lead to any weight reduction, Lucy agreed with her therapist to try to cut these down, initially by agreeing to take no more then 30 laxative tablets a day and then by cutting down her daily 'ration' by five tablets every week. After three weeks of complying with this gradual reduction programme, Lucy decided that she could stop her laxatives altogether; however, after a day without laxatives, she developed rebound oedema and had a setback when she again took 40 laxative tablets a day for three days. The therapist explained to Lucy that she had got 'too ambitious' and that it was vital for her to carry on with the gradual reduction programme. Lucy managed this without any further problems. Once she had stopped her laxative abuse, she began to feel a little less depressed and lethargic and her concentration improved. Her food diary, which she had kept religiously, revealed that she usually ate nothing until mid afternoon, but on her way home from school she would start bingeing on sweets, which she would buy from her pocket money. She would then share the family's evening meal and in the evening withdraw to her room to have a further binge (on foods she had taken from the family's larder). She would induce vomiting after every binge. Her parents, especially her mother, were very critical of Lucy's 'lying and stealing' and threatened to lock the larder and fridge door. At times Lucy herself would implore her mother to do so.

It was discussed with Lucy that her binges were the result of her avoidance of food in the morning and that, if she had some breakfast, she would be less likely to binge so much later on. After much discussion, she agreed to her mother being involved as a co-therapist who would help her to stick to the plan of having breakfast and help her decide on portion size. This was achieved by meeting with Lucy and her mother and by getting her mother to agree that she would try to refrain from comments about Lucy's eating at other times, but would stay around to help Lucy during breakfast. Lucy's breakfasts consisted of a small bowl of cornflakes with milk and a slice of toast and an egg. She found this very difficult at first, and during her first week there were two mornings when she binged during her lunch break at school and then was sick. However, soon she began to find it easier to have breakfast. Her relationship with her mother improved and she could be much more open with her. When Lucy became comfortable with having breakfast on a daily basis, her therapist asked her how she would feel about having a mid-morning snack like a yoghurt or a piece of fruit. Again, Lucy was initially quite worried by this suggestion, but agreed to try. Again, she successfully managed this step. By the time lunch was introduced, Lucy began to notice that she was only bingeing once a day (usually after the evening meal at home) and that these binges were not quite as large as they had been. A further analysis of her food diary revealed that although by now Lucy had a fairly normal daily eating pattern (i.e. she was eating three meals a day plus two snacks), she was still eating relatively little during these meals, and the foods she allowed herself during her meals were mainly health foods. The therapist commented how all the more pleasurable foods (chocolates, ice cream, but also rich cheeses) were contained in Lucy's binge foods, and how during her meals she stuck to fairly safe, boring food. The therapist suggested that Lucy should try to allow herself to eat a chocolate bar on a regular basis and helped Lucy to loosen her rules about the foods she would allow herself to eat during the day. Lucy's weight stabilised at a level of half a stone higher than before, but she was not particularly troubled by this, as the weight gain had occurred slowly. Gradually, Lucy's binges had become less common. They now occurred only two or three times a week. The diary revealed that they occurred mainly in response to emotional triggers, including boredom and loneliness. Problem solving was used to help Lucy think of alternative responses to urges to binge. Cognitive restructuring was started as Lucy had many examples of perfectionist and anorexic attitudes.

Adapting cognitive – behavioural therapy for anorexia nervosa

There is widespread agreement that the standard model of CBT needs considerable modification for use with anorexic patients in order to deal with the often poor motivation of these patients and their need for weight gain (Cooper & Fairburn, 1984; Freeman, 1995). Freeman warns that 'for moderately and severely ill anorexics the treatment is difficult, often repetitive and much more prolonged than for the treatment of depression, anxiety and bulimic disorders.' He also points out that only experienced CBT therapists should take on such a task.

Garner and Bemis (1985) have outlined one possible cognitive–behavioural approach to anorexia nervosa, modified from the approach described by Beck for the treatment of depression, but fail to provide any supporting clinical data. Cooper and Fairburn (1984) used an adaptation of their CBT approach to bulimia nervosa for five patients with anorexia nervosa, with mixed results. Early treatment sessions were devoted to the identification of issues that the patient herself regarded as a problem, typically including such issues as losing control over eating, preoccupation with food and eating, and sensitivity to cold. These problems were discussed with the patient, with particular emphasis being placed on the likely contribution to them of starvation. The need for weight gain was not presented as an important initial step in therapy, and patients were assured that whilst gaining weight they would be helped to maintain control over their eating. In the initial stages of treatment, appointments were frequent, sometimes daily. The patients were given a weight range for their healthy weight and were asked to adhere to a pattern of regular eating comprising preset meals and snacks, and precise instructions were given on their content. The second phase of treatment which closely followed stage two of CBT for bulimia nervosa, was begun only after a significant increase in weight had occurred.

Cognitive–behavioural therapy for obesity

Attempts at weight control for children have focused on the development of healthy, normal eating habits and on increasing exercise levels, in view of concerns that a simplistic dieting approach to intervention may exacerbate obesity through its negative impact upon metabolic rate and that the excessive focus on body shape and dietary intake may trigger eating disorders such as anorexia nervosa and bulimia nervosa. Weight-control interventions for children typically involve a combination of nutritional education, self-monitoring of eating and exercise activities, stimulus control procedures and exercise programmes. Thus, many of the elements described above under CBT for bulimia nervosa can also be used in the treatment of obesity. For example, self-monitoring with a food diary will help to give a good picture of the daily eating pattern and of whether there are any emotional triggers for episodes of over-eating. The 'traffic light system' described by Epstein, Masek and Marshall (1978) can be used to facilitate children's understanding of food groups and high-calorie foods. Using this system, children are taught to classify foods into green (eat freely), amber (eat in moderation) and red (stop, danger) categories. No specified dietary or calory restrictions are imposed.

Advice on how to establish a regular eating pattern and on the use of stimulus control measures may be helpful (see Tables 14.4 & 14.5). Cognitive restructuring may be helpful in reducing black-and-white thinking with regard to dietary lapses. Additionally, it will be important to assess levels of physical exercise, as increased activity levels are one of the best predictors of long-term maintenance of weight control. Regular exercise is linked with increased energy expenditure. In those who are dieting, one effect of exercise may be to limit the decrease in resting metabolic rate that accompanies prolonged caloric restriction. Exercise can also preserve the loss of lean tissue during dieting. Moreover, exercise has many psychological benefits, leading to an improved sense of well-being and enhanced self-confidence and decreasing anxiety and depression. Lastly, it enhances adherence to other weight-control behaviours (Perri et al., 1992).

Overweight children may be teased for their poor performance and be excluded from athletic activities by their peers (Hill, 1993). Many obese children and adolescents thus hate sports. Parents may have unrealistic goals, expecting an hour of exercise to result in noticeable weight loss. Exercise that is too strenuous or uncomfortable may not be repeated. Having said this, the most common reason people fail to exercise is lack of time (Gloag, 1992).

When the main objective is calorie expenditure, exercise can be based primarily on increases in the amount of routine daily activities. Even walking for a few minutes each day, increasing by 5 minutes each day or week, can be useful. With time, this can be increased to 50 or 60 minutes per day. Walking burns off the same number of calories as running the same distance. Walking up stairs burns more calories per minute than vigorous activities like jogging and cycling.

Problem-solving techniques can be used to generate ideas about how to increase daily activities in a structured and pleasurable way: Can the child walk to school or at least part of the distance? If the family lives in a high rise block of flats, can the child walk up the stairs instead of taking a lift? Can the child walk the family dog or run small errands for the parents to the local shops? Using a pedometer whilst walking may help an obese child to increase a sense of achievement. It will also be helpful to get the patient to keep an exercise record with weekly goals.

Dealing with the child or adolescent's weight, dieting and eating and activity patterns is not enough, and attention needs to be paid to what is happening in the wider family in this respect. Obesity runs in families, and family members serve as models, and reinforce and support the acquisition and maintenance of eating and exercise behaviours (Epstein, 1996).

Predictors of treatment outcome

Bulimia nervosa

A consistent finding from different psychological treatment studies of bulimia nervosa is that those with a lower body mass index are less likely to respond to treatment, as are those with more severe eating symptomatology (Garner et al., 1990; Davis, Olmsted & Rockert, 1992; Fahy, Eisler & Russell, 1993; Turnbull et al., 1996). Premorbid obesity may also predict a poorer outcome (Fairburn et al., 1995).

The finding by Turnbull et al. (1996) that a longer duration of bulimia nervosa was associated with a better outcome is perhaps less counterintuitive than it first seems. Especially at the beginning of their disorder, many bulimics begin to binge after a period of 'successful' dieting, and are hoping that, given enough 'willpower', they may be able to return to dieting without bingeing. The message of CBT, which is to cease dieting, is not popular with these patients.

Low self-esteem has also been mentioned as a predictor of poor treatment outcome (Fairburn et al., 1987; 1993c; Baell & Wertheim, 1992). Additionally, comorbid personality disorders are negative prognostic factors (Fichter et al., 1994; Coker et al., 1993; Fahy et al., 1993; Rossiter et al., 1993; Wonderlich et al., 1994); in particular, those with so-called multi-impulse bulimia nervosa have a poor prognosis, even with very intensive treatment (Fichter, Quadflig & Rief, 1994).

One study mentions a highly controlled or discordant family environment as a predictor of poor outcome in group CBT of bulimia nervosa (Blouin *et al.*, 1994).

Anorexia nervosa

There are no studies assessing predictors of outcome after CBT in anorexia nervosa.

Childhood obesity

The best ten-year predictors of outcome from four different studies of the treatment of childhood obesity were weight reduction during the first five years post-treatment and various baseline characteristics, including the eating and exercise environment and availability of support from family and friends (Epstein *et al.*, 1994).

Research into cognitive–behavioural treatment of eating disorders

Bulimia nervosa

In bulimia nervosa, CBT is now very much the first-line treatment of choice (Wilson, 1996). A large number of controlled treatment studies has appeared evaluating CBT against other treatment (psychological and/or drug treatments) administered both individually (Fairburn *et al.*, 1986, 1991, 1993a, 1995; Freeman *et al.*, 1988; Agras *et al.*, 1989; Garner et al., 1993; Thackwray *et al.*, 1993) and in group formats (Yates & Sambrailo, 1984; Kirkley *et al.*, 1985; Lee & Rush, 1986; Wilson *et al.*, 1986; Wolchik, Weiss & Katzman, 1986; Mitchell *et al.*, 1990; Wolf & Crowther, 1992).

Cognitive–behavioural therapy in bulimia nervosa has been found to be more effective than supportive therapy, supportive-expressive therapy, and behaviour therapy (Kirkley *et al.*, 1985; Agras *et al.*, 1989; Fairburn *et al.*, 1993a; Garner *et al.*, 1993; Thackwray *et al.*, 1993; Walsh et al., 1997). Interestingly, interpersonal therapy seems to be as effective as CBT in the longer term (Fairburn *et al.*, 1991; 1995) and may be a useful alternative if CBT fails or is unacceptable.

Drop-out rates for CBT (individual or groups) in bulimia nervosa vary from 0 per cent to 47 per cent with most studies of individual CBT giving drop-out rates between 10 per cent and 30 per cent. Post-treatment abstinence rates range from 25 per cent to 80 per cent, with most studies being somewhere between 30 per cent and 60 per cent. These rates can be maintained for up to five years (Fairburn *et al.*, 1995). Treatment intensity ranges from 9 to 80 hours. When given individually, treatment intensity is usually in the range of approximately 20 sessions.

Cognitive–behavioural therapy is superior to antidepressant medication alone (Agras *et al.*, 1992; Leitenberg *et al.*, 1994; Goldbloom *et al.*, 1995) and a combination of CBT and an antidepressant is superior to antidepressant alone (Mitchell *et al.*, 1990; Agras *et al.*, 1992; Leitenberg *et al.*, 1994; Goldbloom *et al.*, 1995; Walsh *et al.*, 1997). However, there does not seem to be any advantage of the combined treatment (CBT plus antidepressant) over CBT alone (Agras *et al.*, 1992; Leitenberg *et al.*, 1994; Goldbloom *et al.*, 1995) or CBT combined with placebo (Mitchell *et al.*, 1990; Fichter *et al.*, 1991; Walsh *et al.*, 1997).

Unfortunately, CBT has not been evaluated in adolescents with eating disorders, and a recent review by Mitchell *et al.* (1996), which called for a second generation of bulimia treatment studies, suggested that this should be a research priority.

What to do with treatment failures

Despite its broad and durable effects, CBT for bulimia nervosa is 'by no means a panacea: some patients make only a partial response and some patients do not benefit at all' (Fairburn, Agras & Wilson, 1992). What to do with those patients who do not respond to CBT remains a difficult question. Interpersonal therapy may be a useful alternative, as in bulimia nervosa and binge eating disorder it has been shown to be as effective as CBT in the long term (Wilfley *et al.*, 1993; Fairburn *et al.*, 1995). The observations by Peveler and Fairburn (1992) in diabetic bulimics are also promising in this respect as they successfully switched some patients who had not responded to CBT on to interpersonal therapy. However, a controlled study of binge eating disorder found that those who had not responded to CBT fared no better when subsequently given interpersonal therapy (Agras *et al.*, 1995). So the jury on this issue is still out.

Wilson (1996) in an excellent review article, suggests a number of ways in which the scope of CBT could be extended for dealing with recalcitrant cases:

broadening CBT to include an interpersonal focus;

intensifying cognitive restructuring to include an examination of more generic concerns about the patient's self-worth and the nature of interpersonal relationships;

treating comorbid personality disorders by using Linehan's (1993) dialectical behaviour therapy or strategies from this complex package;

using exposure methods in the treatment, which could include exposure to binge foods and prevention of vomiting (Rosen & Leitenberg, 1982) or cue exposure to forbidden foods and prevention of bingeing (Schmidt & Marks, 1989; Jansen, Broekmate & Heymans, 1992).

Another variant of exposure treatment that might be useful in bulimia nervosa is that of 'worry exposure', in which the patient is asked to concentrate on anxiety-provoking thoughts about weight and shape, and to conjure up a detailed mental image of the feared outcome (i.e. massive weight gain), and then to stay with the images/thoughts for approximately half an hour to help reduce the impact of these thoughts and feelings. At the end of the period, cognitive restructuring is used to challenge the problematic thoughts.

Wilson (1996) also points out that, as therapists, we may often feel that we should not and cannot give up on those patients who have failed to respond to treatment. However, some patients may be intractable and there is some evidence that some patients improve following treatment, even if they have not improved during treatment (Fairburn *et al.*, 1995).

Self-care, guided self-care and other minimal CBT interventions in bulimia nervosa
The cost-effectiveness of treatments is an important consideration, especially at times of scarce resources (Koran *et al.*, 1995). Several cognitive–behavioural treatment manuals written for sufferers of bulimia nervosa are now available (Cooper, 1993; Schmidt & Treasure, 1993; Fairburn, 1995) and have been evaluated in open (Schmidt, Tiller & Treasure 1993; Cooper, Coker & Fleming, 1994, 1996) and controlled studies (Treasure et al., 1994, 1996; Thiels *et al.*, submitted). Twenty per cent of bulimic patients fully recover with the help of a self-care book only (Treasure *et al.*, 1994). Compliance with the self-care approach is associated with a better outcome (Troop *et al.*, 1996). Thirty to 50 per cent of patients become symptom free if a few therapist-guided sessions (up to eight) are added *after* self-treatment (sequential treatment) (Treasure *et al.*, 1996) or *concurrently* (guided self-help) (Cooper *et al.*, 1996; Thiels *et al.*, submitted). Patients treated with a minimal intervention involving self-care continue to improve after the end of treatment, with an abstinence rate comparable to that of full CBT (40 per cent symptom free) at follow-up (Treasure *et al.*, 1996; Thiels *et al.*, submitted). These minimal interventions may be less useful for those with a shorter duration and greater severity of illness (Turnbull *et al.*, 1996). To date, none has been evaluated in children and adolescents.

A simplified form of CBT has been developed for primary care (Waller *et al.*, 1996) and seems to benefit a significant proportion of patients.

Anorexia nervosa

In anorexia nervosa, the use of cognitive therapy has been described in only one case series (Cooper & Fairburn, 1984) and one small controlled study (Channon *et al.*, 1989). Freeman et al. compared a conventional intensive inpatient treatment with a day-patient programme along cognitive–behavioural lines in women with severe anorexia nervosa (Freeman, 1995). At three-year follow-up, those treated within the day hospital programme had fewer relapses, fewer re-admissions and more stable weight and better social functioning than those treated within the inpatient model. However, Freeman points out that this cannot necessarily be claimed as a success for CBT as many other factors were involved in the treatment package such that formal CBT may have been irrelevant.

The relative dearth of studies in this area is perhaps not surprising given that the often life-threatening nature of anorexia nervosa makes it necessary to use multifaceted eclectic treatment approaches. Moreover, in young onset anorexia nervosa, family therapy and family counselling seem to be particularly helpful (Russell *et al.*, 1987; Le Grange *et al.*, 1992).

Obesity

In adulthood, obesity is almost untreatable and the overwhelming majority (90–95 per cent) of patients who lose weight during dietary and behavioural treatment return to their baseline weight after five years (Wilson, 1994). In contrast, treatment of childhood obesity can have much better results. Whilst the majority of treatment studies of childhood obesity report reductions in percentage overweight of only around 4–8 per cent (Duffy & Spence, 1993), if the parents are involved in treatment and increase of activity is included in the intervention, post-treatment and long-term results can be much more impressive. Ten years after behavioural family-based treatment 30 per cent of previously obese children were no longer obese and the percentage by which an additional 34 per cent of children were overweight had decreased (Epstein *et al.*, 1994). Direct involvement of at least one parent improves short-term and long-term weight regulation (Epstein, 1996). Whether and how much the addition of cognitive measures adds to the effectiveness of behavioural weight-reduction programmes are as yet uncertain (Duffy & Spence, 1993).

Summary and conclusion

Cognitive–behavioural therapy is the gold standard treatment for bulimia nervosa. However, only 50 per cent of patients fully recover and basic CBT may need to be supplemented with other measures to achieve better abstinence rates. In anorexia nervosa, although cognitive–behavioural techniques have been applied, the evidence supporting their usefulness is much more mixed. In childhood obesity, the involvement of parents and an emphasis on increasing activity levels in addition to nutritional and behavioural measures seem to be crucial in obtaining significant short-term and long-term weight loss.

References

Agras, W.S., Rossiter, E.M., Arnow, B., Schneider, J.A., Telch, C.F., Raeburn, S.D., Bruce, B., Perl, M. & Koran, L.M. (1992). Pharmacologic and cognitive–behavioral treatment for bulimia nervosa: a controlled comparison. *American Journal of Psychiatry*, **149**, 82–7.

Agras, W.S., Schneider, J.A., Arnow, B., Raeburn, S.D. & Telch, C.F. (1989). Cognitive behavioural and response prevention treatments for bulimia nervosa. *Journal of Consulting and Clinical Psychology*, **57**, 215–21.

Agras, W.S., Telch, C.F., Arnow, B., Eldrege, K., Detzer, M.J., Henderson, J. & Marnell, M. (1995). Does interpersonal therapy help patients with binge eating disorder who fail to respond to cognitive–behavioral therapy? *Journal of Consulting and Clinical Psychology*, **63**, 356–60.

Attie, I. & Brooks-Gunn, J. (1989). The development of eating problems in adolescent girls: A longitudinal study. *Developmental Psychology*, **25**, 70–9.

Baell, W.K. & Wertheim, E.H. (1992). Predictors of outcome in the treatment of bulimia nervosa. *British Journal of Clinical Psychology*, **31**, 330–2.

Bhanji, S. & Mattingly, D. (1988). *Medical aspects of anorexia nervosa*. Wright, London.

Blouin, J.H., Carter, J., Blouin, A.G., Tener, L., Schnare-Hayes, K., Zuro, C., Barlow, J. & Perez, E. (1994). Prognostic indicators in bulimia nervosa treated with cognitive behavioral group therapy. *International Journal of Eating Disorders*, **15**, 113–23.

Brooks-Gunn, J. & Warren, M. (1988). The psychological significance of secondary sexual characteristics in nine-to-eleven-year old girls. *Child Development*, **59**, 1061–9.

Channon, S., Da Silva, P., Hemsley, D. & Perkins, R. (1989). A controlled trial of cognitive behavioural and behavioural treatment of anorexia nervosa. *Behaviour Research and Therapy*, **27**, 529–35.

Childress, A.C., Brewerton, T.D., Hodges, E.L. & Jarrell, M.P. (1993). The kids' eating disorder survey (KEDS): a study of middle school students. *The Journal of the American Academy of Child and Adolescent Psychiatry*, **32**, 843–50.

Coker, S., Vize, C., Wade, T. & Cooper, P.J. (1993). Patients with bulimia nervosa who fail to engage in cognitive behavioural therapy. *International Journal of Eating Disorders*, **13**, 35–40.

Collins, M.E. (1991). Body figure perceptions and preferences among preadolescent children. *International Journal of Eating Disorders*, **10**, 199–208.

Cooper, P. (1993). *Bulimia nervosa. A guide to recovery*. Robinson Publishing, London.

Cooper, P.J., Coker, S. & Fleming, C. (1994). Self-help for bulimia: A preliminary report. *International Journal of Eating Disorders*, **16**, 401–4.

Cooper, P.J., Coker, S. & Fleming, C. (1996). An evaluation of the efficacy of supervised cognitive behavioral self-help for bulimia nervosa. *Journal of Psychosomatic Research*, **40**, 281–7.

Cooper, P.J. & Fairburn, C.G. (1984). Cognitive behaviour therapy for anorexia nervosa: Some preliminary findings. *Journal of Psychosomatic Research*, **28**, 493–9.

Davies, E. & Furnham, A. (1986). The dieting and body shape concerns of adolescent females. *Journal of Child Psychology and Psychiatry*, **27**, 417–28.

Davis, R., Olmsted, M.P. & Rockert, W. (1992). Brief group psychoeducation for bulimia nervosa. II Prediction of clinical outcome. *International Journal of Eating Disorders*, **11**, 205–11.

De Silva, P. (1995). Cognitive–behavioural models of eating disorders. In *Handbook of eating disorders: theory, treatment and research* (ed. G. Szmukler, C. Dare & J. Treasure), pp. 141–53. John Wiley, Chichester.

Duffy, G. & Spence, S.H. (1993). The effectiveness of cognitive self-management as an adjunct to a behavioural intervention for childhood obesity: a research note. *Journal of Child Psychology and Psychiatry*, **34**, 1043–50.

Epstein, L.H. (1996). Family-based behavioural interventions for obese children. *International Journal of Obesity Related Metabolic Disorders*, **20**, Supplement 1, S14–21.

Epstein, L., Masek, B. & Marshall, W. (1978). A nutritionally based school program for control of eating in obese children. *Behaviour Therapy*, **9**, 766–78.

Epstein, L.H., Valoski, A., Wing, R.R. & McCurley, J. (1994). Ten-year outcomes of behavioral family-based treatment for childhood obesity. *Health Psychology*, **13**, 373–83.

Fahy, T.A., Eisler, I. & Russell, G.F.M. (1993). Personality disorder and treatment response in bulimia nervosa. *British Journal of Psychiatry* **162**, 765–70.

Fairburn, C.G. (1981). A cognitive behavioural approach to the management of bulimia nervosa. *Psychological Medicine*, **11**, 707–11.

Fairburn, C.G. (1995). *Overcoming binge eating*. Guilford Press, New York.

Fairburn, C.G., Agras, S. & Wilson, G.T. (1992). The research on the treatment of bulimia nervosa: Practical and theoretical implications. In *The biology of feast and famine. Relevance to eating disorders* (ed. G.H. Anderson & S.N Kennedy), pp. 318–40. Academic Press, New York.

Fairburn, C.G., Jones, R., Peveler, R.C., Carr, S.J., Solomon, R.A., O'Connor, M.E., Burton, J. & Hope, R.A. (1991). Three psychological treatments for bulimia nervosa. *Archives of General Psychiatry*, **48**, 463–9.

Fairburn, C.G., Jones, R., Peveler, R.C., Hope, R.A. & O'Connor, M.E. (1993a). Psychotherapy and bulimia nervosa: the longer term effects of interpersonal psychotherapy, behaviour therapy and cognitive behaviour therapy. *Archives of General Psychiatry* **50**, 419–28.

Fairburn, C.G., Kirk, J., O'Connor, M., Anastasiades, P. & Cooper, P.J. (1987). Prognostic factors in bulimia nervosa. *British Journal of Clinical Psychology*, **26**, 223–4.

Fairburn, C.G., Kirk, J., O'Connor, M. & Cooper, P.J. (1986). A comparison of two psychological treatments for bulimia nervosa. *Behaviour Research and Therapy*, **24**, 629–43.

Fairburn, C.G., Marcus, M.D. & Wilson, G.T. (1993b). Cognitive behavioral therapy for binge eating and bulimia nervosa: A comprehensive treatment manual. In *Binge eating: nature, assessment and treatment* (ed. C.G. Fairburn & G.T. Wilson), pp. 361–404. Guilford Press, New York.

Fairburn, C.G., Norman, P.A., Welch, S.L., O'Connor, M.E., Doll, H.A. & Peveler, R.C. (1995). A prospective study of outcome in bulimia nervosa and the long-term effects of three psychological treatments. *Archives of General Psychiatry*, **52**, 304–12.

Fairburn, C.G., Peveler, R.C., Jones, R., Hope, R.A. & Doll, H.A. (1993c). Predictors of 12-month outcome in bulimia nervosa and the influence of attitudes to shape and weight. *Journal of Consulting and Clinical Psychology*, **61**, 696–8.

Fichter, M.M., Leibl, K., Rief, W., Brunner E., Schmidt-Auberger, S. & Engel, R.R. (1991). Fluoxetine versus placebo: a double-blind study with bulimic inpatients undergoing intensive psychotherapy. *Pharmacopsychiatry*, **24**, 1–7.

Fichter, M.M., Quadflig, N. & Rief, W. (1994). Course of multi-impulsive bulimia. *Psychological Medicine*, **24**, 591–604.

Freeman, C. (1995). Cognitive therapy. In *Handbook of eating disorders: theory, treatment and research* (ed. G. Szmukler, C. Dare and J. Treasure), pp. 309–31. John Wiley, Chichester.

Freeman C.P.L., Barry, F., Dunkeld-Turnbull, J. & Henderson, A. (1988) Controlled trial of psychotherapy for bulimia nervosa. *British Medical Journal*, **296**, 521–5.

Garner, D.M. & Bemis, K.M. (1985). Cognitive therapy for anorexia nervosa. In *Handbook of psychotherapy for anorexia nervosa and bulimia* (ed. D.M. Garner & P.E. Garfinkel), pp. 107–46. Guilford Press, New York.

Garner, D.M., Olmsted, M.P., Davis, R., Rockert, W., Goldbloom, D. & Eagle M. (1990). The association between bulimic symptoms and reported psychopathology. *International Journal of Eating Disorders*, **9**, 1–15.

Garner, D.M., Rockert, W., Davis, R., Garner, M.P. & Eagle M. (1993). Comparison of cognitive behavioural and supportive expressive therapy for bulimia nervosa. *American Journal of Psychiatry*, **150**, 37–46.

Gloag, D. (1992). Exercise, fitness and health. *British Medical Journal*, **305**, 377–8.

Goldbloom, D., Olmsted, M., Davis, R. & Shaw, B. (1995) A randomized controlled trial of fluoxetine and individual cognitive behavioural therapy for women with bulimia nervosa: short term outcome. Unpublished manuscript. Department of Psychiatry, University of Toronto.

Gralen, S.J., Levine, M.P., Smolak, L. & Murnen, S.K. (1990). Dieting and disordered eating during early and middle adolescence: do the influences remain the same? *International Journal of Eating Disorders*, **9**, 501–12.

Hill, A.J. (1993). Preadolescent dieting: implications for eating disorders. *International Review of Psychiatry*, **5**, 87–100.

Hill, A.J., Oliver, S. & Rogers, P.J. (1992). Eating in the adult world: the rise of dieting in childhood and adolescence. *British Journal of Clinical Psychology*, **31**, 95–105.

Hill, A.J., Rogers, P.J. & Blundell, J.E. (1989). Dietary restraint in young adolescent girls: a functional analysis. *British Journal of Clinical Psychology*, **28**, 165–76.

Hill, A.J., Weaver, C. & Blundell, J.E. (1990). Dieting concerns of 10-year old girls and their mothers. *British Journal of Clinical Psychology*, **29**, 346–8.

Jansen, A., Broekmate, J. & Heymans, M. (1992). Cue exposure versus self-control in the treatment of binge eating: A pilot study. *Behaviour Research and Therapy*, **30**, 235–41.

Kaplan, A.S. & Garfinkel, P.E. (1993). *Medical issues and the eating disorders*. Brunner/Mazel, New York.

Kirkley, B., Schneider, J.A., Agras, W.S. & Bachman, J.A. (1985). Comparison of two group treatments for bulimia. *Journal of Consulting and Clinical Psychology*, **53**, 43–8.

Koran, L.M., Agras, W.S., Rossiter, E.M., Arnow, B., Schneider, J.A., Telch, C.F., Raeburn, S., Bruce, B., Perl, M. & Kraemer, H.C. (1995). Comparing the cost effectiveness of psychiatric treatments: bulimia nervosa. *Psychiatry Research*, **58**, 13–21.

Lask, B. & Bryant-Waugh, R. (1992). Early-onset anorexia nervosa and related eating disorders. *Journal of Child Psychology and Psychiatry*, **33**, 281–300.

Lee, N.F. & Rush, A.J. (1986). Cognitive-behavioral group therapy for bulimia. *International Journal of Eating Disorders*, **5**, 599–615.

Le Grange, D., Eisler, I., Dare, C. & Russell, G.F.M. (1992). Evaluation of family therapy in anorexia nervosa: a pilot study. *International Journal of Eating Disorders*, **12**, 4, 347–57.

Leitenberg, H., Rosen, J.C., Wolf, J., Vara, L.S., Detzer, M.J. & Srebnik, D. (1994). Comparison of cognitive behavioural therapy and desipramine in the treatment of bulimia. *Behaviour Research and Therapy*, **32**, 37–48.

Linehan, M. (1993). *Cognitive–behavioral treatment of borderline personality disorder*. Guilford Press, New York.

Loro, A.D. (1984). Binge eating: a cognitive-behavioral treatment approach. In *The binge–purge syndrome. Diagnosis, treatment, and research* (ed. R.C. Hawkins, W.J. Fremouw & P.F. Clement). Springer, New York.

Maloney, M.J., McGuire, L., Daniels, S.R. & Specker, B. (1989). Dieting behaviour and eating attitudes in children. *Pediatrics*, **84**, 482–9.

Mitchell, J.E., Hoberman, H.N., Peterson, C.B., Mussell, M. & Pyle, R. L. (1996). Research on the psychotherapy of bulimia nervosa: Half empty or half full. *International Journal of Eating Disorders*, **20**, 219–29.

Mitchell, J.E., Pyle, R.L., Eckert, E.D., Hatsukmi, D., Pomery, C. & Zimmerman, R. (1990). A comparison study of antidepressants and structured intensive group psychotherapy in the treatment of bulimia nervosa. *Archives of General Psychiatry*, **47**, 149–57.

Mitchell, J.E., Pyle, R.L., Pomery, C., Zollman, M., Crosby, R., Seim, H., Eckert, E.D. & Zimmerman, R. (1993). Cognitive-behavioral group psychotherapy of bulimia nervosa: Importance of logistical variables. *International Journal of Eating Disorders*, **14**, 277–87.

Olmsted, M.P., Kaplan, A.S. & Rockert, W. (1994). Rate and prediction of relapse in bulimia nervosa. *American Journal of Psychiatry*, **151**, 738–43.

Patton, G.C., Johnson-Sabine, E., Wood, K., Mann, A.H. & Wakeling, A. (1990). Abnormal eating attitudes in London schoolgirls – a prospective epidemiological study: outcome at twelve month follow-up. *Psychological Medicine*, **20**, 383–94.

Perri, M.G., Nezu, A.M. & Viegener, B.J. (eds.) (1992). Increasing exercise and physical activity. In *Improving the long-term management of obesity. Theory, research and clinical guidelines*, pp. 185–212. Wiley & Sons, New York.

Peveler, R.C. & Fairburn, C.G. (1992). The treatment of bulimia nervosa in patients with diabetes mellitus. *International Journal of Eating Disorders*, **11**, 45–53.

Rosen, J.C. & Leitenberg, H. (1982). Bulimia nervosa: treatment with exposure and response prevention. *Behavior Therapy*, **13**, 117–24.

Rossiter, E.M., Agras, W.S., Telch, C.F. & Schneider, J.A. (1993). Cluster B personality disorder characteristics predict outcome in the treatment of bulimia nervosa. *International Journal of Eating Disorders*, **13**, 349–58.

Russell, G.F.M., Szmukler, G., Dare, C. & Eisler, I. (1987). An evaluation of family therapy in anorexia nervosa and bulimia nervosa. *Archives of General Psychiatry*, **44**, 1047–56.

Schmidt, U. & Marks, I. (1989). Exposure and prevention of binges versus exposure plus prevention of vomiting: A crossover study. *Journal of Nervous and Mental Disease*, **177**, 259–66.

Schmidt, U., Tiller, J. & Treasure, J. (1993). Self-treatment of bulimia nervosa – A pilot study. *International Journal of Eating Disorders*, **13**, 273–7.

Schmidt, U. & Treasure, J. (1993). *Getting better bit(e) by bit(e)*. Lawrence Erlbaum Associates, London.

Sharpe, C.W. & Freeman, C.P.L. (1993). The medical complications of anorexia nervosa. *British Journal of Psychiatry*, **162**, 452–62.

Steel, Z.P., Farag, P.A. & Blaszczynski, A.P. (1995). Interrupting the binge–purge cycle in bulimia: The use of planned binges. *International Journal of Eating Disorders*, **18**, 199–208.

Telch, C.F., Agras, W.S., Rossiter, E.M., Wilfley, D. & Kenardy, J. (1990). Group cognitive–behavioral treatment for the non-purging bulimic: An initial evaluation. *Journal of Consulting and Clinical Psychology*, **58**, 629–35.

Thackwray, D.E., Smith, M.C., Bodfish, J.W. & Meyers, A.W. (1993). A comparison of behavioral and cognitive–behavioral interventions for bulimia nervosa. *Journal of Consulting and Clinical Psychology*, **61**, 639–45.

Thiels, C., Schmidt, U., Treasure, J., Garthe, R. & Troop, N. (submitted). Guided self-change for bulimia nervosa incorporating a self-treatment manual.

Treasure, J. & Schmidt, U. (1997). *Clinician's guide to getting better bit(e) by bit(e)*. Lawrence Erlbaum Associates, Hove, Sussex.

Treasure, J., Schmidt, U., Troop, N., Tiller, J. & Todd, G. (1994). First step in managing bulimia nervosa – a controlled trial of a therapeutic manual. *British Medical Journal*, **308**, 686–9.

Treasure, J., Schmidt, U., Troop, N., Tiller, J., Todd, G. & Turnbull, S. (1996). Sequential treatment for bulimia nervosa incorporating a self-care manual. *British Journal of Psychiatry*, **68**, 94–8.

Treasure, J. & Szmukler, G. (1995). Medical complications of chronic anorexia nervosa. In *Handbook of eating disorders: theory, treatment and research* (ed. G. Szmukler, C. Dare & J. Treasure), pp. 197–220. John Wiley, Chichester.

Troop, N., Schmidt, U., Tiller, J., Todd, G., Keilen, M. & Treasure, J. (1996). Compliance with a self-directed treatment manual for bulimia nervosa: Predictors and outcome. *Journal of Clinical Psychology*, **35**, 435–8.

Turnbull, S., Treasure, J., Schmidt, U., Troop, N., Tiller, J. & Todd, G. (1996). Predictors of short- and long-term outcome of bulimia nervosa. *International Journal of Eating Disorders*, **21**, 17–22.

Wadden, T.A., Foster, G.D., Stunkard, A.J. & Linowitz, J.R. (1989). Dissatisfaction with weight and figure in obese girls: discontent but not depression. *International Journal of Obesity*, **13**, 89–97.

Waller, D., Fairburn, C.G., McPherson, A., Kay, R., Lee, A. & Nowell, T. (1996). Treating bulimia nervosa in primary care – a pilot study. *International Journal of Eating Disorders*, **19**, 99–103.

Walsh, B.T., Wilson, G.T., Loeb, K., Pike, K. & Devlin, M.J. (1997). Pharmacological and psychological treatment of bulimia nervosa. *Journal of Psychiatry*, **154**, 523–31.

Ward, A., Troop, N., Todd, G. & Treasure, J. (1996). To change or not to change – 'How' is the question? *British Journal of Medical Psychology*, **69**, 139–46.

Wardle, J. & Beales, S. (1986). Restraint, body image and food attitudes in children from 12 to 18 years. *Appetite*, **7**, 209–17.

Wardle, J. & Marsland, L. (1990). Adolescent concerns about weight and eating: a social–developmental perspective. *Journal of Psychosomatic Research*, **34**, 377–91.

Wilfley, D.E., Agras, W.S., Telch, C.F., Rossiter, E.M., Schneider, J.A., Cole, A.G., Sifford, L.A. & Raeburn, S.D. (1993). Group cognitive–behavioral therapy and group interpersonal psychotherapy for the nonpurging bulimic: a controlled comparison. *Journal of Consulting and Clinical Psychology*, **61**, 296–305.

Wilson, G.T. (1994). Behavioral treatment of childhood obesity: theoretical and practical implications. *Health Psychology*, **13**, 371–2.

Wilson, G.T. (1996). Treatment of bulimia nervosa: When CBT fails. *Behaviour Research and Therapy*, **34**, 197–212.

Wilson, G.T., Eldredge, K.L., Smith, D. & Niles, B. (1991). Cognitive behavioral treatment of bulimia nervosa: a controlled evaluation. *Behaviour Research and Therapy*, **29**, 579–83.

Wilson, G.T., Rossiter, E., Kleinfels, E.I. & Lindholm., L. (1986). Cognitive behavioral treatment of bulimia nervosa: a controlled evaluation. *Behaviour Research and Therapy*, **24**, 277–88.

Wolchik, S.A., Weiss, L. & Katzman, M.A. (1986). An empirically validated, short-term psychoeducational group treatment program for bulimia. *International Journal of Eating Disorders*, **5**, 21–34.

Wolf, E.M. & Crowther, J.H. (1992). An evaluation of behavioral and cognitive–behavioral group intervention for the treatment of bulimia nervosa in women. *International Journal of Eating Disorders*, **11**, 3–16.

Wonderlich, S.A., Fullerton, D., Swift, W.J. & Klein, M.H. (1994). Five year outcome from eating disorders: Relevance of Personality Disorders. *International Journal of Eating Disorders*, **15**, 233–43.

Yates, A.J. & Sambrailo, F. (1984). Bulimia nervosa: A descriptive and therapeutic study. *Behaviour Research and Therapy*, **5**, 503–17.

15
Summary and overview

Philip Graham

Definitional issues

Reviewing the contributions to this book, one is first struck by the point made by Tammie Ronen in her introductory chapter: there is a wide diversity of techniques considered to be components of CBT. It appears there are core procedures, such as those described by Richard Harrington in his chapter on depression, which aim to alter distorted thought processes. But around these there is a cluster of other techniques. Parent management training, described by Jo Douglas for pre-school children and by Veira Bailey in relation to older children with conduct disorders, is more directly behaviourally orientated, with the cognitive element limited to helping parents under-stand the rationale of the therapy. The social skills training described by Sue Spence has a great deal in common with other varieties of interpersonal therapies, focusing parti-cularly on the improvement of social relationships through building up understanding of the rules of social behaviour and rehearsing them. In contrast, van der Krol and his colleagues focus in their treatment of hyperactivity on developing new cognitive links to behaviour by defining problematic situations in which coping is assisted by a specified cognitive set aiming at greater reflectivity. Ulrike Schmidt points to a similar approach in bulimia. Using yet another framework, Bill Yule, in considering cognitive treatment for PTSD, describes a cognitive approach in which reliving a traumatic situation through recapturing specific memories is the basis for achieving control over unpleasant flashbacks.

The justification for grouping these diverse techniques under the heading of 'cogni-tive behaviour therapy' lies in the fact that all of them involve an attempt to change behaviour through the mediation of cognitive processes. But is this a satisfactory defi-nition of CBT? Surely psychodynamic therapies also involve the mediation of cognitive processes and, although behaviour change as a goal is sometimes viewed somewhat ambivalently by psychodynamic therapists, the latter are certainly interested in such changes as an outcome of their therapies. The distinction between CBT and psychodynamic therapies, therefore, has to be drawn more precisely. Both may require emergence into consciousness of thoughts and feelings hitherto outside the realm of immediate awareness. But CBT involves systematic testing of the success of behavioural techniques in the real world in a way that psychodynamic therapy does not. Both types of therapists can be proved wrong by their clients or patients and thus can claim their therapies to be scientifically based, but whereas cognitive–behaviour therapists can be proved wrong in the living room, in the classroom or on the street ('Your technique did not work for me. My behaviour did not change.'), psychodynamic therapists are more likely to be proved wrong in the consulting room ('Your insight or interpretation was unhelpful to me.').

From the outset, an important feature of the behavioural therapies has been their grounding in theory validated by empirical investigation. Pavlov and Skinner provided theoretical models which were tested, extended and applied in clinical situations with at least some modest success. CBT has been developed at the same time as the field of cognitive psychology has greatly flourished, and one might expect this relatively new science to provide a similar theoretical underpinning. The scientific foundations of CBT in different psychological domains have been well discussed by Gelder (1977). In fact, links between cognitive psychology and clinical practice sometimes appear rather tenuous, though significant attempts have been made to strengthen them (Stein & Young, 1992). Teasdale and Barnard (1993) have, for example, developed new theoretical models to help explain the interplay between emotional (especially depressive) experience and behaviour. Further conceptual and experimental work is required to place such studies in a developmental framework so that they can be made more applicable to children and adolescents.

Evidence for effectiveness

The most thorough and systematic review of the effectiveness of the behavioural psychotherapies for children (Target & Fonagy, 1996) concludes that these are effective, and that they are more effective than non-behavioural therapies. Nevertheless, one must concede that the evidence for effectiveness presented in some of these chapters is far from overwhelming. In some conditions (depressive and obsessional disorders and bulimia are examples) it is reasonable to assume, by extrapolating from work with adults and adding results from a small number of trials with adolescents, that CBT is indeed significantly effective. In other conditions, such as ADHD, it seems clear that existing techniques, although initially promising, do not add significantly to other measures such as medication. In some, such as anxiety and conduct disorders, although there are a number of studies with promising results, final judgement on evidence for effectiveness must be suspended until more conclusive trials have been carried out. In particular, evidence on medium-term and long-term effectiveness is lacking. Of course, as clinical experience increases, and evaluative studies become more numerous, the effectiveness of these forms of therapy will doubtless become more clearly established. One might, for example, expect CBT to be more effective than medication in preventing recurrence because it provides a technique for dealing with the impact of life stress that could be helpful when new problems arise in a way that medication would not. Evidence in this respect is lacking in relation to children and young people. There is a further problem, discussed by Weisz *et al.* (1995), in the fact that many studies of effectiveness have been carried out on volunteers or subjects recruited through newspaper advertisements rather than on clinic cases. Evaluation of treatments carried out on such subjects shows them to be more effective than those carried out on regular clinic attenders, perhaps because the latter are more severely impaired. One therefore needs to be cautious in generalising from results of trials carried out with non-clinic subjects.

A major problem for therapists is the ambivalence of their clients or patients towards change and therefore towards attendance. There is one component of CBT that is of particular interest here. The techniques involved in motivational interviewing, described by van Bilsen and Wilke, are of great relevance, and may be of wider applicability than in the context of alcohol and substance abuse in which they describe them. If behavioural techniques such as motivational interviewing can be demonstrated to be effective methods of helping impaired but unmotivated individuals, adults or children, this would have far-reaching significance.

Ethical issues

Motivating the unmotivated raises ethical issues. Indeed, the use of CBT more generally has provoked ethical concern in a number of ways. These have recently been considered by a working party of the Royal College of Psychiatrists, which has produced a useful document (Royal College of Psychiatrists, 1997). A number of issues discussed by the working party affect both adults and children, but there is also a section specifically concerned with children and adolescents. The Working Party Report, amongst other matters, discusses consent issues, with emphasis on the need to involve children in the consent procedures as far as is possible. The special needs of children arising from their dependency, immaturity, difficulties in understanding and problems in communicating should be taken fully into account.

Combined approaches

Finally, the contributors, without exception, make clear that CBT is only likely to be effective when it forms one component of multi-modal therapy. The amount of benefit to the subject is therefore likely to be related to the effectiveness of the other therapies applied, and this in turn will depend at least to some degree on the skill of other therapists and agents of change such as social workers. The degree to which the therapist applying CBT can work co-operatively with others in the field is therefore an important ingredient of success.

Nevertheless, it is clear from the contributions to this book that CBT provides a significant advance in our therapeutic armamentarium, an advance particularly notable for its emphasis on improving reasoning and thought processes. In an irrational world, any advance that combats unreason is surely to be strongly welcomed, from whichever direction it may come.

References

Gelder, M. (1977). The scientific foundations of cognitive behaviour therapy. In *Science and practice of cognitive behaviour therapy* (ed. D.M. Clarke & C.G. Fairbairn), pp. 27–46. Oxford University Press, Oxford.

Royal College of Psychiatrists (1997). *Guidelines to good practice in the use of behavioural and cognitive treatments*. Report of a Working Party of the Royal College of Psychiatrists. Royal College of Psychiatrists, London.

Stein, D.J. & Young, J.E. (eds.) (1992). *Cognitive science and clinical disorders*. Academic Press, San Diego.

Target, M. & Fonagy, P. (1996). The psychological treatment of child and adolescent psychiatric disorders. In *What Works for Whom?* (ed. A. Roth & P. Fonagy), pp. 263–320. Guilford Press, New York and London.

Teasdale, J.D. & Barnard, P.J. (1993). *Affect: cognition and change*. Lawrence Erlbaum, Hove, UK.

Weisz, J.R., Donenburg, G.R., Han, S.S. & Weiss, B. (1995). Bridging the gap between laboratory and clinic in child and adolescent psychotherapy. *Journal of Consulting and Clinical Psychology*, **63**, 688–701.

Index

286